T0249794

Changing Paradigms in Breast Cancer Diagnosis and Treatment

Editor

KELLY K. HUNT

SURGICAL ONCOLOGY CLINICS OF NORTH AMERICA

www.surgonc.theclinics.com

Consulting Editor
TIMOTHY M. PAWLIK

January 2018 • Volume 27 • Number 1

ELSEVIER

1600 John F. Kennedy Boulevard • Suite 1800 • Philadelphia, Pennsylvania, 19103-2899

http://www.theclinics.com

SURGICAL ONCOLOGY CLINICS OF NORTH AMERICA Volume 27, Number 1
January 2018 ISSN 1055-3207, ISBN-13: 978-0-323-56659-9

Editor: John Vassallo (j.vassallo@elsevier.com)
Developmental Editor: Meredith Madeira

Surgical Oncology Clinics of North America (ISSN 1055-3207) is published quarterly by Elsevier Inc., 360 Park Avenue South, New York, NY 10010-1710. Months of publication are January, April, July, and October. Business and Editorial Offices: 1600 John F. Kennedy Blvd., Ste. 1800, Philadelphia, PA 19103-2899. Customer Service Office: 3251 Riverport Lane, Maryland Heights, MO 63043. Periodicals postage paid at New York, NY and additional mailing offices. Subscription prices are $296.00 per year (US individuals), $505.00 (US institutions) $100.00 (US student/resident), $337.00 (Canadian individuals), $638.00 (Canadian institutions), $205.00 (Canadian student/resident), $418.00 (foreign individuals), $638.00 (foreign institutions), and $205.00 (foreign student/resident). Foreign air speed delivery is included in all *Clinics* subscription prices. All prices are subject to change without notice. **POSTMASTER**: Send address changes to *Surgical Oncology Clinics of North America,* Elsevier Health Science Division, Subscription Customer Service, 3251 Riverport Lane, Maryland Heights, MO 63043. **Customer Service: 1-800-654-2452 (US and Canada). 314-447-8871 (outside US and Canada). Fax: 314-447-8029. E-mail: journalscustomerservice-usa@elsevier.com (for print support); journalsonline support-usa@elsevier.com (for online support).**

Reprints. For copies of 100 or more, of articles in this publication, please contact the Commercial Reprints Department, Elsevier Inc., 360 Park Avenue South, New York, New York 10010-1710. Tel. 212-633-3874; Fax: 212-633-3820; E-mail: reprints@elsevier.com.

Surgical Oncology Clinics of North America is covered in *MEDLINE/PubMed (Index Medicus)* and *EMBASE/ Excerpta Medica, Current Contents/Clinical Medicine,* and *ISI/BIOMED.*

Contributors

CONSULTING EDITOR

TIMOTHY M. PAWLIK, MD, MPH, PhD, FACS, FRACS (Hon)
Professor and Chair, Department of Surgery, The Urban Meyer III and Shelley Meyer Chair for Cancer Research, Professor of Surgery, Oncology, Health Services Management and Policy, The Ohio State University, Wexner Medical Center, Columbus, Ohio, USA

EDITOR

KELLY K. HUNT, MD, FACS
Hamill Foundation Distinguished, Professor of Surgery in Honor of Dr. Richard G. Martin, Sr. Chair, Department of Breast Surgical Oncology, The University of Texas MD Anderson Cancer Center, Houston, Texas, USA

AUTHORS

REBECCA AFT, MD, PhD
Professor of Surgery, Department of Surgery, Washington University in St. Louis, St Louis, Missouri, USA

SARAH L. BLAIR, MD
Professor, Department of Surgery, Division of Surgical Oncology, UC San Diego Health, Moores Cancer Center, La Jolla, California, USA

KRISTEN P. BRODERICK, MD
Assistant Professor of Surgery, Department of Plastic and Reconstructive Surgery, Johns Hopkins University, Baltimore, Maryland, USA

BRITTANY M. CAMPBELL, BS
Medical Student, Department of Surgery, Duke University Medical Center, Durham, North Carolina, USA

LUBNA N. CHAUDHARY, MD, MS
Assistant Professor, Department of Medicine, Division of Hematology/Oncology, Medical College of Wisconsin, Milwaukee, WI, USA

MELISSA B. DAVIS, PhD
Research Scientist, Henry Ford Cancer Institute, Detroit, Michigan, USA

AMY C. DEGNIM, MD
Department of Surgery, Mayo Clinic, Rochester, Minnesota, USA

SARAH M. DESNYDER, MD, FACS
Assistant Professor, Breast Surgical Oncology, The University of Texas MD Anderson Cancer Center, Houston, Texas, USA

MOHAMMAD EGHTEDARI, MD, PhD
Assistant Professor of Clinical Radiology, Department of Radiology, Breast Imaging Section, UC San Diego Health, Moores Cancer Center, La Jolla, California, USA

SIMONA MARIA FRAGOMENI, MD
Division of Gynecologic Oncology, Multidisciplinary Breast Center, Catholic University of the Sacred Heart Rome, Rome, Italy

KRISTALYN GALLAGHER, DO, FACOS
Assistant Professor, Department of Surgery, Breast Surgical Oncology and Oncoplastics, The University of North Carolina at Chapel Hill, Chapel Hill, North Carolinas, USA

STEPHANIE GRAY, MD
Resident in General Surgery, Department of Surgery, The University of North Carolina at Chapel Hill, Chapel Hill, North Carolina, USA

JULIE GROSSMAN, MD
Resident Physician, Department of Surgery, Washington University in St. Louis, St Louis, Missouri, USA

MEHRAN HABIBI, MD, MBA
Assistant Professor, Department of Surgery, Johns Hopkins University, Baltimore, Maryland, USA

BRUCE G. HAFFTY, MD
Professor, Department of Radiation Oncology, Rutgers Cancer Institute of New Jersey, New Brunswick, USA

E. SHELLEY HWANG, MD, MPH
Vice Chair of Research and Professor, Department of Surgery, Chief, Breast Surgical Oncology, Duke University Medical Center, Durham, North Carolina, USA

LISA K. JACOBS, MD, MSPH
Associate Professor, Department of Surgery, Johns Hopkins University, Baltimore, Maryland, USA

JACQUELINE S. JERUSS, MD, PhD
Division of Anatomic Pathology, Department of Pathology, Director, Breast Care Center and Breast Surgical Oncology Fellowship, Division of Surgical Oncology, Associate Professor, Department of Surgery, University of Michigan, Ann Arbor, Michigan, USA

TARI A. KING, MD, FACS
Associate Chair for Multidisciplinary Oncology, Department of Surgery, Brigham and Women's Hospital, Chief of Breast Surgery, Dana-Farber/Brigham and Women's Cancer Center, Anne E. Dyson Associate Professor of Surgery in the Field of Women's Cancers, Harvard Medical School, Boston, Massachusetts, USA

AMANDA KONG, MD, MS
Associate Professor, Department of Surgery, Medical College of Wisconsin, Milwaukee, Wisconsin, USA

CHRISTINE LARONGA, MD, FACS
Department of Breast Oncology, Moffitt Cancer Center, Tampa, Florida, USA

CYNTHIA MA, MD, PhD
Associate Professor, Department of Medicine, Washington University in St. Louis, St Louis, Missouri, USA

ANITA MAMTANI, MD
Chief Resident, Department of Surgery, Beth Israel Deaconess Medical Center, Clinical Fellow in Surgery, Harvard Medical School, Boston, Massachusetts, USA

KATHLEEN MARULANDA, MD, MS
Resident in General Surgery, Department of Surgery, The University of North Carolina at Chapel Hill, Chapel Hill, North Carolina, USA

ELIZABETH A. MITTENDORF, MD, PhD
Associate Professor, Deputy Chair of Research, Department of Breast Surgical Oncology, The University of Texas MD Anderson Cancer Center, Houston, Texas, USA

LISA A. NEWMAN, MD, MPH
Director, Breast Oncology Program, Department of Surgery, Henry Ford Health System, Henry Ford Cancer Institute, Director, International Center for the Study of Breast Cancer Subtypes, Detroit, Michigan, USA

NISHA OHRI, MD
Assistant Professor, Department of Radiation Oncology, Rutgers Cancer Institute of New Jersey, New Brunswick, USA

HAYDEE OJEDA-FOURNIER, MD
Professor of Clinical Radiology, Department of Radiology, Breast Imaging Section, UC San Diego Health, Moores Cancer Center, La Jolla, California, USA

TUYA PAL, MD, FACMG
Department of Medicine, Vanderbilt University Medical Center, Vanderbilt-Ingram Cancer Center, Nashville, Tennessee, USA

JENNIFER K. PLICHTA, MD, MS
Assistant Professor, Department of Surgery, Duke University Medical Center, Durham, North Carolina, USA

BENJAMIN POWERS, MD
Department of Breast Oncology, Moffitt Cancer Center, Tampa, Florida, USA

JENNIFER M. RACZ, MD, MBA
Department of Surgery, Mayo Clinic, Rochester, Minnesota, USA

CHANTAL REYNA, MD
Assistant Professor, Breast Surgical Oncology, The University of Texas MD Anderson Cancer Center, Houston, Texas, USA

JULIE ROBLES, MD
General Surgery Resident, Department of Surgery, UC San Diego, San Diego, California, USA

KELLY J. ROSSO, MD
Department of Breast Surgical Oncology, The University of Texas MD Anderson Cancer Center, Houston, Texas, USA

ANDREW SCIALLIS, MD
Division of Anatomic Pathology, Department of Pathology, University of Michigan, Ann Arbor, Michigan, USA

MOHAMAD E. SEBAI, MBBS
Postdoctoral Fellow, Department of Surgery, The Johns Hopkins University School of
Medicine, Baltimore, Maryland, USA

ALASTAIR M. THOMPSON, BSc (Hons), MBChB, MD, FRCSEd (Gen)
Department of Breast Surgical Oncology, The University of Texas MD Anderson Cancer
Center, Houston, Texas, USA

CATHERINE TSAI, MD
General Surgery Resident, Department of Surgery, UC San Diego, San Diego, California,
USA

ANNA WEISS, MD
Department of Breast Surgical Oncology, Brigham and Women's Hospital, Boston,
Massachusetts, USA

K. HOPE WILKINSON, MD, MS
Department of Surgery, Division of Surgical Oncology, Medical College of Wisconsin,
Milwaukee, WI, USA

Contents

no further management. DBT is used in the screening and diagnostic setting, and for guidance of wire localization or core biopsy, performing more accurately in the dense breast.

Breast cancer staging concisely summarizes disease status, creating a framework for assessing and relaying prognostic information. The fundamental concepts and components of breast cancer staging are reviewed. The AJCC *Cancer Staging Manual*, which includes traditional anatomic factors, now includes additional tumor characteristics: tumor grade, estrogen receptor status, progesterone receptor status, human epidermal growth factor receptor 2 status, and (when available) multigene panel testing from the primary tumor. With these updates, staging provides the most reliable system for accurately predicting patient outcome. When the AJCC eighth edition guidelines are adopted, they will more closely reflect tumor biology.

The management of ductal carcinoma in situ (DCIS) has traditionally followed the evidence base for invasive breast cancer using surgery, radiation therapy, and drug therapy to remove the DCIS from the breast and reduce the risk of recurrence for both DCIS and invasive breast cancer. Because of concerns regarding the overtreatment of DCIS, randomized controlled trials have been established to test the outcomes (invasive breast cancer outcomes and patient-reported outcome measures) of active surveillance compared with guideline-concordant care for low-risk (for progression) DCIS. These strategies are undergoing rigorous evaluation to evaluate alternatives to the current management of DCIS.

Invasive lobular carcinoma (ILC) is the second most common type of breast cancer, with a unique pathogenesis and distinct clinical biology. ILCs display a characteristic loss of E-cadherin, are largely estrogen receptor positive, HER2 negative, and low to intermediate grade. These features portend a favorable prognosis, but there is a tendency for late recurrences and atypical metastases. ILCs tend to be insidious and infiltrative, which can pose a challenge for diagnosis, and emerging data suggest they may have a propensity for a differing response to standard therapies.

In the era of personalized medicine, there has been significant progress regarding the molecular analysis of breast cancer subtypes. Research efforts have focused on how classification of subtypes could provide information on prognosis and influence treatment planning. Although much is known about the impact of different molecular subtypes on disease-specific survival, more recent studies have investigated the role of the different molecular subtypes on local-regional recurrence. This is an area of active study, and in recent years there has been significant progress. This article describes outcomes among disease subtypes to aid in optimal surgical decision making to improve local-regional control.

Neoadjuvant endocrine therapy (NET) can be effective at downstaging patients with estrogen receptor–positive tumors and identifying those tumors that are endocrine sensitive and resistant. The optimal prognostic markers for stratification are under investigation. Use of NET will allow the identification of patients with estrogen receptor–positive tumors who might benefit from additional treatment and allow better understanding of endocrine resistance.

Progress in the treatment of triple-negative breast cancer remains an important challenge. Given the aggressive biology and high risk of distant recurrence, systemic chemotherapy is warranted in most patients. Neoadjuvant chemotherapy benefits patients with locally advanced disease by downsizing the tumor and increasing the probability of breast-conserving surgery. Clinical and pathologic responses provide important prognostic information, which makes neoadjuvant therapy an attractive approach for all patients with triple-negative breast cancer. Clinical research in the neoadjuvant setting is focused on improvement in pathologic complete response rates and outcomes of patients with residual disease.

The goal of breast-conserving surgery is to excise the tumor with negative margins while achieving a successful cosmetic result. Although it is not feasible to have reexcision rates of zero, several techniques have been described to reduce the need for a return to the operating room. When rates of reexcision are high, consideration should be given to using one or more of these techniques. It is critical that reexcision rates are tracked when new techniques are implemented to ensure progress. In addition, attention must be paid to ensure that cosmetic outcomes remain optimal.

Oncoplastic surgery of the tissue defect from partial mastectomy should be considered for all patients. It can result in significant asymmetries, from scar contraction and skin tethering to alterations in the nipple areolar complex location. Indications, risks, and benefits are discussed. Optimal procedures are described, considering resected specimen volume, primary tumor location, tumor to breast size ratio, and the impact on the nipple areolar complex. Indications for plastic surgery consultation and joint surgery are discussed. Surgical management includes incision planning, preservation of the nipple areolar complex pedicle and position, patient positioning, incision location, and recovery.

Adjuvant whole-breast irradiation (WBI) after lumpectomy has been an established standard of care for decades. Standard-fractionation WBI delivered over 5 to 7 weeks can achieve durable tumor control with low toxicity but can be inconvenient for patients and cost-ineffective. Hypofractionated WBI can be completed in 3 to 4 weeks and, based on long-term randomized data, is the preferred standard of care in select patients. Accelerated partial-breast irradiation can be delivered using even shorter treatment regimens. Although the available data on accelerated partial-breast irradiation are more limited, early results suggest it is an effective alternative to WBI in select patients.

Lymphedema is a chronic, progressive disease with no curative treatment. Breast cancer therapy is the most common cause of secondary lymphedema in the developed world. Treatment includes nonsurgical and surgical strategies. Conservative measures are reserved for subclinical lymphedema. Surgical options are divided into physiologic (to restore function) and reductive (to remove diseased tissue). Early-stage disease is managed with physiologic procedures. Reductive treatment is reserved for moderate to severe staged disease owing to high morbidity. Surgical options effectively decrease edema and improve quality of life. However, further research is necessary to best establish management of lymphedema.

Breast cancer mortality rates are higher in African American compared with white American women. Disproportionately rising incidence rates, coupled with higher rates of biologically aggressive disease among African Americans is resulting in a widening of the mortality disparity. Higher rates of triple-negative breast cancer among African American women, as well as women from western sub-Saharan Africa, has prompted questions regarding the role of African ancestry as a marker of hereditary susceptibility for specific disease phenotypes. Advances in germline genetics, as well as somatic tumor genomic research, hold great promise in the effort to understand the biology of breast cancer variations between different population subsets.

SURGICAL ONCOLOGY
CLINICS OF NORTH AMERICA

RELATED INTEREST

Radiologic Clinics, June 2017 (Vol. 55, Issue 3)
Breast Imaging
Sarah M. Friedewald, *Editor*
Available at: www.radiologic.theclinics.com

THE CLINICS ARE AVAILABLE ONLINE!
Access your subscription at:
www.theclinics.com

Foreword

Innovation in the Diagnosis and Management of Breast Cancer

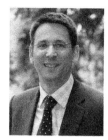

Timothy M. Pawlik, MD, MPH, PhD, FACS, FRACS (Hon)
Consulting Editor

This issue of the *Surgical Oncology Clinics of North America* is devoted to highlighting the integration of new knowledge and surgical innovation into the diagnosis and management of breast cancer. The guest editor is Kelly Hunt, MD, FACS. Dr Hunt is Professor and Chair of the Department of Breast Surgical Oncology at The University of Texas MD Anderson Cancer Center. Her expertise in the treatment of patients with breast cancer is nationally and internationally recognized. Dr Hunt has played a pivotal role in numerous breast cancer trials, and her own research has provided some of the most important novel clinical data in the field of breast cancer over the last two decades. In fact, Dr Hunt's career has centered on the fostering of new knowledge, advocacy of clinical trials, and innovation in surgical management of patients with breast cancer. As such, Dr Hunt is ideally suited to be the guest editor of this important issue of the *Surgical Oncology Clinics of North America*.

The issue covers a number of important topics, including genetic testing, management of high-risk lesions, as well as novel technologies in breast imaging and innovations in surgical and adjuvant decision making. The issue touches on such important topics as intraoperative margin assessment, management of nodal disease, and timing of systemic therapies. To accomplish such a comprehensive and thorough state-of-the-art review on this wide range of topics, Dr Hunt used an incredible group of authors who are respective leaders in their field. As you will note in reading this issue, Dr Hunt and her colleagues strongly demonstrate the importance and progress that have been made in the area of the diagnosis and management of breast cancer. I would like to

Surg Oncol Clin N Am 27 (2018) xiii–xiv
https://doi.org/10.1016/j.soc.2017.10.002
1055-3207/18/© 2017 Published by Elsevier Inc.

surgonc.theclinics.com

thank Dr Hunt and her colleagues for an excellent issue of the *Surgical Oncology Clinics of North America* and for taking on such an important topic.

Timothy M. Pawlik, MD, MPH, PhD, FACS, FRACS (Hon)
Department of Surgery
The Ohio State University
Wexner Medical Center
395 West 12th Avenue, Suite 670
Columbus, OH 43210, USA

E-mail address:
Tim.Pawlik@osumc.edu

Preface

Integrating New Knowledge and Surgical Innovation into the Diagnosis and Management of Breast Cancer

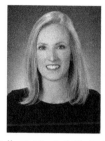

Kelly K. Hunt, MD, FACS
Editor

Anyone currently practicing in the field of breast oncology would certainly agree that there have been major advances in all aspects of breast cancer diagnosis and treatment over the last decade and even over the last few years. In order to offer our patients the best chance for long-term survival and the best quality of life, we must constantly evaluate the new knowledge and innovations in order to learn how best to incorporate them into our practice. In this issue of the *Surgical Oncology Clinics of North America*, we examine the changing paradigms in breast cancer diagnosis and treatment. The contributing authors have provided tremendous expertise across many areas of breast cancer diagnosis and treatment from genetic testing to management of high-risk lesions, new technologies in breast imaging, modifications in the breast cancer staging system, potential deescalation of therapies for ductal carcinoma in situ, treatment algorithms for management of lobular breast cancer, incorporating molecular subtypes into the decision making regarding local regional therapy, use of different systemic therapies in the neoadjuvant setting based on approximated subtypes, understanding how intraoperative margin assessment can reduce the need for reexcision in breast-conserving surgery, expanding the use of breast reconstruction and oncoplastic techniques, moving beyond the "whole breast radiation fits all after lumpectomy" strategy to include newer techniques in different populations, surgical strategies for management of lymphedema, and finally, understanding how genomics and big data can help us to reduce breast cancer disparities and improve outcomes locally and globally.

Surg Oncol Clin N Am 27 (2018) xv–xvi
https://doi.org/10.1016/j.soc.2017.10.001
1055-3207/18/© 2017 Published by Elsevier Inc.

This compilation of articles provides the reader with the most current evidence across the spectrum of breast oncology that can be utilized in patient management today and in the foreseeable future. Each contribution provides a critical review of the published literature with current guidelines and recommendations and identification of gaps in knowledge. The authors also describe novel technologies and ongoing clinical trials that will provide further evidence to further refine our practice in the coming years. It is critical that we continue to evaluate our diagnostic and treatment strategies in order to personalize the care that we provide and minimize the cost, inconvenience, and above all morbidity that our patients experience. I am grateful to all of the contributing authors for their excellent contributions and hope that the readers of these articles are inspired to embrace new concepts that will provide the optimal care for their patients and are challenged to consider new ideas that can further improve the prevention, detection, and treatment of our patients with breast cancer.

Kelly K. Hunt, MD, FACS
Department of Breast Surgical Oncology
The University of Texas MD Anderson Cancer Center
1400 Pressler Street
Unit 1434
Houston, TX 77030
USA

E-mail address:
khunt@mdanderson.org

Considerations in Testing for Inherited Breast Cancer Predisposition in the Era of Personalized Medicine

Benjamin Powers, MD[a], Tuya Pal, MD[b], Christine Laronga, MD[a,*]

KEYWORDS

- Inherited breast cancer syndromes • Surgical considerations
- Personalized medicine • Germline mutation

KEY POINTS

- Multigene panel testing has led to an increase in the number of individuals (both affected and unaffected by cancer) being identified with a germline mutation (ie, pathogenic variant).
- Surgeons are often at the forefront of point of service for individuals at risk for inherited cancer syndromes and must stay current with identifying these at-risk individuals.
- Provision of care through a multidisciplinary team, inclusive of genetic counseling before and after testing, is imperative to appropriately counsel and manage individuals with inherited cancer syndromes.
- Surveillance and management of individuals is personalized based on the gene in which the pathogenic variant is identified, often in conjunction with the personal and family cancer history.

INTRODUCTION

Breast cancer remains the most common cancer and the second leading cause of death affecting women in 2017.[1] Women in the United States have a 12% lifetime risk of developing breast cancer,[2] with an increase in breast cancer incidence from 2004 to 2013, exclusively caused by increasing rates among nonwhite women.[3]

Studies of families have shown that the risk of breast cancer increases with the number of affected relatives.[4] Although most breast cancers are sporadic, 5% to

Disclosures: Dr C. Laronga is on the Speaker's Bureau at Genomic Health and receives royalties from Up-To-Date. Drs B. Powers and T. Pal have nothing to disclose.
[a] Department of Breast Oncology, H. Lee Moffitt Cancer Center, 10920 N. Mckinley Drive, Tampa, FL 33612, USA; [b] Department of Medicine, Vanderbilt University Medical Center, Vanderbilt-Ingram Cancer Center, Nashville, TN, USA
* Corresponding author.
E-mail address: christine.laronga@moffitt.org

10% of cases are caused by a germline mutation (which may also be referred to as a pathogenic variant) in an inherited cancer gene leading to hereditary cancer predisposition.[5] Mutations in these genes lead to a significantly higher risk of developing breast and other cancers compared with cancer risks among women with sporadic breast cancer.[6]

Over the last few years, important technological advances realized through next-generation sequencing (NGS) technologies coupled with the loss of the ability to patent genes have led to greatly decreased costs for genetic testing. NGS-based tests have led to paradigm shifts in genetic testing, enabling clinicians to test for multiple conditions simultaneously (called multigene panel testing) compared with the prior phenotype-directed approaches with sequential testing of 1 condition at a time through the use of Sanger sequencing. With the increasing use of multigene panel tests, the genetic counseling and testing landscape has continued to rapidly evolve. Furthermore, with the identification of more high-risk individuals, the hope is that this information may be leveraged to improve cancer outcomes and influence evidence-based screening, diagnosis, and treatment of patients with breast cancer. Despite the considerable technological advances in genetic testing, the surgical clinic remains the primary locus for identification and management of many of these high-risk patients.[7] However, lack of identification coupled with barriers in access and use of genetic services remain significant challenges to achieving equity through risk reduction strategies.[8,9] Furthermore, many busy surgeons lack the time needed to appropriately counsel patients regarding risk assessment, testing, and results interpretation, and some also have limited proficiency and lack formal training in genetics. These factors may lead them to recommend prophylactic surgery regardless of the gene in which the pathogenic variant (or even a variant of uncertain significance [VUS]) is encountered.

This article focuses on identification of individuals at high risk for inherited breast cancer and referral to (and/or conduct of) genetic counseling and testing for hereditary cancer syndromes, if appropriate. Referral in the context of a newly diagnosed patient with breast cancer or a suspected unaffected high-risk patient for further genetic evaluation is outlined. In addition, approaches for management of specific moderate-penetrance to high-penetrance hereditary breast cancer syndromes are reviewed.

IDENTIFICATION OF HIGH-RISK INDIVIDUALS

Identification of high-risk individuals is predicated on knowledge of the extent and magnitude of breast cancer risk factors and is a multistep process involving a multidisciplinary team of health care professionals. Multiple associations and societies have produced recommendations for screening for genetic predisposition to cancer. Based on recommendations from the National Comprehensive Cancer Network (NCCN), US Preventive Services Task Force, and the National Accreditation Program for Breast Centers (NAPBC), individuals at high risk for hereditary cancer should be offered genetic counseling.[10–12] Although the definition of high risk carries a subjective component, because patients may interpret personal risk differently, there remains an onus on clinicians to provide patients with an accurate assessment of risk to best equip the patients in the informed decision-making process.

The starting point in surgical practice for identification of high-risk (genetic and nongenetic) individuals is the clinical history and physical examination (**Table 1**). Clinical history should include a 3-generation family pedigree of any cancer occurrence and age at diagnosis, inclusive of both the maternal and paternal lineage, as well as all relatives given that family structure is also an important consideration when

Table 1

Indications for genetic counseling referral

Personal History		Personal + Family History Risk Factors		Family History Risk Factors
No history: Breast cancer		➡ (arrow)		with known mutation in a cancer susceptibility gene in family
			or	≥ 2 Breast cancer primaries in same individual
			or	≥ 2 Breast cancer primaries same side of family with 1 person diagnosed <50yrs
			or	1st/2nd degree relative with Breast cancer <45yrs
			or	family history of Ovarian cancer
			or	Male Breast Cancer
			or	≥3 of the following cancers in any combination: breast, colon, kidney, pancreatic, prostate, melanoma, sarcoma, adrenocortical, brain tumors, leukemia, diffuse gastric cancer, endometrial, thyroid
		Personal History of Ovarian cancer		
		Personal History of Pancreatic cancer		and Ashkenazi Jewish ancestry
			or	1 Breast cancer ≤50yrs
			or	1 Ovarian cancer
			or	1 Pancreatic cancer
		Personal History of 2 of these (1 <45yrs): sarcoma or brain tumor or leukemia or lung bronchoaveolar		
		Personal history of adrenocortical cancer		
		Large head circumference and: thyroid cancer or endometrial cancer or multiple GI harmatoma polyps or mucocutaneous lesions		
History: Breast cancer	if:	with known inherited gene mutation		
	or	Breast cancer <50yrs (Triple Negative Cancer <60yrs)		
	or	2 Breast cancer primaries in same person		
	or	Pancreatic cancer any age		
	or	Male Breast cancer		
Any Age if:		1. Ashkenazi Jewish ancestry or	or	≥1 close relative with Breast cancer ≤50yrs or Ovarian Cancer any age
		2. personal history of: pancreatic, prostate, melanoma, sarcoma, adrenocortical, leukemia, diffuse gastric cancer, colon, endometrial, thyroid, kidney	or	≥3 of the following cancers in any combination: breast, pancreatic, prostate, melanoma, sarcoma, adrenocortical, brain tumors, leukemia, diffuse gastric cancer, colon, endometrial, thyroid, kidney
			or	≥2 close relative with Breast cancer and/or Pancreatic cancer any age

determining risk. Identification of breast cancer in a first-degree relative nearly doubles the risk in an individual and has been observed in approximately 13% of patients with breast cancer. The elements of risk factors for breast cancer span across categories of demographic, reproductive, and biological, and environmental risk factors (**Table 2**). Because most breast cancers are hormone receptor positive, many of these risk factors are hormonally driven.

The timeline for patient referral for genetic counseling is based on the clinical context. Undiagnosed patients who present with symptoms or signs of breast cancer should first undergo appropriate steps for diagnosis of cancer, including imaging studies and tissue biopsy. Once a cancer diagnosis has been made, the timeline to

Table 2 Elements of breast cancer risk		
Category	**Factor**	**Comments**
Demographics	Female sex Increasing age	
Ethnicity/race	White	Increased incidence of *BRCA1/BRCA2* mutations in Ashkenazi Jewish descent
BMI*	Obesity Obesity	Postmenopausal: all races/ethnicities White: any age
Reproductive history*	Younger age at menarche Lower parity Age at first live birth Age at menopause	Age <11 y Nulliparous: highest risk Age >30 y Older
Exogenous factors*	Estrogen/progestin therapy Alcohol consumption	Current or past; especially combination use >10 y Weekly, >3 servings
Miscellaneous	Genetic predisposition Prior thoracic radiation Prior breast biopsy with mammary dysplasia Prior breast biopsies Breast density	<30 y of age Lobular carcinoma in situ, atypical ductal hyperplasia, atypical lobular hyperplasia, flat epithelia atypia Risk increase with number of biopsies; cyst aspiration not included

Abbreviation: BMI, body mass index.

refer for genetic counseling and consider testing becomes short, because this information may contribute to surgical decision making. If the patient has no evidence suggestive of breast cancer, it still remains important to identify and offer the patient a nonurgent genetic counseling referral, given that the results may alter the clinical surveillance and management of the patient (ie, through early detection or prevention of cancer).

Given the wide variation in magnitude of cancer risk as well as cancer spectrum based on the gene in which a mutation is identified, the American Society of Clinical Oncology has consistently used 3 criteria since 1996 for proceeding with genetic testing[1]: the individual has a personal or family history suggestive of a cancer genetic susceptibility condition,[2] the test can be adequately interpreted, and[3] the results will aid in the diagnosis or influence the medical or surgical management of the patient or family members.[13] Although these criteria were developed at a time when testing was limited to 1 or 2 genes, they have become increasingly important because multigene panel testing is becoming the norm in many practices, leading to complex conversations with patients regarding management strategies if a pathogenic variant is identified. Keeping abreast of all of the inherited breast cancer genes and their respective cancer spectra contained within the various multigene panels is a challenge to most practicing surgeons. This challenge has made it even more imperative for surgeons to become familiar with the criteria for referral for genetic counseling and testing.

Among patients without a personal history or current diagnosis of breast cancer, several familial risk stratification tools are available to determine the need for in-depth genetic counseling, including the Ontario Family History Assessment Tool, Manchester Scoring System, Referral Screening Tool, Pedigree Assessment Tool, and

FHS-7.[12] The US Preventive Services Task Force listed these tools as clinical predictors to determine which women should undergo referral for genetic counseling because of increased risk for *BRCA* mutations.[11] Furthermore, they recommend against general breast cancer risk assessment models such as the National Cancer Institute Breast Cancer Risk Assessment Tool (based on the Gail model), which are not designed to stratify based on inherited risk in order to identify those who should receive genetic counseling or *BRCA* testing. The NCCN also has criteria for appropriate referrals for further genetic evaluation according to personal risk factors, personal and/or family history risk factors, and family history risk factors.[10]

GENETIC COUNSELING

The National Society of Genetic Counselors (NSGC) has enumerated several components of genetic counseling.[14] Broadly, the aim of genetic counseling is to discuss the benefits, limitations, and risks of genetic testing. This process involves communicating often complex biomedical and statistical issues at the core of genetic testing into a language that patients can understand. This dialogue forms the foundation for the patients to make informed decisions about proceeding with genetic testing and management of risk in their health care. In addition, the counseling process serves to describe the link between testing options for cancer and the goals of early detection and management. The NCCN guidelines highly recommend both pretest and posttest counseling when results are disclosed.[10] Furthermore, the NAPBC has included access to a credentialed genetic counselor to perform both pretest and posttest counseling as a standard component of each breast center's certification.[12]

Per NCCN and NAPBC guidelines, pretest counseling includes collection of a comprehensive family history; evaluation of the patient's cancer risk; generating a differential diagnosis and educating the patient on the penetrance of inheritance patterns; variable expressivity and the possibility of genetic heterogeneity; preparing the patient for possible outcomes of testing, including positive, negative, and uncertain findings; and obtaining informed consent. Posttest counseling centers discussion on the results of the genetic test and the recommended referrals for management options. In addition, the aim is to interpret the results in the context of personal and family history of cancer, providing opportunities to inform and test potential at-risk family members, and providing available resources such as online information or brochures for further reading, disease-specific support groups, and possible research studies (**Table 3**).[15]

Genetic counseling should also include a discussion of testing sensitivity and specificity, inconclusive genetic results, and variants of uncertain clinical significance. In addition, the NSGC has highlighted that attending to the psychosocial issues involved in genetic testing is a vital aspect of care that underpins health care behavior changes. Therefore, "genetic counseling is best offered in the context of a multidisciplinary team, which would include experts in genetic counseling, surgery, oncology, social work, nursing oncology, and psychology."[14]

GENETIC TESTING

The decision to proceed with genetic testing should be based on whether the test is clinically indicated and will affect clinical management of the patient, the results can be adequately interpreted, and (of paramount importance) patient preference. Given the complexity of communicating genetic concepts and information, it is only possible for patients to make an informed decision about testing once the pros and cons have been explained to them in an understandable way. Among patients presenting in the

Table 3
Lifetime cancer risk of common hereditary cancer syndromes

Column 1	General Population Risk (%)	BRCA1 (%)	BRCA2 (%)	TP53 (%)	PTEN (%)	PALB2 (%)	CDH1 (%)	ATM (%)	CHEK2 (%)
Breast	10–12	87	84	44–95	85	33–58	39–52	15–52	28–48
Ovarian	1.1	63	27	—	—	—	—	—	—
Melanoma	2–3.5	—	Increased	—	6	—	—	—	—
Endometrial	2.3–2.6	—	—	—	19–28	—	—	—	—
Colorectal	3–5	—	—	3–19	9–16	—	—	—	Increased
Thyroid	0.6–1.8	—	—	—	21–35	—	—	—	—
Bone Sarcoma	0.1	—	—	3–14	—	—	—	—	—
Soft Tissue Sarcoma	0.3	—	—	10–31	—	—	—	—	—
Brain	0.5	—	—	10–30	—	—	—	—	—
Gastric	0.6	—	—	—	—	—	Increased	—	—
Pancreatic	1.0	—	7	2–19	—	Increased	—	Increased	—
Prostate	12.8	16	20	—	—	—	—	—	—
Renal	1.2–2.1	—	—	—	15–34	—	—	—	—
Adrenocortical	—	—	—	Increased	—	—	—	—	—

context of a new breast cancer diagnosis, there is urgency in offering them genetic counseling and testing as appropriate, given that this information may inform medical or surgical management.[16]

In the context of a known family mutation, a negative test result in a family member unaffected with cancer is highly reassuring and considered informative in most cases. In contrast, when the first person in the family to be tested is an individual unaffected with cancer, there remain limitations in the interpretation of a negative result because it is not possible to distinguish between a true-negative and an uninformative result. A true-negative is someone not at risk for an inherited cancer (ie, a pathogenic variant has been previously identified in the family and accounts for the cancer phenotype observed in the family, and the individual tested does not have this previously identified mutation). An uninformative result means that an informative (or best testable) individual in the family was tested and not identified to have any pathogenic variant that explains the personal and family cancer history (suggesting that the pathogenic variant leading to cancer in this high-risk family may not have been discovered yet) or there is no living affected (best testable) family member available to test and confirm the existence of a pathogenic variant. Consequently, when suspicion of a hereditary syndrome is high, a negative result is not reassuring and should be interpreted as uninformative and management should be guided by family history. It is important to identify these patients upfront when initial testing is ordered, to set their expectations that, even if their tests do not identify a pathogenic variant, they will remain at high risk based on personal and/or family history. In these circumstances, it is also important to encourage testing among affected family members, if available, because this has the potential to clarify this type of uninformative result.

In circumstances in which multiple family members are affected, recommendations are first to test the family member with the youngest age at diagnosis, and those with bilateral disease, multiple primary cancers, or other cancers associated with the syndrome or most closely related to the patient.[11] In cases in which there is no living relative with the cancer in question, consideration may be given to testing first-degree or second-degree family members with other cancers thought to be related to the genetic mutation under suspicion. Although there are significant limitations in testing unaffected family members, it should be considered when no affected family member is available.

Genetic testing approaches may be grouped into targeted testing for mutations associated with a specific hereditary risk syndrome or more broadly approached with multigene panel testing through NGS-based technology that simultaneously analyzes a set of genes that are associated with multiple phenotypes.[17,18] When considering genetic testing options, it is important to consider the presenting phenotype, including the patient's personal and family cancer history, and physical examination. In this context, it is appropriate to test for specific genes based on a phenotype-directed approach or, alternatively, test through a multigene panel test while ensuring that the genes based on the patient's presenting phenotype are included. In cases of high suspicion that lack distinguishing features of a single inherited cancer syndrome, multigene panel testing provides a more expansive approach to hereditary syndrome identification and may be the best option. However, when testing through a multigene panel approach, it remains important to explain to the patient that some of the genes included on the panel have uncertain or even unproven associations with cancer risks and/or that there is a lack of evidence-based guidelines; furthermore, it is important to discuss the range of cancer risks of genes included on these tests, including those with moderate versus high penetrance, which carry substantial differences in management guidelines. In addition, it is important to discuss the high likelihood of identifying a VUS result with testing for more genes, and that this type of result does not inform medical management.

Furthermore, there may be a role for multigene panel testing in individuals who have tested negative (indeterminate) for a single syndrome but whose personal or family history remains suggestive of an inherited susceptibility. Because commercially available tests differ in the specific genes analyzed (as well as classification of variants and many other factors), choosing the specific laboratory and test panel is important. Multigene testing can include intermediate-penetrant (moderate-risk) genes. For many of these genes, there are limited data on the degree of cancer risk and there are no clear guidelines on risk management for carriers of these mutations.[10] As stated earlier, it is particularly important to recognize that not all genes included on available multigene tests are necessarily clinically actionable, leaving surgeons with a conundrum of surveillance and management decisions. In these circumstances, it remains critical to evaluate the evidence when providing management recommendations, given that there are harms to both overtreatment and undertreatment. Furthermore, there have been attempts by commercial laboratories to provide decision support to facilitate delivery of care to these patients, which can also result in misinformation. For example, several laboratories currently indicate that the lifetime risk for breast cancer among women with a germline mutation in the ATM gene is up to 60%, which is a level of risk at which risk-reducing mastectomy would be a consideration. However, this risk level is misleading given that it is a single allele (the 7279 C>G pathogenic variant) that has been established to confer this level of risk, and individuals with other pathogenic variants in the ATM gene have ∼30% lifetime risk of breast cancer.[19] This type of information on test reports has high potential to be misinterpreted and lead to universal recommendations for bilateral mastectomy without the patients being given correct information about their cancer risks based on the specific ATM mutations with which they were identified.

As is the case with high-risk genes, it is possible that the risks associated with moderate-risk genes may not be entirely caused by that gene alone but may be influenced by gene/gene or gene/environment interactions. In addition, certain mutations in a gene may pose higher or lower risk than other mutations in that same gene. Therefore, it may be difficult to use a known mutation alone to assign risk for relatives. In many cases, the information from testing for moderate penetrance genes does not change risk management compared with that based on family history alone. Mutations in many breast cancer susceptibility genes involved in DNA repair may be associated with rare autosomal recessive conditions.[20] Thus when these are identified, it is important to review the phenotype of the autosomal recessive condition and the carrier frequency, and advise the patient about carrier testing options, particularly among family members in their childbearing years. There is an increased likelihood of finding VUS when testing for mutations in multiple genes. It is for these and other reasons that multigene panel testing is ideally offered in the context of pretest and posttest counseling by individuals with professional genetics expertise.

In addition, genetic testing is often complicated by results that reveal a VUS, which occurs in roughly 10% to 13% of white patients who undergo BRCA gene sequencing.[21] Women of African descent have been noted to have higher rates of VUS, although populations that are genetically distinct or undertested may not show the VUS seen in the reference white/European population.[22] A VUS result is typically a missense mutation that is not involved in messenger RNA processing. For these results, it is important to determine the number of times the particular variant has been detected, whether it has been reported with another deleterious BRCA gene mutation, whether it is tracking with the cancer in the family, conservation of the change across species, the region of the gene in which the change is located, change in the base pair that does not change the amino acid, or whether additional data based on functional studies are available.[23] Genetic variants that do not track with cancer, are seen with a proven deleterious mutation, are not conserved across species, are located in a region of the gene not known to have important functional significance, and have been evaluated through functional studies that suggest the change does not affect function are less likely to be of clinical significance to the patient. Understanding these concepts (or referring their patients to credentialed or certified genetics professionals) is paramount to surgeons because a recent study showed that 24% to 50% (high-volume vs low-volume cancer practices) of surgeons managed a VUS as they would a pathogenic mutation of BRCA1/BRCA2.[10] As the majority stakeholders in referral or ordering of genetic testing for patients with newly diagnosed breast cancer, surgeons must keep abreast of the current increase in genetic information. They must order testing for the right patients with the correct genes in a timely fashion, and accurately interpret results of genetic testing to appropriately guide treatment decisions such as risk-reducing mastectomy.

HIGHLY PENETRANT GENETIC SYNDROMES
BRCA1/BRCA2

It has now been roughly 20 years since the discovery of the BRCA genes, BRCA1 and BRCA2, both of which encode for proteins involved in tumor suppression.[24] This breakthrough allowed the identification of patients with hereditary breast and ovarian cancer syndrome. BRCA1 and BRCA2 mutations comprise almost all hereditary breast cancers and these individuals are at a significantly increased risk of breast and ovarian cancer.[6,25,26] Initial epidemiologic studies suggested a lifetime risk for BRCA1 carriers as high as 87% and BRCA2 as high as 84%.[27,28] However, given that the sample population contained patients with a significant number of cancer diagnoses, bias likely existed favoring highly penetrant gene variants that resulted in an overestimation of the lifetime risk.[29] Subsequent meta-analysis has suggested that the risk of breast cancer from BRCA1 ranges from 57% to 65%, and the risk from BRCA2 from 45% to 49%.[29] Regarding ovarian cancer, the risk for BRCA1 is 40% and these tumors are typically epithelial in origin, high grade, and advanced stage at diagnosis. The risk of ovarian cancer for BRCA2 is 18%. For hereditary families with both breast and ovarian cancers, more than 90% are likely caused by mutations in the BRCA1/BRCA2 genes.[6] Additional risks among BRCA mutation carriers include male breast cancer, prostate cancer, and pancreatic cancer, with BRCA2 conferring higher risks for these cancers than BRCA1.

Pitfalls to risk identification of BRCA carriers include small biological family size, which may decrease sensitivity. In addition, in the rare cases of prophylactic operations that remove the susceptible organs or death before onset, the true incidence of the cancer remains unknown and this can hamper BRCA risk identification.[30]

BRCA1 and BRCA2 are autosomal dominant genes; they may be inherited from either parent, resulting in the need for a complete 3-generation (maternal and paternal) family history. BRCA1 and BRCA2 mutations are rare in most populations, although much more common in certain populations. In the Ashkenazi Jewish population, 1 in 40 individuals carries 1 of 3 main disease-causing mutations, compared with an estimated prevalence of 1 in 300 for BRCA1 and 1 in 800 for BRCA2 in general populations.[31]

There has been a great deal of research into the tumor biology associated with BRCA1/BRCA2 mutation carriers. Although BRCA2-associated breast cancers are clinically comparable with sporadic cancers (estrogen receptor positive), *BRCA1*-related breast cancers are often more aggressive, show higher histologic grade, and are triple negative (estrogen receptor negative, progesterone receptor negative, and HER2 negative), with reports of *BRCA1* mutation ranging from 8.5% to 28% in patients with triple-negative breast cancer.[11,32–34]

Unlike other hereditary cancer syndromes, models exist to estimate the likelihood of identifying a mutation in the *BRCA1* or *BRCA2* genes. For example, the BRCAPRO statistical model and associated software estimate the likelihood of a germline mutation of *BRCA1* or *BRCA2* using family history and Bayes theorem.[35] As well as the predictive benefits, the limitations of the models and interpretation in the appropriate context should be noted. Penetrance of *BRCA1* and *BRCA2* have been variable and there may be additional genetic or environmental factors that play a role.

BRCA mutation–positive patients should undergo specific risk management strategies to optimize outcomes. Specifically, breast cancer screening guidelines have been proposed by the NCCN and are updated biannually.[10] Current recommendations include, but are not limited to, a discussion of risk-reducing mastectomies with women who are *BRCA* carriers. Patients should be counseled that there is a 90% to 95% reduction in breast cancer risk following prophylactic mastectomy.[35–39] In addition, reconstructive options should be proposed and plastic surgery consultation provided. Limited data exist regarding chemoprevention for *BRCA* carriers; however, because the mean cumulative lifetime risks for contralateral breast cancer have been estimated at 83% for *BRCA1* carriers and 62% for *BRCA2* carriers, efforts have been made to use chemoprevention as a strategy.[40] The Hereditary Breast Cancer Clinical Study Group reported that tamoxifen showed a statistically significant protective effect, with an odds ratio (OR) of 0.38 (95% confidence interval [CI], 0.19–0.74) against contralateral breast cancer among *BRCA1* mutation carriers, although no statistically significant difference was seen for patients with *BRCA2* (OR, 0.63; 95% CI, 0.20–1.50).[41] Some reports have shown the benefit of risk-reducing salpingo-oophorectomy, with a significant reduction in ovarian cancer for women who underwent prophylactic surgery compared with those who underwent close surveillance.[42,43] Oral contraceptives with estrogen and progestin have shown mixed results, with a protective effect against ovarian cancer in some studies but not in others.[44–46]

In addition to prevention strategies, another consideration is treatment of *BRCA* mutation–positive patients with breast cancer and involves usage of targeted agents such as poly (ADP-ribose) polymerase (PARP) inhibitors and platinum-based therapies.[47,48] PARP inhibitors are currently US Food and Drug Administration approved for *BRCA*-related ovarian cancer and are currently in clinical trials for breast cancer.

TP53/Li-Fraumeni Syndrome

Li-Fraumeni syndrome (LFS) is a very rare cancer syndrome thought to be responsible for approximately 1% of breast cancers.[49] The syndrome is associated with germline mutations in the *TP53* gene. LFS encompasses a breadth of cancer types and is viewed as a hereditary predisposition to cancer in general occurring at any point in an individual's lifetime. The cumulative lifetime cancer incidence nears 100%.[50] Mutations in the *TP53* gene, a tumor suppressor gene, comprise most LFS cases.[51–53] The more common LFS tumors, referred to as component tumors, include osteosarcomas, chondrosarcomas, soft tissue sarcomas, breast cancer, brain tumors, leukemia, and adrenocortical carcinomas, with typical onset of a cancer in childhood.[53] The component tumors are thought to account for 63% to 77% of cancer diagnoses in individuals with LFS.[54–58]

Regarding breast cancer, it is the most common tumor in p53 mutation carriers, as well as the most common second cancer diagnosis. Recent epidemiologic studies have suggested that although soft tissue tumors are most common among the very young and older patients with LFS, breast cancer was the most common diagnosis among those aged 18 to 44 years.[56] On histology, breast cancers are most commonly invasive ductal carcinomas.[55]

LFS was first identified in 1988 through examining 24 kindreds.[55] Subsequent efforts to broaden criteria to identify families with p53 mutations were reported by Birch and colleagues[58] in 1994, who identified LFS-like (LFL) families. Nevertheless, a noted drawback is that both classic and LFL criteria rely on family history and do not capture patients with potential de novo germline p53 mutations, which have been estimated to be from 7% to 20%.[54]

In 2001, Chompret and colleagues[57] developed criteria for identifying patients likely to carry p53 mutations and included criteria that address families who display a collection of component tumors but also address individuals whose personal histories are suggestive of p53 mutation even in the absence of a suggestive family history. The Chompret criteria were designed to include individuals who may potentially carry de novo p53 mutations. Estimates place mutations in p53 at 50% to 70% for the classic definition, 21% to 40% for the LFL definition, and 20% for Chompret.[55,58–64]

Studies that have examined overall cancer risk in p53 mutation carriers show that the risk of developing cancer by 15 to 20 years of age is 12% to 42%, by age 40 to 45 years is 52% to 66%, by age 50 years is 80%, and by age 85 years is 85%.[57,63–66] When stratified by sex, female p53 mutation carriers have a higher lifetime cancer risk compared with male carriers.[57,63,66] Individuals with LFS are also more likely to develop multiple primary tumors.[67]

Patients at risk for breast cancer should undergo a detailed discussion of risk management strategies and surveillance (**Table 4**).[11] Of note, recent articles have suggested that enhanced screening protocols may detect early-stage disease and potentially lead to improved outcomes in patients with LFS, commonly referred to as the Toronto protocol.[68–70] The surveillance protocol included physical examinations, laboratory studies, and imaging with ultrasonography, brain MRI, and rapid total-body MRI scans to minimize radiation exposure. A prospective, observational study of 8 families with LFS who were followed either with enhanced surveillance (n = 18) or routine institutional follow-up care (n = 16; 1 patient with LFS was in both groups) showed a significant difference in overall survival at 3 years, with 100% survival in the surveillance group, and 21% in the group without enhanced surveillance.[70]

Although there are no data for patients with LFS regarding risk reduction surgery, NCCN guidelines recommend discussion on a case-by-case basis.[10] However, breast cancer remains the first and second most common cancer affecting patients with TP53 and, thus consideration for risk-reducing surgery is reasonable. For family members of patients with LFS, breast cancer screening should begin between age 20 and 25 years or, if younger than 20 years, at the age of the earliest known breast cancer in the family. Breast screening recommendations in LFS mirror those for BRCA-related breast and ovarian cancer syndrome management and vary with patient age. For women aged 20 to 29 years, annual breast MRI screening with contrast is preferred, or mammogram if MRI is not available. For women aged 30 to 75 years, annual mammogram and breast MRI screening with contrast is recommended. An individualized approach is recommended for women more than 75 years old. Screening for other component cancers should be performed in the setting of a multidisciplinary genetics clinical service.

Table 4
Screening recommendations and management strategies

	Recommend Breast MRI	Age to Begin (y)	Recommend Prophylactic BSO	Age (y)	Recommend Prophylactic Mastectomy	Other Recommendations
Intervention Based on Pathogenic Variant Alone	BRCA1 BRCA2 TP53 PTEN PALB2 CDH1 CHEK2 ATM	25 25 20 30 30 30 40 40	BRCA1 BRCA2	35–45 or when identified at later age	BRCA1 BRCA2 TP53 PTEN CDH1	1. BRCA2: annual skin examination, pancreatic screen if fam history 2. TP53: annual rapid total-body MRI, skin examination, neurologic examination, CBC, UA; colonoscopy q 2–5 y starting age 25 y 3. PTEN: annual thyroid and transvaginal US and skin examination starting age 30 y, colonoscopy and renal US q 2y starting age 40 y 4. CDH1: EGD 5. CHEK2: colonoscopy q 5 y
Insufficient Data for Intervention Based on Pathogenic Variant Alone	—	—	PALB2	—	ATM CHEK2 PALB2	ATM: can consider mastectomy based on addition of family history

Abbreviations: BSO, bilateral salpingo-oophorectomy; CBC, complete blood count; EGD, esophagogastroduodenoscopy; q, every; UA, urinalysis; US, ultrasonography.

In the context of a breast cancer diagnosis, detection of a *TP53* mutation may refine surgical treatment, with some patients choosing to undergo bilateral mastectomy to reduce risks of a second primary breast cancer. Furthermore, studies have suggested that radiation treatment as part of a primary cancer treatment may increase the risks of subsequent cancers among individuals with germline *TP53* mutations.[71,72] The NCCN practice guidelines state that "Therapeutic radiation treatment for cancer should be avoided when possible"[10] among patients with LFS. A recent French study of more than 400 patients with LFS reported a high rate (43%) of multiple primary cancers, most of which were cancers that developed following an initial cancer diagnosis.[72] Treatment records were available on a subset of patients who received radiation treatment of their first tumor, which showed that 30% developed secondary tumors in the radiation field, within 2 to 26 years (mean, 10.7 years) following their initial cancer treatment.[72] Therefore, caution is advised before offering surgical choices that are contingent on subsequent radiation administration for completion of standard of care.

PTEN/Cowden Syndrome

The *PTEN* hamartoma tumor syndrome (PHTS) is a rare hereditary cancer syndrome arising from germline mutations in *PTEN* (phosphate and tensin homolog), a tumor suppressor gene. These mutations manifest in a spectrum of clinical disorders characterized by overgrowth in different organ systems. PHTS encompasses Cowden syndrome (CS), Bannayan-Riley-Ruvalcaba syndrome, adult Lhermitte-Duclos disease, Proteus and Proteus-like syndrome, and autism spectrum disorders with macrocephaly.[73–77]

The best studied of these is CS, an autosomal dominant disorder with an incidence of approximately 1 in 200,000, although, given the difficulty of diagnosis, it may be underestimated.[78,79] The initial estimated penetrance of *PTEN* mutation was roughly 80%, although expanded criteria have decreased that figure to approximately 25%.[79–81] Although *PTEN* mutations are the most common, mutations in other genes, such as *SDHx* and *KILLIN*, have been reported in small cohorts of patients.[81,82]

The lifetime risk for breast cancer for women diagnosed with CS has been estimated at 25% to 50%, with an average age of 38 to 50 years at diagnosis.[83] The lifetime breast cancer risk for *PTEN* hamartoma syndrome ranged from 67% to 85% in 3 studies, with increased risk beginning around the age of 30 years.[84–86] Additional studies have shown that women with PTEN mutations and a breast cancer diagnosis have a 29% risk of a secondary breast cancer within 10 years.[87]

Patients with suspicion of CS/PHTS should be assessed with a detailed history that should explore both benign and malignant conditions associated with the syndrome and a physical examination with attention to skin and oral mucosa for hamartomas, breast, and thyroid gland.[10] The classic feature of CS is development of multiple hamartomas of the skin and mucosa. A thorough physical examination, including head circumference measurement and examination for skin manifestations, is an important component of assessing for CS. However, a lack of hamartomas does not exclude CS.

In 1995 the International Cowden Consortium produced the first diagnostic criteria for CS.[79] Since that time, criteria have evolved and been modified. Of note, the criteria are used to assess the need for further risk assessment and genetic testing but are not intended to serve as clinical diagnostic criteria. Given the complexity and degree of variability in CS, making a formal diagnosis is difficult except in the most obvious of cases. In cases of high suspicion, a negative genetic test result may be uninformative for the patient and her family. In contrast, a positive result or VUS in an individual without classic features of CS can lead to uncertainty regarding how aggressive to be about screening and prevention measures.

The highest risk of cancer associated with CS is for female breast cancer, with estimates of cancer risk ranging from 25% to 85%. Other cancers comprising CS include thyroid cancer, with a risk of 3% to 38%, and endometrial cancer, with a risk of 5% to 28%. In addition, renal cell cancer with a risk estimate of 34%, melanoma with a risk of 6%, and colorectal cancer with a risk of 9% have also been reported.[74,84]

As such, patients with PTEN (CS) should undergo specific risk management strategies to optimize outcomes (see **Table 4**). Recommendations are for annual breast MRI starting at age 30 years followed by consideration of risk-reducing surgery.[10] In addition, annual thyroid ultrasonography, transvaginal ultrasonography, and a skin survey should likewise begin at age 30 years. Colonoscopy and renal ultrasonography scans begin at age 40 years and should be performed every 2 years.

Other High-Penetrance Genes

PALB2

PALB2 (partner and localizer of BRCA2) is a Fanconi anemia gene that was initially identified as a protein involved in BRCA2 genome caretaker functions and subsequently showed interaction with BRCA1.[87,88] Fanconi anemia arises when germline loss-of-function mutations are biallelic, although monoallelic mutations are associated with breast and pancreatic cancer.[89] Studies have shown that 1% to 3% of women with breast cancer possess a PALB2 mutation.[90,91]

The lifetime breast cancer risk in women with a PALB2 mutation is 14% by age 50 years and 35% by age 70 years; however, the risk also increases with increasing number of relatives affected with breast cancer.[89] Breast cancer risk by age 70 years for those with no first-degree relatives with breast cancer was 33%, compared with 58% in those with 2 first-degree relatives.[89] Contralateral breast cancer was reported in 10% of PALB2 carriers and the 10-year survival among PALB2 carriers with breast cancer was 48%, compared with 72% in BRCA1 mutation carriers and 75% in noncarriers.[91] Thus, there are suggestions that PALB2 mutations may be associated with aggressive breast cancer.

NCCN recommendations include annual mammogram for PALB2 mutation carriers beginning at age 30 years and that additional consideration should be given to breast MRI screening (see **Table 4**).[10,20] The NCCN also recommends consideration of risk-reducing mastectomy. However, because of an uncertain association between PALB2 and increased ovarian cancer risk, there is no recommendation to consider salpingo-oophorectomy as a risk reduction strategy at this time.[92,93]

CDH1

In 1998, linkage analysis suggested that germline mutations in CDH1, which encodes the tumor suppressor protein E-cadherin, were associated with hereditary diffuse gastric cancer.[94] A year later, CDH1 mutations were also shown to be associated with lobular breast cancer.[95] Studies have shown the lifetime risk for breast cancer to be 39% to 52%.[96–98] Pertaining to lobular breast cancer, updated clinical guidelines state that established criteria for CDH1 genetic testing include a personal or family history of diffuse gastric cancer and lobular breast cancer with 1 diagnosed before 50 years of age. Consideration of genetic testing should be given with a history of bilateral lobular breast cancer or family history of 2 or more cases of lobular breast cancer before age 50 years.[99] The NCCN recommends annual mammogram, or consideration of a breast MRI, starting at age 30 years and considering earlier screening in patients with a family history of early-onset breast cancer (see **Table 4**).[10] In addition, risk-reducing mastectomy should be discussed with patients with *CDH1*.

MODERATE PENETRANCE GENES
ATM

Biallelic germline mutations of the ataxia telangiectasia (*ATM*) gene cause ataxia telangiectasia, a pediatric neurologic disorder associated with telangiectasias; immunodeficiency; sensitivity to ionizing radiation; and a 20% to 30% lifetime risk of lymph, gastric, breast, nervous, skin, and other cancers.[99,100]

The association between *ATM* genetic variants and breast cancer risk is not fully clarified. Studies have reported a risk of breast cancer ranging from 15% to 52%.[19,101–104] A recent meta-analysis showed that the lifetime risk of breast cancer for *ATM* mutation carriers was 38% compared with carriers of the c.7271T>G missense mutation, who have a 69% risk of breast cancer by age 70 years.[19]

The NCCN recommends annual screening mammogram for women with an *ATM* gene mutation beginning at age 40 years and consideration of annual breast MRI (see **Table 4**). In addition, mastectomy may be considered based on family history.[10] Although there has been concern that radiation exposure in heterozygous carriers may increase breast cancer risk, there is insufficient evidence of an association at this time. A meta-analysis reported that radiation therapy is not contraindicated in patients with a heterozygous *ATM* mutation.[19] Thus, per current NCCN guidelines, *ATM* heterozygosity (ie, an individual with a single pathogenic variant in the *ATM* gene) is not a contraindication to receipt of radiation therapy in the context of a breast cancer diagnosis.

Breast cancer has long been linked with the *ATM* gene, which is fairly well known and characterized given that biallelic mutations are causative of ataxia telangiectasia, a childhood-onset progressive neurologic disorder associated with telangiectasias, immunodeficiency, sensitivity to ionizing radiation, and increased risks for malignancies (primarily leukemias and lymphomas). Approximately 1% to 3% of the general population may be heterozygous carriers of an *ATM* mutation.[186,187] Studies on the association of *ATM* heterozygous mutations on breast cancer risk have conflicting results, although the 2 largest provide the most convincing evidence of an association.[188,189] The risk is estimated at 15% to 52%, and the relative increase in risk may be even higher for women younger than 50 years.[188–192] *ATM* mutations have been found to cosegregate in several families with multiple cases of pancreatic cancer. Stomach, ovarian, bladder, and colon cancer risks may also be increased, although the evidence of a strong association is less compelling.[189,192] Although breast cancer risk is modest, it has been proposed that *ATM* carriers may need different approaches to treatment o.

CHEK2

CHEK2 (cell cycle checkpoint kinase 2) genes are involved in protein signaling related to DNA double-strand breaks. In a study of patients with breast cancer and a strong family history of breast or ovarian cancer but without *BRCA*, a *CHEK2* mutation was detected in 5%.[105] This mutation is more frequent in northern and eastern European populations.[106] The lifetime risk for breast cancer in women with a *CHEK2* mutation ranges from 28% to 37% and is higher in women with stronger family histories of breast cancer than in those without.[107,108] The specific *CHEK2* variant, 110delC, has been shown to increase breast cancer risk by more than 2-fold when stratified by age and sex.[109] Another study showed that heterozygous 1100delC carriers have a higher risk of developing ER-positive breast cancer, and therefore may be considered for chemoprevention with tamoxifen.[110,111]

The NCCN recommends annual mammogram starting at age 40 years for women with a *CHEK2* mutation and consideration of annual breast MRI (see **Table 4**).[10] For *CHEK2*, no data exist regarding the benefit of risk-reducing mastectomy for women, although, given the context of family history, it may be considered. As for colorectal cancer, recommendations are for colonoscopy every 5 years, and are adjusted based on colonoscopy findings and family history.

NEWER GENES WITHOUT A PROVEN ASSOCIATION WITH BREAST CANCER

The *RAD51* family of genes is involved in DNA damage repair via the homologous recombination pathway. Although *RAD51C* and *RAD51D* have been shown to be associated with increased risk for ovarian cancer, there is currently insufficient evidence that they are associated with increased breast cancer risk.[11] Patients with *RAD51C* and *RAD51D* mutations should be managed as average-risk patients.[11] However, they are at an increased risk for ovarian cancer and consideration for risk-reducing bilateral salpingo-oophorectomy is reasonable.[112,113]

SUMMARY

With nascent advances in genomic technologies, genetic counseling and testing for inherited cancer predisposition is rapidly evolving. The dissemination of next-generation multigene sequencing panels will continue to provide an opportunity for the identification of genetic aberrations for patients at high risk for cancer. However, the identification of those patients involves surgeon awareness and a thorough clinical evaluation, including a systemic history and physical examination. In concert with a rigorous 3-generation family history, high-risk patients can be identified and decisions based on currently available evidence can then be made regarding further counseling and use of genetic testing to identify hereditary breast cancer syndromes. As research unveils additional cancer susceptibility genes, further work regarding the interpretation and implementation of clinical management plans will be needed. Surgeons, therefore, must keep abreast of these advances and, at the minimum, refer patients to genetic services for in-depth evaluation for risk assessment, testing, and results interpretation. For most surgeons, having a well-established multidisciplinary team comprising genetic counselors, oncologists, psychosocial experts, other specialists (plastic surgeons, dermatology, gastroenterology, gynecology), and imagers vested in inherited cancer syndromes is imperative. The advances in genomic testing bring forth an exciting time, with surgeons at the front lines of identification and management of many of these high-risk individuals. However, the tremendous potential for genomic testing to prevent disease and positively affect health can only be realized if patient testing and follow-up care are guided by evidence-based recommendations, and accessible across all segments of the population.

REFERENCES

1. Siegel RL, Miller KD, Jemal A. Cancer statistics, 2017. CA Cancer J Clin 2017; 67(1):7–30.
2. American Cancer Society. Breast cancer facts & figures 2013-2014, 2013.
3. DeSantis CE, Fewewa SA, Goding Sauer A, et al. Breast cancer statistics, 2015: convergence of incidence rates between black and white women. CA Cancer J Clin 2016;66(1):31–42.

4. Collaborative Group on Hormonal Factors in Breast Cancer. Familial breast cancer: collaborative reanalysis of individual data from 52 epidemiological studies including 58,209 women with breast cancer and 101,986 women without the disease. Lancet 2001;358(9291):1389–99.
5. van der Groep P, Bouter A, van der Zanden R, et al. Distinction between hereditary and sporadic breast cancer on the basis of clinicopathological data. J Clin Pathol 2006;59(6):611–7.
6. Kleibl Z, Kristensen VN. Women at high risk of breast cancer: molecular characteristics, clinical presentation and management. Breast 2016;28:136–44.
7. McCarthy AM, Bristol M, Domchek SM, et al. Health care segregation, physician recommendation, and racial disparities in BRCA1/2 testing among women with breast cancer. J Clin Oncol 2016;34(22):2610–8.
8. Cragun D, Weidner A, Lewis C, et al. Racial disparities in BRCA testing and cancer risk management across a population-based sample of young breast cancer survivors. Cancer 2017;123(13):2497–505.
9. Forman AD, Hall MJ. Influence of race/ethnicity on genetic counseling and testing for hereditary breast and ovarian cancer. Breast J 2009;15(Suppl 1): S56–62.
10. National Comprehensive Cancer Network. Genetic/familial high-risk assessment: breast and ovarian (Version 2.2017). Available at: https://www.nccn.org/professionals/physician_gls/pdf/genetics_screening.pdf. Accessed March 23, 2017.
11. Moyer VA, US Preventive Services Task Force. Risk assessment, genetic counseling, and genetic testing for BRCA-related cancer in women: U.S. Preventive Services Task Force recommendation statement. Ann Intern Med 2014;160(4): 271–81.
12. Available at: https://www.facs.org/quality-programs/napbc/standards/components.
13. American Society of Clinical Oncology. American Society of Clinical Oncology policy statement update: genetic testing for cancer susceptibility. J Clin Oncol 2003;21:2397–406.
14. Berliner JL, Fay AM. Risk assessment and genetic counseling for hereditary breast and ovarian cancer: recommendations of the National Society of Genetic Counselors. J Genet Couns 2007;16:241–60.
15. Pal T, Vadaparampil ST. Genetic risk assessments in individuals at high risk for inherited breast cancer in the breast oncology care setting. Cancer Control 2012;19(4):255–66.
16. Robson ME, Bradbury AR, Arun B, et al. American Society of Clinical Oncology policy statement update: genetic and genomic testing for cancer susceptibility. J Clin Oncol 2015;33(31):3660–7.
17. LaDuca H, Stuenkel AJ, Dolinsky JS, et al. Utilization of multigene panels in hereditary cancer predisposition testing: analysis of more than 2,000 patients. Genet Med 2014;16(11):830–7.
18. Kurian AW, Hare EE, Mills MA, et al. Clinical evaluation of a multiple-gene sequencing panel for hereditary cancer risk assessment. J Clin Oncol 2014; 32(19):2001–9.
19. van Os NJ, Roeleveld N, Weemaes CM, et al. Health risks for ataxia-telangiectasia mutated heterozygotes: a systematic review, meta-analysis, and evidence-based guideline. Clin Genet 2016;90:105–17.
20. Tung N, Domchek SM, Stadler Z, et al. Counselling framework for moderate-penetrance cancer-susceptibility mutations. Nat Rev Clin Oncol 2016;13(9): 581–8.

21. Hall MJ, Reid JE, Burbidge LA, et al. BRCA1 and BRCA2 mutations in women of different ethnicities undergoing testing for hereditary breast-ovarian cancer. Cancer 2009;115(10):2222–33.
22. Pal T, Bonner D, Kim J, et al. Early onset breast cancer in a registry-based sample of African American women: BRCA mutation prevalence, and other personal and system-level clinical characteristics. Breast J 2013;19(2):189–92.
23. Slavin TP, Niell-Swiller M, Solomon I, et al. Clinical application of multigene panels: challenges of next-generation counseling and cancer risk management. Front Oncol 2015;5:208.
24. King M-C. "The race" to clone BRCA1. Science 2014;343(6178):1462–5.
25. Risch HA, McLaughlin JR, Cole DE, et al. Prevalence and penetrance of germline BRCA1 and BRCA2 mutations in a population series of 649 women with ovarian cancer. Am J Hum Genet 2001;68(3):700–10.
26. Narod SA, Offit K. Prevention and management of hereditary breast cancer. J Clin Oncol 2005;23(8):1656–63.
27. Ford D, Easton DF, Bishop DT, et al. Risks of cancer in BRCA1-mutation carriers. Breast Cancer Linkage Consortium. Lancet 1994;343(8899):692–5.
28. Ford D, Easton DF, Stratton M, et al. Genetic heterogeneity and penetrance analysis of the BRCA1 and BRCA2 genes in breast cancer families. The Breast Cancer Linkage Consortium. Am J Hum Genet 1998;62(3):676–89.
29. Chen S, Parmigiani G. Meta-analysis of BRCA1 and BRCA2 penetrance. J Clin Oncol 2007;25(11):1329–33.
30. Weitzel JN, Lagos VI, Cullinane CA, et al. Limited family structure and BRCA gene mutation status in single cases of breast cancer. JAMA 2007;297(23): 2587–95.
31. American College of Obstetricians and Gynecologists, ACOG Committee on Practice Bulletins–Gynecology, ACOG Committee on Genetics, Society of Gynecologic Oncologists. ACOG practice bulletin no. 103: hereditary breast and ovarian cancer syndrome. Obstet Gynecol 2009;113:957–66.
32. Whittemore AS. Risk of breast cancer in carriers of BRCA gene mutations. N Engl J Med 1997;337:788–9.
33. Fostira F, Tsitlaidou M, Papadimitriou C, et al. Prevalence of BRCA1 mutations among 403 women with triple-negative breast cancer: implications for genetic screening selection criteria: a Hellenic Cooperative Oncology Group study. Breast Cancer Res Treat 2012;134:353–62.
34. Gonzalez-Angulo AM, Timms KM, Liu S, et al. Incidence and outcome of BRCA mutations in unselected patients with triple receptor-negative breast cancer. Clin Cancer Res 2011;17:1082–9.
35. Antoniou AC, Hardy R, Walker L, et al. Predicting the likelihood of carrying a BRCA1 or BRCA2 mutation: validation of BOADICEA, BRCAPRO, IBIS, Myriad and the Manchester scoring system using data from UK genetics clinics. J Med Genet 2008;45:425–31.
36. Hartmann LC, Sellers TA, Schaid DJ, et al. Efficacy of bilateral prophylactic mastectomy in BRCA1 and BRCA2 gene mutation carriers. J Natl Cancer Inst 2001; 93:1633–7.
37. Rebbeck TR, Friebel T, Lynch HT, et al. Bilateral prophylactic mastectomy reduces breast cancer risk in BRCA1 and BRCA2 mutation carriers: the PROSE Study Group. J Clin Oncol 2004;22:1055–62.
38. Meijers-Heijboer H, van Geel B, van Putten WL, et al. Breast cancer after prophylactic bilateral mastectomy in women with a BRCA1 or BRCA2 mutation. N Engl J Med 2001;345:159–64.

39. Mavaddat N, Peock S, Frost D, et al. Cancer risks for BRCA1 and BRCA2 mutation carriers: results from prospective analysis of EMBRACE. J Natl Cancer Inst 2013;105:812–22.
40. Gronwald J, Tung N, Foulkes WD, et al. Tamoxifen and contralateral breast cancer in BRCA1 and BRCA2 carriers: an update. Int J Cancer 2006;118:2281–4.
41. Narod SA, Brunet JS, Ghadirian P, et al. Tamoxifen and risk of contralateral breast cancer in BRCA1 and BRCA2 mutation carriers: a case-control study. Hereditary Breast Cancer Clinical Study Group. Lancet 2000;356:1876–81.
42. Kauff ND, Satagopan JM, Robson ME, et al. Risk-reducing salpingo-oophorectomy in women with a BRCA1 or BRCA2 mutation. N Engl J Med 2002;346:1609–15.
43. Rebbeck TR, Lunch HT, Neuhausen SL, et al. Prophylactic oophorectomy in carriers of BRCA1 or BRCA2 mutations. N Engl J Med 2002;346:1616–22.
44. Modan B, Hartge P, Hirsh-Yechezkel G, et al. Parity, oral contraceptives, and the risk of ovarian cancer among carriers and noncarriers of a BRCA1 or BRCA2 mutation. N Engl J Med 2001;345:235–40.
45. Narod SA, Risch H, Moslehi R, et al. Oral contraceptives and the risk of hereditary ovarian cancer. Hereditary Ovarian Cancer Clinical Study Group. N Engl J Med 1998;339:424–8, 55.
46. Narod SA, Dubé MP, Klihn J, et al. Oral contraceptives and the risk of breast cancer in BRCA1 and BRCA2 mutation carriers. J Natl Cancer Inst 2002;94:1773–9.
47. Domagala P, Hybiak J, Rys J, et al. Pathological complete response after cisplatin neoadjuvant therapy is associated with the downregulation of DNA repair genes in BRCA1-associated triple-negative breast cancers. Oncotarget 2016;7(42):68662–73.
48. Schouten PC, Dackus GM, Marchetti S, et al. A phase I followed by a randomized phase II trial of two cycles carboplatin-olaparib followed by olaparib monotherapy versus capecitabine in BRCA1- or BRCA2-mutated HER2-negative advanced breast cancer as first line treatment (REVIVAL): study protocol for a randomized controlled trial. Trials 2016;17(1):293.
49. Sidransky D, Tokino T, Helzlsouer K, et al. Inherited p53 gene mutations in breast cancer. Cancer Res 1992;52(10):2984–6.
50. Mai PL, Best AF, Peters JA, et al. Risks of first and subsequent cancers among TP53 mutation carriers in the National Cancer Institute Li-Fraumeni syndrome cohort. Cancer 2016;122(23):3673–81.
51. Lane DP. Cancer. p53, guardian of the genome. Nature 1992;358:15–6.
52. Levine AJ. p53, the cellular gatekeeper for growth and division. Cell 1997;88:323–31.
53. Gonzalez KD, Noltner KA, Buzin CH, et al. Beyond Li Fraumeni syndrome: clinical characteristics of families with p53 germline mutations. J Clin Oncol 2009;27:1250–6.
54. Li FP, Fraumeni JF Jr, Mulvihill JJ, et al. A cancer family syndrome in twenty-four kindreds. Cancer Res 1988;48:5358–62.
55. Nichols KE, Malkin D, Garber JE, et al. Germ-line p53 mutations predispose to a wide spectrum of early-onset cancers. Cancer Epidemiol Biomarkers Prev 2001;10:83–7.
56. Hwang SJ, Lozano G, Amos CI, et al. Germline p53 mutations in a cohort with childhood sarcoma: sex differences in cancer risk. Am J Hum Genet 2003;72:975–83.

57. Chompret A, Abel A, Stoppa-Lyonnet D, et al. Sensitivity and predictive value of criteria for p53 germline mutation screening. J Med Genet 2001;38:43–7.
58. Birch JM, Hartley AL, Tricker KJ, et al. Prevalence and diversity of constitutional mutations in the p53 gene among 21 Li-Fraumeni families. Cancer Res 1994;54: 1298–304.
59. Varley JM, Evans DG, Birch JM. Li-Fraumeni syndrome—a molecular and clinical review. Br J Cancer 1997;76:1–14.
60. Frebourg T, Barbier N, Yan YX, et al. Germ-line p53 mutations in 15 families with Li- Fraumeni syndrome. Am J Hum Genet 1995;56:608–15.
61. Brugières L, Gardes M, Moutou C, et al. Screening for germ line p53 mutations in children with malignant tumors and a family history of cancer. Cancer Res 1993;53:452–5.
62. Varley JM, McGown G, Thorncraft M, et al. Germ-line mutations of TP53 in Li-Fraumeni families: an extended study of 39 families. Cancer Res 1997;57: 3245–52.
63. Chompret A, Brugières L, Ronsin M, et al. P53 germline mutations in childhood cancers and cancer risk for carrier individuals. Br J Cancer 2000;82:1932–7.
64. Le Bihan C, Moutou C, Brugières L, et al. ARCAD: a method for estimating age-dependent disease risk associated with mutation carrier status from family data. Genet Epidemiol 1995;12:13–25.
65. Wu CC, Shete S, Amos CI, et al. Joint effects of germ-line p53 mutation and sex on cancer risk in Li-Fraumeni syndrome. Cancer Res 2006;66:8287–92.
66. Hisada M, Garber JE, Fung CY, et al. Multiple primary cancers in families with Li-Fraumeni syndrome. J Natl Cancer Inst 1998;90:606–11.
67. Villani A, Tabori U, Schiffman J, et al. Biochemical and imaging surveillance in germline TP53 mutation carriers with Li-Fraumeni syndrome: a prospective observational study. Lancet Oncol 2011;12(6):559–67.
68. Masciari S, Van den Abbeele AD, Diller LR, et al. F18-Fluorodeoxyglucose-positron emission tomography/computed tomography screening in Li-Fraumeni syndrome. JAMA 2008;299(11):1315–9.
69. Monsalve J, Kapur J, Malkin D, et al. Radiographics: a review. Imaging of cancer predisposition syndromes in children, vol. 31(1). Radiological Society of North America; 2011. p. 263–80.
70. Henry E, Villalobos V, Million L, et al. Chest wall leiomyosarcoma after breast-conservative therapy for early-stage breast cancer in a young woman with Li-Fraumeni syndrome. J Natl Compr Canc Netw 2012;10:939–42.
71. Kast K, Krause M, Schuler M, et al. Late onset Li-Fraumeni syndrome with bilateral breast cancer and other malignancies: case report and review of the literature. BMC Cancer 2012;12:217.
72. Bougeard G, Renaux-Petel M, Flaman JM, et al. Revisiting Li-Fraumeni syndrome from TP53 mutation carriers. J Clin Oncol 2015;33:2345–52.
73. Pilarski R. Cowden syndrome: a critical review of the clinical literature. J Genet Couns 2009;18:13–27.
74. Eng C. PTEN hamartoma tumor syndrome (PTHS). GeneReviews 2009.
75. Pilarski R, Stephens JA, Noss R, et al. Predicting PTEN mutations: an evaluation of Cowden syndrome and Bannayan-Riley-Ruvalcaba syndrome clinical features. J Med Genet 2011;48:505–12.
76. Eng C. PTEN hamartoma tumor syndrome (PTHS). GeneReviews 2001.
77. Nelen MR, Padberg GW, Peeters EA, et al. Localization of the gene for Cowden disease to chromosome 10q22-23. Nat Genet 1996;13:114–6.

78. Pilarski R, Eng C. Will the real Cowden syndrome please stand up (again)? Expanding mutational and clinical spectra of the PTEN hamartoma tumour syndrome. J Med Genet 2004;41:323–6.

79. Mester J, Charis E. PTEN hamartoma tumor syndrome. Handb Clin Neurol 2015; 132:129–37.

80. Tan MH, Mester J, Peterson C, et al. A clinical scoring system for selection of patients for PTEN mutation testing is proposed on the basis of a prospective study of 3042 probands. Am J Hum Genet 2011;88:42–56.

81. Bennett KL, Mester J, Eng C. Germline epigenetic regulation of KILLIN in Cowden and Cowden-like syndrome. JAMA 2010;304:2724–31.

82. Hobert JA, Eng C. PTEN hamartoma tumor syndrome: an overview. Genet Med 2009;11:687–94.

83. Tan MH, Mester JL, Ngeow J, et al. Lifetime cancer risks in individuals with germline PTEN mutations. Clin Cancer Res 2012;18:400–7.

84. Nieuwenhuis MH, Kets CM, Murphy-Ryan M, et al. Cancer risk and genotype-phenotype correlations in PTEN hamartoma tumor syndrome. Fam Cancer 2014;13:57–63.

85. Bubien V, Bonnet F, Brouste V, et al. High cumulative risks of cancer in patients with PTEN hamartoma tumour syndrome. J Med Genet 2013;50:255–63.

86. Ngeow J, Eng C. PTEN hamartoma tumor syndrome: clinical risk assessment and management protocol. Methods 2015;77-78:11–9.

87. Xia B, Sheng Q, Nakanishi K, et al. Control of BRCA2 cellular and clinical functions by a nuclear partner, PALB2. Mol Cell 2006;22:719–29.

88. Antoniou AC, Casadei S, Heikkinen T, et al. Breast cancer risks in families with mutations in PALB2. N Engl J Med 2014;7:497–506.

89. Sy SM, Huen MS, Zhu Y, et al. PALB2 regulates recombinational repair through chromatin association and oligomerization. J Biol Chem 2009;284:18302–10.

90. Zhang F, Ma J, Wu J, et al. PALB2 links BRCA1 and BRCA2 in the DNA-damage response. Curr Biol 2009;19:524–9.

91. Cybulski C, Kluzniak W, Huzarski T, et al. Clinical outcomes in women with breast cancer and a PALB2 mutation: a prospective cohort analysis. Lancet Oncol 2015;16:638–44.

92. Basham VM, Lipscombe JM, Ward JM, et al. BRCA1 and BRCA2 mutations in a population-based study of male breast cancer. Breast Cancer Res 2002;4:R2.

93. Norquist BM, Harrell MI, Brady MF, et al. Inherited mutations in women with ovarian carcinoma. JAMA Oncol 2016;2(4):482–90.

94. Guilford P, Hopkins J, Harraway J, et al. E-cadherin germline mutations in familial gastric cancer. Nature 1998;392:402–5.

95. Keller G, Vogelsang H, Becker I, et al. Diffuse type gastric and lobular breast carcinoma in a familial gastric cancer patient with an E-cadherin germline mutation. Am J Pathol 1999;155:337–42.

96. Kaurah P, MacMillan A, Boyd N, et al. Founder and recurrent CDH1 mutations in families with hereditary diffuse gastric cancer. JAMA 2007;297:2360–72.

97. Pharoah PD, Guilford P, Caldas C. Incidence of gastric cancer and breast cancer in CDH1 (E-cadherin) mutation carriers from hereditary diffuse gastric cancer families. Gastroenterology 2001;121:1348–53.

98. van der Post RS, Vogelaar IP, Carneiro F, et al. Hereditary diffuse gastric cancer: updated clinical guidelines with an emphasis on germline CDH1 mutation carriers. J Med Genet 2015;52(6):361–74.

99. Choi M, Kipps T, Kurzrock R. ATM mutations in cancer: therapeutic implications. Mol Cancer Ther 2016;15(8):1781–91.

100. Renwick A, Thompson D, Seal S, et al. ATM mutations that cause ataxia-telangiectasia are breast cancer susceptibility alleles. Nat Genet 2006;38: 873–5.
101. Thompson D, Duedal S, Kirner J, et al. Cancer risks and mortality in heterozygous ATM mutation carriers. J Natl Cancer Inst 2005;97:813–22.
102. Ahmed M, Rahman N. ATM and breast cancer susceptibility. Oncogene 2006; 25:5906–11.
103. Morrell D, Cromartie E, Swift M. Mortality and cancer incidence in 263 patients with ataxia-telangiectasia. J Natl Cancer Inst 1986;77:89–92.
104. Bueno RC, Canevari RA, Villacis RA, et al. ATM down-regulation is associated with poor prognosis in sporadic breast carcinomas. Ann Oncol 2014;25(1): 69–75.
105. Walsh T, Casadei S, Coats KH, et al. Spectrum of mutations in BRCA1, BRCA2, CHEK2, and TP53 in families at high risk of breast cancer. JAMA 2006;295: 1379–88.
106. Gage M, Wattendorf D, Henry LR. Translational advances regarding hereditary breast cancer syndromes. J Surg Oncol 2012;105(5):444–51.
107. Cybulski C, Wokolorczyk D, Jakubowska A, et al. Risk of breast cancer in women with a CHEK2 mutation with and without a family history of breast cancer. J Clin Oncol 2011;29:3747–52.
108. Weischer M, Bojesen SE, Ellervik C, et al. CHEK2*1100delC genotyping for clinical assessment of breast cancer risk: meta-analyses of 26,000 patient cases and 27,000 controls. J Clin Oncol 2008;26(4):542–8.
109. Naslund-Koch C, Nordestgaard BG, Bojesen SE. Increased risk for other cancers in addition to breast cancer for CHEK2*1100delC heterozygotes estimated from the Copenhagen General Population Study. J Clin Oncol 2016;34:1208–16.
110. Schmidt MK, Hogervorst F, van Hien R, et al. Age- and tumor subtype-specific breast cancer risk estimates for CHEK2*1100delC carriers. J Clin Oncol 2016; 34:2750–60.
111. Cybulski C, Huzarski T, Byrski T, et al. Estrogen receptor status in CHEK2-positive breast cancers: implications for chemoprevention. Clin Genet 2009; 75(1):72–8.
112. Loveday C, Turnbull C, Ruark E, et al. Germline RAD51C mutations confer susceptibility to ovarian cancer. Nat Genet 2012;44:475–6.
113. Song H, Dicks E, Ramus SJ, et al. Contribution of germline mutations in the RAD51B, RAD51C, and RAD51D genes to ovarian cancer in the population. J Clin Oncol 2015;33:2901–7.

When Does Atypical Ductal Hyperplasia Require Surgical Excision?

Jennifer M. Racz, MD, MBA, Amy C. Degnim, MD*

KEYWORDS

- Atypical ductal hyperplasia • Epithelial proliferative lesion • Surgical excision
- Core needle biopsy

KEY POINTS

- Surgical excision remains the standard of care following a core needle biopsy diagnosis of atypical ductal hyperplasia (ADH), particularly in the presence of an associated mass lesion and radiologic-pathologic discordance.
- Recent research efforts have attempted to identify a favorable subgroup of patients with ADH at low risk of upgrade in order to allow the selection of women who may avoid surgical excision and be safely observed with minimal risk of a missed invasive carcinoma.
- Long-term counseling of women with ADH should include some discussion of long-term breast cancer risk, surveillance strategies, and options for prevention therapy.

INTRODUCTION

Atypical ductal hyperplasia (ADH) is an epithelial proliferative lesion of the mammary terminal duct lobular units that shows both cytologic atypia and architectural changes that are similar in appearance to ductal carcinoma in situ (DCIS). Given that the size and extent of the lesion are smaller, involving only 1 or 2 ducts and measuring less than 2 mm, it does not meet the criteria for DCIS. ADH is identified in 8% to 17% of all core needle breast biopsy specimens.[1,2] Because ADH may coexist with DCIS, and its distinction from DCIS is partly quantitative, it is sometimes not possible to distinguish these two lesions in the limited samples provided by core needle biopsy; therefore, sampling error is an issue relevant in core biopsies showing ADH. In addition, multiple studies of surgical excision of core biopsy sites showing ADH have reported upgrade rates of 4% to 54%.[3–48] For this reason, surgical excision has been the standard approach; recent research is intended to define which women with ADH may not require surgical excision.

Disclosure: The authors have nothing to disclose.
Department of Surgery, Mayo Clinic, 200 First Street Southwest, Rochester, MN 55905, USA
* Corresponding author.
E-mail address: degnim.amy@mayo.edu

SAMPLING ERROR WITH CORE NEEDLE BIOPSY

Before the early 1990s, the recommended evaluation of a suspicious breast abnormality noted on either clinical examination or mammography involved a surgical breast biopsy.[49] Subsequently, less invasive alternatives to open breast biopsy, including stereotactic and ultrasonography-guided core needle biopsy, were evaluated and shown to have a high degree of diagnostic accuracy, thereby reducing the need for surgical intervention.[50–53] However, the shift to percutaneous core needle biopsy led to the introduction of new concerns in the diagnosis and management of breast lesions; more specifically, the designation of certain breast lesions as being high risk for underestimation or a missed diagnosis of malignancy.[54] These concerns were appropriate because there are several factors that can lead to underestimation of cancer using the percutaneous needle biopsy approach, especially undersampling and the challenges of pathologic diagnosis.

First, the targeted lesion may be completely missed or only a portion of the lesion removed, therefore introducing the possibility of sampling error.[55] The primary strategy to reduce sampling error has been to obtain a larger tissue sample, either with more core samples[11,56–58] or with larger gauge core needles. Several studies have shown that the extent of tissue sampling by needle biopsy is related to the frequency of missed cancer diagnosis, with higher upgrade rates for smaller-gauge biopsy needles (ie, 14-gauge needle vs 11-gauge vacuum-assisted biopsy devices), a smaller number of core samples submitted, and larger mammographic lesions.[14,16,59]

Pathologic diagnosis is also more challenging even if a lesion is completely removed. The fragmentation of the specimen into multiple small pieces increases the difficulty in making a definitive histologic diagnosis.[60] This issue is also ameliorated by the use of larger cores obtained by vacuum assistance, such that the lesion histology is less fragmented than with smaller core samples. The main strategy to counteract this issue is to assess concordance between the radiologic and pathologic findings on core biopsy, which is endorsed by both the American College of Radiology[61] and the American Society of Breast Surgeons, as explained later.

RADIOLOGIC-PATHOLOGIC CONCORDANCE

Concordance between radiologic and pathologic findings on core needle biopsy is required in current practices that perform percutaneous needle biopsy and is an integral step in determining further management and surveillance. Agreement or consistency between clinical, imaging, and pathologic findings is referred to as concordance. Radiologic-pathologic concordance assessment consists of joint evaluation of the mammographic and histologic findings, usually involving both radiologists and pathologists, to ensure that the histologic findings are plausible to explain the mammographic lesion. The surgeon is also an important part of the multidisciplinary team that characterizes modern breast care and should contribute to the concordance assessment of breast core needle biopsy results.[62–65]

Concordance assessment requires review of the original diagnostic mammograms showing the abnormality, and also the postbiopsy imaging, in order to assess whether the biopsy marker is located at the site of the original lesion. The histologic findings as described by the pathologist are then interpreted in the context of the clinical and imaging findings to determine whether they are all in agreement. Ideally, concordance determination is performed with input from the radiologist, pathologist, and the surgeon. Surgical excision is indicated if findings are discordant or if there is concern that the target lesion was not sampled adequately. When surgical excision is recommended, the goal is to remove the biopsy site and the original imaging lesion that led to the core needle biopsy in order to rule out the presence of an existing malignancy. Concordance assessment is particularly important in patients with borderline breast lesions (ie, ADH, lobular neoplasia [atypical lobular hyperplasia or lobular carcinoma in situ], papillary lesions, radial scars/complex sclerosing lesions, fibroepithelial lesions [with or without cellular stroma], columnar cell lesions [columnar cell hyperplasia or flat epithelial atypia], spindle cell lesions, and mucocelelike lesions). In general, surgical excision should be performed for a core needle biopsy showing atypia in the presence of a palpable mass or for mass lesions noted on imaging. Specific recommendations for surgical excision of ADH are discussed later.

ATYPICAL DUCTAL HYPERPLASIA

ADH is recognized as not only a marker for an increased long-term risk of breast cancer but also as a nonobligate precursor lesion that shares molecular similarities to DCIS and invasive breast cancer.[66] The concern that ADH may progress to carcinoma, coupled with reports that ADH found on core needle biopsy of a mammographic abnormality can be associated with an upgrade rate to noninvasive and invasive breast cancer in 10% to 31% of cases, has resulted in the practice of routine surgical excision of all ADH lesions. At present, surgical excision remains the standard of care following a core needle biopsy showing ADH.[67]

CRITERIA FOR CONSERVATIVE MANAGEMENT

Although surgical excision remains the standard of care following a core biopsy diagnosis of ADH, given that most ADH cases diagnosed by percutaneous biopsy are not upgraded to cancer, routine excision may represent overtreatment. Therefore, recent research efforts have attempted to identify factors associated with a low risk of cancer upgrade, in order to define a favorable subgroup of women who may avoid surgical excision with minimal risk of a missed invasive carcinoma.

Early studies identified risk factors associated with increased likelihood of upgrade. Such factors identified included: age ($\geq$50 years),[17] ADH involving greater than or equal to 3 foci,[15,19,68,69] use of conventional 14-gauge automated needle instead of larger devices,[3,12,16,70] lesion size on imaging greater than 10 mm,[29] and presence of a mass lesion on imaging.[3,70]

From these studies, multivariate models have been proposed to identify low-risk subgroups of patients who might safely forego surgical excision. The earliest of these was that proposed by Forgeard and colleagues,[24] who suggested that women with the combined features of less than or equal to 2 foci of ADH in microcalcifications, lesion size less than 6 mm with incomplete removal, or lesion size between 6 and 21 mm had a 4% risk of a missed invasive carcinoma. In 2008, Ko and colleagues[13] reported features associated with cancer upgrade by multivariate analysis, including age greater than 50 years, microcalcification on mammography, size on imaging greater than 15 mm, the presence of a palpable lesion, and focal ADH. Using these factors, a scoring system was developed to predict malignancy, and a subset of probably benign lesions was identified with a less than 2% risk of upgrade to malignancy at follow-up surgical excision.

In 2011, Nguyen and colleagues[71] published criteria by which ADH lesions found on core biopsy could be triaged according to the risk of upgrade to an associated carcinoma. In this series of 140 patients, several factors were significantly correlated with a higher rate of upgrade to carcinoma, including (1) removal of less than 95% of calcifications in the absence of an associated mass, (2) involvement of 2 or more terminal duct lobular units, (3) the presence of significant cytologic atypia, and (4) the presence of necrosis. They concluded that ADH without these features, regardless of extent of involvement or terminal duct lobular units (with the exception of the presence of a mass lesion), was associated with a minimal risk of upgrade to carcinoma (<3%), and as a result mammographic follow-up may be appropriate. Of note, the patients in this series underwent image-guided vacuum-assisted biopsy with larger probes (9 or 11 gauge) rather than the conventional 14-gauge needle.

Similar criteria were also recently reported by Pena and colleagues[72] from the Benign Breast Disease Cohort at Mayo Clinic. In this series of 399 patients, the overall upgrade rate was 16.1%. The report similarly concluded that the features on core biopsy most strongly associated with upgrade were imaging-estimated percentage of the lesion removed, individual cell necrosis, and number of ADH foci. Using these criteria, upgrade rates as low as 5.0% could be achieved in women with no necrosis and either 1 focus with greater than or equal to 50% removal, or more than 1 focus with greater than or equal to 90% removal of the lesion.

The long-term safety of prospectively omitting surgical excision was recently reported by Menen and colleagues[73] in the low-risk subgroup of women defined by the criteria of Nguyen and colleagues.[71] In this series of 175 patients who all fit the low-risk criteria, 125 were observed and 50 underwent excision; 6 women developed breast cancer in the surgery group compared with 7 cancers in the observed group. Although there was no difference between the observed and excised groups with regard to the total number of breast cancer events, approximately 75% of cancer events occurred in the ipsilateral breast, with most outside of the index site. Interestingly, 76.8% of patients in the observation group did not receive chemoprevention. These data suggest that observation, rather than surgical excision, following a core biopsy diagnosis of ADH may be a safe option in a select subgroup of patients meeting the radiologic and histologic criteria discussed earlier; however, prospective validation of this approach in a larger multi-institutional sample is recommended before implementing this into routine patient care.

Caution with omitting surgical excision is further highlighted by the results reported by Deshaies and colleagues.[3] In this large retrospective study of 422 cases of ADH, 6 factors independently associated with cancer upgrade were identified: severe ADH, mammography for ipsilateral symptoms, mammographic lesions other than microcalcifications alone, codiagnosis of papilloma, use of a 14-gauge needle for biopsy, and ADH diagnosis performed by pathologists with low-volume. Out of the 422 biopsies, 128 did not present any of these 6 characteristics, but the upgrade frequency at surgery was substantial (17.2% compared with 31.3% for the whole group). Thus the investigators were unable to identify a subgroup of patients in whom excision could confidently be omitted with a low risk of upgrade. Notably, this study did not include the proportion of the lesion removed with needle biopsy, which seemed to be a key factor in the other models discussed earlier that succeeded in identifying a low-risk subgroup.

ADDITIONAL FACTORS TO CONSIDER

For women with ADH diagnosed by core needle biopsy, surgical excision is not the only relevant clinical decision in patient management. For these women, estimating their long-term breast cancer risk is important in order to advise on surveillance and prevention strategies. However, commonly used breast cancer risk models such as the Gail model and the Tyrer-Cuzick model do not predict risk very accurately for individual women with atypical hyperplasia.[74] For this reason, absolute risk estimation is recommended. Based on data from the Mayo Clinic and Nashville Cohorts, risk is approximately 1% per year in women with ADH.[75,76] The Partners Cohort has found a higher risk for women with ADH, approximately 1.7% per year.[77] In contrast, recent data from the Breast Cancer Surveillance Consortium found a lower annual average risk of breast cancer in women with ADH, only 0.6% per year, although they included only invasive breast cancer events and excluded DCIS.[78]

Further work is ongoing to optimize accurate risk assessment in women with ADH. Another factor shown to stratify risk in women with ADH is the number of foci of ADH present within the benign breast biopsy specimen, with increasing risk associated with increasing foci of atypia, observed in both the Mayo Clinic and Nashville Cohorts.[79,80] This finding was challenged by the Nurses' Health Study, in which the number of foci of ADH did not significantly affect later breast cancer risk.[81] Risk estimation is relevant, because a lifetime risk of greater than 25% indicates use of MRI for breast cancer screening, whereas risk below that threshold does not.[82]

Regardless of the means used to estimate long-term breast cancer risk in women with ADH, prevention therapy should be discussed. In younger women with an anticipated long life expectancy and long at-risk period for breast cancer, prevention therapy should be strongly recommended, because their cumulative risk is almost certainly greater than 25%. In older women with competing morbidity, prevention therapy is unlikely to make any impact on survival and will have minimal benefit for quality of life, because most breast cancers that develop are likely to be hormonally sensitive. However, prevention therapy should be recommended for most women with ADH, because their long-term risk is substantial and prevention medications result in a 70% reduction in breast cancer risk.[77,83–86]

SUMMARY

Surgical excision remains the standard of care following a core needle biopsy diagnosis of ADH, particularly in the presence of an associated mass lesion and radiologic-pathologic discordance. However, recent research efforts have attempted to identify a favorable subgroup of patients with ADH at low risk of upgrade in order to allow the selection of women who may avoid surgical excision and be safely observed with minimal risk of a missed invasive carcinoma. Data suggest that women who meet the following criteria are likely to have a less than 5% chance of a missed cancer:

- No mass lesion or discordance
- Removal of greater than or equal to 90% of calcifications at the time of core needle biopsy
- Involvement of less than or equal to 2 terminal duct lobular units
- Absence of individual cell necrosis

Although promising, almost all of these data have been in retrospective studies, with only 1 single-institution prospective study in a limited number of women. Therefore, the standard approach remains surgical excision until further prospective studies confirm the validity of these criteria. Long-term counseling of women with ADH should include some discussion of long-term breast cancer risk, surveillance strategies, and options for prevention therapy.

REFERENCES

1. McGhan LJ, Pockaj BA, Wasif N, et al. Atypical ductal hyperplasia on core biopsy: an automatic trigger for excisional biopsy? Ann Surg Oncol 2012;19(10): 3264–9.

2. Pearlman MD, Griffin JL. Benign breast disease. Obstet Gynecol 2010;116(3): 747–58.
3. Deshaies I, Provencher L, Jacob S, et al. Factors associated with upgrading to malignancy at surgery of atypical ductal hyperplasia diagnosed on core biopsy. Breast 2011;20(1):50–5.
4. Fajardo LL, Pisano ED, Caudry DJ, et al. Stereotactic and sonographic large-core biopsy of nonpalpable breast lesions: results of the Radiologic Diagnostic Oncology Group V study. Acad Radiol 2004;11(3):293–308.
5. Fuhrman GM, Cederbom GJ, Bolton JS, et al. Image-guided core-needle breast biopsy is an accurate technique to evaluate patients with nonpalpable imaging abnormalities. Ann Surg 1998;227(6):932–9.
6. Lin PH, Clyde JC, Bates DM, et al. Accuracy of stereotactic core-needle breast biopsy in atypical ductal hyperplasia. Am J Surg 1998;175(5):380–2.
7. Liberman L, Dershaw DD, Glassman JR, et al. Analysis of cancers not diagnosed at stereotactic core breast biopsy. Radiology 1997;203(1):151–7.
8. Gadzala DE, Cederbom GJ, Bolton JS, et al. Appropriate management of atypical ductal hyperplasia diagnosed by stereotactic core needle breast biopsy. Ann Surg Oncol 1997;4(4):283–6.
9. Moore MM, Hargett CW 3rd, Hanks JB, et al. Association of breast cancer with the finding of atypical ductal hyperplasia at core breast biopsy. Ann Surg 1997;225(6):726–31 [discussion: 731–3].
10. Meyer JE, Smith DN, Lester SC, et al. Large-core needle biopsy of nonpalpable breast lesions. JAMA 1999;281(17):1638–41.
11. Jackman RJ, Burbank F, Parker SH, et al. Atypical ductal hyperplasia diagnosed at stereotactic breast biopsy: improved reliability with 14-gauge, directional, vacuum-assisted biopsy. Radiology 1997;204(2):485–8.
12. Jang M, Cho N, Moon WK, et al. Underestimation of atypical ductal hyperplasia at sonographically guided core biopsy of the breast. AJR Am J Roentgenol 2008; 191(5):1347–51.
13. Ko E, Han W, Lee JW, et al. Scoring system for predicting malignancy in patients diagnosed with atypical ductal hyperplasia at ultrasound-guided core needle biopsy. Breast Cancer Res Treat 2008;112(1):189–95.
14. Houssami N, Ciatto S, Ellis I, et al. Underestimation of malignancy of breast core-needle biopsy: concepts and precise overall and category-specific estimates. Cancer 2007;109(3):487–95.
15. Wagoner MJ, Laronga C, Acs G. Extent and histologic pattern of atypical ductal hyperplasia present on core needle biopsy specimens of the breast can predict ductal carcinoma in situ in subsequent excision. Am J Clin Pathol 2009;131(1): 112–21.
16. Sohn V, Arthurs Z, Herbert G, et al. Atypical ductal hyperplasia: improved accuracy with the 11-gauge vacuum-assisted versus the 14-gauge core biopsy needle. Ann Surg Oncol 2007;14(9):2497–501.
17. Chae BJ, Lee A, Song BJ, et al. Predictive factors for breast cancer in patients diagnosed atypical ductal hyperplasia at core needle biopsy. World J Surg Oncol 2009;7:77.
18. Zhao L, Freimanis R, Bergman S, et al. Biopsy needle technique and the accuracy of diagnosis of atypical ductal hyperplasia for mammographic abnormalities. Am Surg 2003;69(9):757–62 [discussion: 762].
19. Sneige N, Lim SC, Whitman GJ, et al. Atypical ductal hyperplasia diagnosis by directional vacuum-assisted stereotactic biopsy of breast microcalcifications. Considerations for surgical excision. Am J Clin Pathol 2003;119(2):248–53.

20. Graesslin O, Antoine M, Chopier J, et al. Histology after lumpectomy in women with epithelial atypia on stereotactic vacuum-assisted breast biopsy. Eur J Surg Oncol 2010;36(2):170–5.
21. Eby PR, Ochsner JE, DeMartini WB, et al. Frequency and upgrade rates of atypical ductal hyperplasia diagnosed at stereotactic vacuum-assisted breast biopsy: 9- versus 11-gauge. AJR Am J Roentgenol 2009;192(1):229–34.
22. Lourenco AP, Mainiero MB, Lazarus E, et al. Stereotactic breast biopsy: comparison of histologic underestimation rates with 11- and 9-gauge vacuum-assisted breast biopsy. AJR Am J Roentgenol 2007;189(5):W275–9.
23. Ingegnoli A, d'Aloia C, Frattaruolo A, et al. Flat epithelial atypia and atypical ductal hyperplasia: carcinoma underestimation rate. Breast J 2010;16(1):55–9.
24. Forgeard C, Benchaib M, Guerin N, et al. Is surgical biopsy mandatory in case of atypical ductal hyperplasia on 11-gauge core needle biopsy? A retrospective study of 300 patients. Am J Surg 2008;196(3):339–45.
25. Teng-Swan Ho J, Tan PH, Hee SW, et al. Underestimation of malignancy of atypical ductal hyperplasia diagnosed on 11-gauge stereotactically guided Mammotome breast biopsy: an Asian breast screen experience. Breast 2008;17(4):401–6.
26. Travade A, Isnard A, Bouchet F, et al. Non-palpable breast lesions and core needle biopsy with Mammotome 11G: is surgery required in patients with atypical ductal hyperplasia? J Radiol 2006;87(3):307–10.
27. Winchester DJ, Bernstein JR, Jeske JM, et al. Upstaging of atypical ductal hyperplasia after vacuum-assisted 11-gauge stereotactic core needle biopsy. Arch Surg 2003;138(6):619–22 [discussion: 622–3].
28. Gal-Gombos EC, Esserman LE, Recine MA, et al. Large-needle core biopsy in atypical intraductal epithelial hyperplasia including immunohistochemical expression of high molecular weight cytokeratin: analysis of results of a single institution. Breast J 2002;8(5):269–74.
29. Jackman RJ, Birdwell RL, Ikeda DM. Atypical ductal hyperplasia: can some lesions be defined as probably benign after stereotactic 11-gauge vacuum-assisted biopsy, eliminating the recommendation for surgical excision? Radiology 2002;224(2):548–54.
30. Adrales G, Turk P, Wallace T, et al. Is surgical excision necessary for atypical ductal hyperplasia of the breast diagnosed by Mammotome? Am J Surg 2000;180(4):313–5.
31. Burak WE Jr, Owens KE, Tighe MB, et al. Vacuum-assisted stereotactic breast biopsy: histologic underestimation of malignant lesions. Arch Surg 2000;135(6):700–3.
32. Darling ML, Smith DN, Lester SC, et al. Atypical ductal hyperplasia and ductal carcinoma in situ as revealed by large-core needle breast biopsy: results of surgical excision. AJR Am J Roentgenol 2000;175(5):1341–6.
33. Cangiarella J, Waisman J, Symmans WF, et al. Mammotome core biopsy for mammary microcalcification: analysis of 160 biopsies from 142 women with surgical and radiologic followup. Cancer 2001;91(1):173–7.
34. Brem RF, Behrndt VS, Sanow L, et al. Atypical ductal hyperplasia: histologic underestimation of carcinoma in tissue harvested from impalpable breast lesions using 11-gauge stereotactically guided directional vacuum-assisted biopsy. AJR Am J Roentgenol 1999;172(5):1405–7.
35. Rizzo M, Lund MJ, Oprea G, et al. Surgical follow-up and clinical presentation of 142 breast papillary lesions diagnosed by ultrasound-guided core-needle biopsy. Ann Surg Oncol 2008;15(4):1040–7.

36. Gendler LS, Feldman SM, Balassanian R, et al. Association of breast cancer with papillary lesions identified at percutaneous image-guided breast biopsy. Am J Surg 2004;188(4):365–70.

37. Valdes EK, Tartter PI, Genelus-Dominique E, et al. Significance of papillary lesions at percutaneous breast biopsy. Ann Surg Oncol 2006;13(4):480–2.

38. Renshaw AA, Derhagopian RP, Tizol-Blanco DM, et al. Papillomas and atypical papillomas in breast core needle biopsy specimens: risk of carcinoma in subsequent excision. Am J Clin Pathol 2004;122(2):217–21.

39. Sohn V, Porta R, Brown T. Flat epithelial atypia of the breast on core needle biopsy: an indication for surgical excision. Mil Med 2011;176(11):1347–50.

40. Lavoue V, Roger CM, Poilblanc M, et al. Pure flat epithelial atypia (DIN 1a) on core needle biopsy: study of 60 biopsies with follow-up surgical excision. Breast Cancer Res Treat 2011;125(1):121–6.

41. Chivukula M, Bhargava R, Tseng G, et al. Clinicopathologic implications of "flat epithelial atypia" in core needle biopsy specimens of the breast. Am J Clin Pathol 2009;131(6):802–8.

42. Subhawong AP, Subhawong TK, Khouri N, et al. Incidental minimal atypical lobular hyperplasia on core needle biopsy: correlation with findings on follow-up excision. Am J Surg Pathol 2010;34(6):822–8.

43. Shah-Khan MG, Geiger XJ, Reynolds C, et al. Long-term follow-up of lobular neoplasia (atypical lobular hyperplasia/lobular carcinoma in situ) diagnosed on core needle biopsy. Ann Surg Oncol 2012;19(10):3131–8.

44. Renshaw AA, Derhagopian RP, Martinez P, et al. Lobular neoplasia in breast core needle biopsy specimens is associated with a low risk of ductal carcinoma in situ or invasive carcinoma on subsequent excision. Am J Clin Pathol 2006;126(2):310–3.

45. Karabakhtsian RG, Johnson R, Sumkin J, et al. The clinical significance of lobular neoplasia on breast core biopsy. Am J Surg Pathol 2007;31(5):717–23.

46. Brem RF, Lechner MC, Jackman RJ, et al. Lobular neoplasia at percutaneous breast biopsy: variables associated with carcinoma at surgical excision. AJR Am J Roentgenol 2008;190(3):637–41.

47. Rendi MH, Dintzis SM, Lehman CD, et al. Lobular in-situ neoplasia on breast core needle biopsy: imaging indication and pathologic extent can identify which patients require excisional biopsy. Ann Surg Oncol 2012;19(3):914–21.

48. Murray MP, Luedtke C, Liberman L, et al. Classic lobular carcinoma in situ and atypical lobular hyperplasia at percutaneous breast core biopsy: outcomes of prospective excision. Cancer 2013;119(5):1073–9.

49. Parker SH. Percutaneous large core breast biopsy. Cancer 1994;74(1 Suppl):256–62.

50. Parker SH, Lovin JD, Jobe WE, et al. Stereotactic breast biopsy with a biopsy gun. Radiology 1990;176(3):741–7.

51. Gisvold JJ, Goellner JR, Grant CS, et al. Breast biopsy: a comparative study of stereotaxically guided core and excisional techniques. AJR Am J Roentgenol 1994;162(4):815–20.

52. Parker SH, Lovin JD, Jobe WE, et al. Nonpalpable breast lesions: stereotactic automated large-core biopsies. Radiology 1991;180(2):403–7.

53. Liberman L, Fahs MC, Dershaw DD, et al. Impact of stereotaxic core breast biopsy on cost of diagnosis. Radiology 1995;195(3):633–7.

54. Ghosh K, Melton LJ 3rd, Suman VJ, et al. Breast biopsy utilization: a population-based study. Arch Intern Med 2005;165(14):1593–8.

55. Burbank F. Stereotactic breast biopsy of atypical ductal hyperplasia and ductal carcinoma in situ lesions: improved accuracy with directional, vacuum-assisted biopsy. Radiology 1997;202(3):843–7.

56. Jackman RJ, Nowels KW, Shepard MJ, et al. Stereotaxic large-core needle biopsy of 450 nonpalpable breast lesions with surgical correlation in lesions with cancer or atypical hyperplasia. Radiology 1994;193(1):91–5.

57. Jackman RJ, Burbank F, Parker SH, et al. Stereotactic breast biopsy of nonpalpable lesions: determinants of ductal carcinoma in situ underestimation rates. Radiology 2001;218(2):497–502.

58. Zografos GC, Zagouri F, Sergentanis TN, et al. Minimizing underestimation rate of microcalcifications excised via vacuum-assisted breast biopsy: a blind study. Breast Cancer Res Treat 2008;109(2):397–402.

59. Green S, Khalkhali I, Azizollahi E, et al. Excisional biopsy of borderline lesions after large bore vacuum-assisted core needle biopsy- is it necessary? Am Surg 2011;77(10):1358–60.

60. Corben AD, Edelweiss M, Brogi E. Challenges in the interpretation of breast core biopsies. Breast J 2010;16(Suppl 1):S5–9.

61. American College of Radiology. American College of Radiology practice parameter for the performance of ultrasound-guided percutaneous breast interventional procedures. 2017. Available at: https://www.acr.org/~/media/96DB6A439 6D242848418CB6E83B55EFE.pdf. Accessed March 29, 2017.

62. Johnson NB, Collins LC. Update on percutaneous needle biopsy of nonmalignant breast lesions. Adv Anat Pathol 2009;16(4):183–95.

63. Landercasper J, Linebarger JH. Contemporary breast imaging and concordance assessment: a surgical perspective. Surg Clin North Am 2011;91(1):33–58.

64. Masood S, Rosa M. Borderline breast lesions: diagnostic challenges and clinical implications. Adv Anat Pathol 2011;18(3):190–8.

65. American Society of Breast Surgeons. Position statement on concordance assessment of image-guided breast biopsies and management of borderline or high-risk lesions. 2011. Available at: https://www.breastsurgeons.org/new_layout/about/statements/PDF_Statements/Concordance_Assessment.pdf. Accessed March 14, 2017.

66. Ma XJ, Salunga R, Tuggle JT, et al. Gene expression profiles of human breast cancer progression. Proc Natl Acad Sci U S A 2003;100(10):5974–9.

67. National Comprehensive Cancer Network. NCCN guidelines version 1.2016 breast cancer screening and diagnosis. Available at: https://www.nccn.org/professionals/physician_gls/pdf/breast-screening.pdf. Accessed March 14, 2017.

68. Kohr JR, Eby PR, Allison KH, et al. Risk of upgrade of atypical ductal hyperplasia after stereotactic breast biopsy: effects of number of foci and complete removal of calcifications. Radiology 2010;255(3):723–30.

69. Allison KH, Eby PR, Kohr J, et al. Atypical ductal hyperplasia on vacuum-assisted breast biopsy: suspicion for ductal carcinoma in situ can stratify patients at high risk for upgrade. Hum Pathol 2011;42(1):41–50.

70. Youk JH, Kim EK, Kim MJ. Atypical ductal hyperplasia diagnosed at sonographically guided 14-gauge core needle biopsy of breast mass. AJR Am J Roentgenol 2009;192(4):1135–41.

71. Nguyen CV, Albarracin CT, Whitman GJ, et al. Atypical ductal hyperplasia in directional vacuum-assisted biopsy of breast microcalcifications: considerations for surgical excision. Ann Surg Oncol 2011;18(3):752–61.

72. Pena A, Shah SS, Fazzio RT, et al. Multivariate model to identify women at low-risk of cancer upgrade after a core needle biopsy diagnosis of atypical ductal hyperplasia. Breast Cancer Res Treat 2017;164(2):295–304.
73. Menen RS, Ganesan N, Bevers T, et al. Long-term safety of observation in selected women following core biopsy diagnosis of atypical ductal hyperplasia. Ann Surg Oncol 2017;24(1):70–6.
74. Pankratz VS, Hartmann LC, Degnim AC, et al. Assessment of the accuracy of the Gail model in women with atypical hyperplasia. J Clin Oncol 2008;26(33):5374–9.
75. Hartmann LC, Degnim AC, Santen RJ, et al. Atypical hyperplasia of the breast–risk assessment and management options. N Engl J Med 2015;372(1):78–89.
76. Degnim AC, Visscher DW, Radisky DC, et al. Breast cancer risk by the extent and type of atypical hyperplasia. Cancer 2016;122(19):3087–8.
77. Coopey SB, Mazzola E, Buckley JM, et al. The role of chemoprevention in modifying the risk of breast cancer in women with atypical breast lesions. Breast Cancer Res Treat 2012;136(3):627–33.
78. Menes TS, Kerlikowske K, Lange J, et al. Subsequent breast cancer risk following diagnosis of atypical ductal hyperplasia on needle biopsy. JAMA Oncol 2017;3(1):36–41.
79. Degnim AC, Visscher DW, Berman HK, et al. Stratification of breast cancer risk in women with atypia: a Mayo cohort study. J Clin Oncol 2007;25(19):2671–7.
80. Hartmann LC, Radisky DC, Frost MH, et al. Understanding the premalignant potential of atypical hyperplasia through its natural history: a longitudinal cohort study. Cancer Prev Res (Phila) 2014;7(2):211–7.
81. Collins LC, Baer HJ, Tamimi RM, et al. The influence of family history on breast cancer risk in women with biopsy-confirmed benign breast disease: results from the Nurses' Health Study. Cancer 2006;107(6):1240–7.
82. Saslow D, Boetes C, Burke W, et al. American Cancer Society guidelines for breast screening with MRI as an adjunct to mammography. CA Cancer J Clin 2007;57(2):75–89.
83. Fisher B, Costantino JP, Wickerham DL, et al. Tamoxifen for prevention of breast cancer: report of the National Surgical Adjuvant Breast and Bowel Project P-1 Study. J Natl Cancer Inst 1998;90(18):1371–88.
84. Fisher B, Costantino JP, Wickerham DL, et al. Tamoxifen for the prevention of breast cancer: current status of the National Surgical Adjuvant Breast and Bowel Project P-1 Study. J Natl Cancer Inst 2005;97(22):1652–62.
85. Cuzick J, DeCensi A, Arun B, et al. Preventive therapy for breast cancer: a consensus statement. Lancet Oncol 2011;12(5):496–503.
86. Goss PE, Ingle JN, Ales-Martinez JE, et al. Exemestane for breast-cancer prevention in postmenopausal women. N Engl J Med 2011;364(25):2381–91.

Tomosynthesis in Breast Cancer Imaging

How Does It Fit into Preoperative Evaluation and Surveillance?

Mohammad Eghtedari, MD, PhD[a], Catherine Tsai, MD[b],
Julie Robles, MD[b], Sarah L. Blair, MD[c],
Haydee Ojeda-Fournier, MD[a],*

KEYWORDS

- Breast cancer • Digital mammography • Digital breast tomosynthesis
- Breast imaging • Diagnostic breast imaging • Mammography
- Image-guided interventions

KEY POINTS

- Digital breast tomosynthesis is a quasi-three-dimensional radiograph mammogram with radiation dose well below the maximum allowed by the Mammography Quality Standards Act.
- Digital breast tomosynthesis has been shown to increase the number of breast cancers detected while lowering the callback rates when compared with full-field digital mammography.
- Availability of digital breast tomosynthesis–guided breast interventions allows for the minimally invasive sampling of lesions detected with this new modality.
- Digital breast tomosynthesis shows increase in the detection of sclerosing papillary lesions and scars; however, fewer cysts and fibroadenomas are called back for evaluation.

INTRODUCTION

Screening mammography has been shown in multiple, long-term, randomized clinical trials to decrease breast cancer mortality rates by 30% and possibly more.[1–6] These randomized clinical trials were started 40 years ago and used screen-film mammography. In 2005, the Food and Drug Administration (FDA) approved the use of

Disclosure Statement: The authors have nothing to disclose.
[a] Department of Radiology, Breast Imaging Section, UC San Diego Health, Moores Cancer Center, 3855 Health Sciences Drive, #0846, La Jolla, CA 92093-0846, USA; [b] Department of Surgery, University of California San Diego, 9500 Gilman drive, La Jolla, CA 92093-0846, USA; [c] Department of Surgery, Division of Surgical Oncology, UC San Diego Health, Moores Cancer Center, 3855 Health Sciences Drive, La Jolla, CA 92093-0846, USA
* Corresponding author.
E-mail address: hojeda@ucsd.edu

full-field digital mammography (FFDM) and since then, most mammographic units in the United States are FFDM. The DIMIST trial[7] showed that there was no difference in breast cancer detection between screen-film mammography and FFDM except in three groups of women: (1) those younger than 50 years old, (2) those with dense breast tissue, and (3) premenopausal or perimenopausal women. In that subgroup of women, FFDM found more cancers. Both screen-film mammography and FFDM use x-ray to create a two-dimensional (2D) image of the breast. The main limitation of 2D mammography is that the entire volume of tissue is displayed as a planar image with tissue overlap. In dense breasts, the overlap may obscures masses, the so-called masking effect.[8] In 2011, the FDA approved the first digital breast tomosynthesis (DBT) unit. Since then, additional vendors have obtained FDA approval for commercial DBT units. DBT overcomes the overlapping of tissue limitation of 2D mammography by generating images of the breast in planes.

In addition to screening for breast cancer, x-ray mammography is used to evaluate patients presenting with breast clinical findings as the first-line imaging modality in patients 30 years old or older. Mammography is also used in the preoperative- and postoperative evaluation of patients with breast cancer and for image guidance in patients requiring wire localization or biopsy of nonpalpable breast lesions that are not seen on ultrasound. DBT has rapidly been adopted in clinical practices across the United States because it detects more invasive breast cancers and reduces the callback rate. DBT is also used in the diagnostic setting and is referred to as a better mammogram, which is specifically true in the evaluation of patients with dense breast tissue.

This article reviews the technology used to create a DBT study, summarizes recent clinical studies, and focuses on the utility of DBT in the preoperative evaluation and surveillance of patients.

TECHNIQUE

DBT, first described by Niklason and colleagues[9] in 1997, reconstructs a tomographic quasi-three-dimensional (3D) radiographic image of the breast by applying a mathematical algorithm to a few low-dose 2D projection images. Reconstructed 3D images are superior to 2D mammograms mainly because they provide blurring of the tissue above and below the selected plane lowering the effect of overlapping breast tissue. A composite 2D image, which looks like a conventional FFDM image, can also be generated from the projection images, the so-called synthetic view.

In DBT, the breast is compressed against a detector while the x-ray tube rotates around the breast in an arc and captures a series of 2D images that are known as projections.[10,11] Because of the limited angular rotation of the x-ray tube, the z-resolution of the 3D (ie, perpendicular to the detector surface) is worse than that of in-plane resolution. However, even this limited z-resolution seems to be sufficient to lower the superimposition of breast tissue resulting in better cancer detection and lower callback rates as reported in the literature.

The FDA has approved the following DBT systems with the year approved shown in parenthesis: Hologic Selenia Dimensions (2011), GE SenoClaire (2014), Siemens Mammomat Inspiration (2015), Fujifilm ASPIRE Cristalle (2017), and GE Senographe Pristina (2017). Most DBT machines use similar components, such as a full-field digital detector, breast compression mechanism, and an x-ray tube mounted on an arm that rotates around the compressed static breast. The x-ray tube may rotate continuously (Hologic, Bedford, MA, USA and Siemens, Malvern, MA, USA) or may rotate in steps (GE, Waukesha, WI, USA). The detector is usually static; however, Hologic Selenia uses a rotating detector. The angular range of rotation of the x-ray tube is 15° acquiring 15 projections for (Hologic, Bedford, MA, USA and Fujifilm, Torrance, CA, USA), 25° acquiring nine projections for GE, and 50° acquiring 25 images for (Siemens malvern, PA, USA).[10,12] Hologic and Siemens use a filtered back projection algorithm; this is the same algorithm that is used to reconstruct computed tomography images. However, the GE machines use an iterative method to reconstruct 3D images. The optimal parameters, such as the number of projections and the extent of angular rotation to obtain DBT, are the subject of continued debate.

Because of the limited number of projection images, reconstructed DBT images are prone to artifacts.[13] The most common artifact is the repeated and shifted projection of a high-density object, such as calcification and metallic markers on adjacent images, the "zippering" artifact. Mathematical algorithms are suggested to minimize this artifact.[14] Another artifact is truncation artifact that generates bright horizontal lines at the edge of the reconstructed image.

Because tomosynthesis enables separation of tissue in the z-axis, one may conclude that the DBT would not require the breast to be compressed. Förnvik and colleagues[15] investigated the effect of reduced compression on the breast during DBT by allowing three radiologists to subjectively rate the quality of visualizing glandular tissue on DBT obtained with full compression and reduced compression; they concluded that the reviewer radiologists significantly preferred the DBT obtained with full compression. Compression of the breast spreads the glandular tissue, reduces the scattering of photons, decreases the dose to the breast, and reduces motion artifact. Therefore, all DBT machines use a breast compression mechanism similar to FFDM.

Fig. 1 shows images from a DBT study including a thin slice and a thick slab. In a different patient, the standard 2D and the synthetic craniocaudal views are shown in a heterogeneously dense breast. DBT vendors have gained FDA approval, or are in the process of gaining approval, to have the synthetic view replace the 2D view, a move that will further decrease radiation dose from DBT.

Radiation Dose

The radiation dose of a DBT is the summation of the absorbed glandular tissue dose (AGD) from all low-dose projections.[16] The estimated AGD for a standard breast size during DBT has been reported to be in the range of 1.74 to 1.9 mGy, which is lower than the Mammography Quality Standards Act limit of 3 mGy per view.[17] Paulis and colleagues[18] calculated the radiation exposure of breasts undergoing DBT using GE SenoClaire and compared it with FFDM and concluded that the AGD was lower with DBT as compared with FFDM for breast thickness more than 50 mm and was equivalent between DBT and FFDM when the thickness of the breast was 50 mm or less. Shin and colleagues[19] calculated AGD for 149 subjects who underwent mammography with both FFDM and DBT and concluded that mediolateral oblique projection DBT with craniocaudal projection FFDM resulted in maximum detection of lesions with minimal increase in AGD when compared with conventional FFDM obtained in craniocaudal and mediolateral oblique projections.

Svahn and colleagues[17] compared the dose of radiation of DBT with that of FFDM and concluded that the dose for obtaining each view between DBT and FFDM is comparable; however, the glandular dose increases up to 2.23 times when two-view DBT is obtained along with FFDM. Synthetic 2D images, which are reconstructed from projection images, reduce the total glandular dose when they are substituted for FFDM.

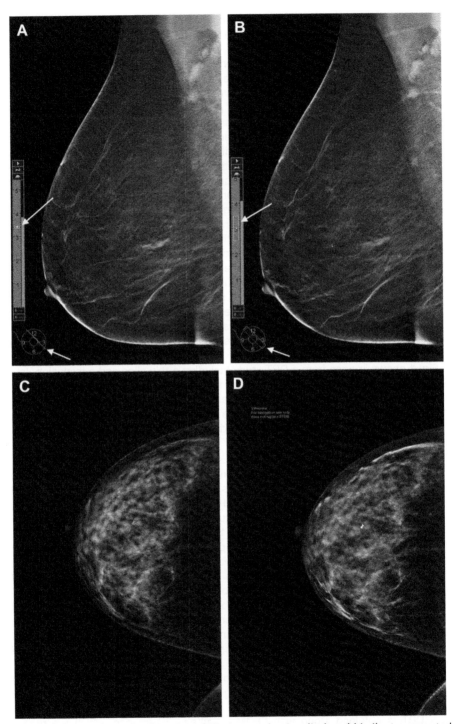

Fig. 1. The DBT study is a combination of 2D views and a cine displayed (similar to computed tomography) stack of slices or slabs. (*A*) Single DBT slice. Note the navigation sidebar on the

Breast Density

Heterogeneously dense and extremely dense breast tissue decreases the sensitivity of mammograms and increases the chance of developing an interval cancer despite mammographic screening.[20] A meta-analysis of screen-detected cancers in more than 10,000 subjects with dense breast tissue who underwent mainly biennial mammography using both DBT and FFDM demonstrated detection of an additional 3.9 cancers per 1000 screens when DBT was used. Houssami[21] suggested that based on the reported literature on the performance of DBT in dense breasts, patients with dense breast tissue may not need an "adjunct" screening method if DBT is used. A review article by Destounis and colleagues[22] shows that the greatest reduction in call-back rate happens when DBT is used for women with dense breast tissue and in those younger than 50 years old. Overall, it seems that the benefit of DBT for women with dense breast tissue is related to both increasing the sensitivity of mammogram to detect cancer and reducing callback rate.

Contraindications to Digital Breast Tomosynthesis

There is no absolute contraindication for breast tomosynthesis; however, it is found that the deleterious effect of silicone implants in obscuring findings is more prominent for DBT as compared with FFDM.[23] Another factor that may limit the application of DBT is related to the longer exposure time during DBT as compared with FFDM and the fact that the x-ray tube rotates around the patient's breast. Therefore, patients with severe kyphosis and those with limited mobility may not be ideal candidates for DBT. In these types of patients, comfort is the limiting factor for performing DBT.

CLINICAL TRIALS
STORM Trial

Several clinical trials have been performed to study the diagnostic utility of DBT when used in conjunction with 2D mammography screening. Although there are few trials to date on this new modality of breast imaging, studies generally show a significant improvement in diagnostic accuracy with the addition of DBT to conventional screening methods.

The STORM[24] trial was a large prospective study that compared 2D mammography with DBT to 2D mammography alone. The patient population comprised of 7292 asymptomatic Italian women aged 48 and older at standard risk for breast cancer. A total of 59 cancers were detected from this population, 39 were detected using conventional 2D mammography. An additional 20 cancers were detected when DBT was used with 2D mammography. There were no cancers detected with 2D only that were not detected with combination study (DBT with 2D mammography modality). The results also showed that there was a decrease in false positives when DBT was used in conjunction with 2D mammography compared with mammography alone (36% compared with 18%). This study showed that the addition of DBT in screening a

---

left side of the image is a thin bar on both the slice number and the anatomic diagram (*arrows*). (*B*) In comparison, a slab is a thicker volume represented by a bar rather than line on the navigation tools (*arrows*). The slices allows for better margin analysis, whereas the slabs are better at identifying calcifications. (*C*) 2D craniocaudal view mammogram obtained at the time of combination study (2D and DBT) in a heterogeneously dense breast. (*D*) For comparison the synthetic view generated from the DBT data, which is FDA approved in some vendors to completely replace the 2D portion of the examination.

population of asymptomatic women at average risk of breast cancer could increase the detection of breast cancer while decreasing the rate of false-positive results.

TOMMY Trial

The TOMMY trial[25] was a multicenter retrospective reading study that compared the diagnostic performance among three separate reading arms of the study: conventional 2D mammography alone versus 2D mammography with DBT versus synthetic 2D mammography with DBT in women 47 to 73 years old. Synthetic 2D mammograms were created using existing software that created 2D images from single DBT scans, simulating a conventional 2D image. The readers in the study consisted of radiologists, advanced practitioner radiographers, and breast clinicians that had a track record of high-volume film reading and met minimum experience criteria. The readers assessed level of suspicion for cancer for each lesion and recorded decisions to recall or not. Readers also made assessments of lesion visibility, extent, density, and discrimination. The results showed that there was a significant improvement in specificity when DBT was used in conjunction with 2D images or synthetic images compared with 2D images alone. This result was observed irrespective of mammographic density, age, tumor size, and dominant radiologic feature and in invasive carcinoma and ductal carcinoma in situ (DCIS).

In a substudy of the TOMMY trial, the main radiologic features were assessed in the three reading arms. It was observed that DBT was more advantageous for lesions in which a mass was the main radiologic feature rather than microcalcifications. Tomosynthesis facilitated detection of stellate lesions, which tend to have greater desmoplastic reaction, resulting in more spiculated lesions. However, there was also an increase in detection of benign lesions with tomosynthesis, including radial scars and complex sclerosing lesions (discussed later), increasing false positives that may lead to a higher negative biopsy rate. However, disadvantages of identifying these lesions may be outweighed by the increased detection of malignant lesions.

It is well known that dense breast tissue increases the risk of breast cancer, and that dense breasts make imaging interpretation more difficult. Another substudy of the TOMMY trial showed that although there is a high degree of variation in observed breast density between image readers, commercially available software can provide a more reliable assessment of breast density. Comparing reader assessments of lesions with various breast densities, there was a significant improvement in sensitivity in women with breast density greater than 50% when DBT is used in conjunction with 2D mammography.

Clinical Performance Reader Trials

A recent radiologist performance study by Rafferty and colleagues[26] found that the diagnostic accuracy for combined DBT and 2D mammography was superior to that of 2D mammography alone. The increase in sensitivity was the largest in cases of invasive cancers. It was thought that DBT reduced tissue superimposition, rendering lesions more visible, especially for masses, asymmetries, and areas of architectural distortion. When lesions were broken down into calcification or noncalcification lesions, nearly all the gain in reader performance was attributable to noncalcification cases. The study also showed that recall rates for noncancer cases for all readers was significantly decreased with the addition of DBT, similar to results seen in the STORM trial. This study concluded that given the emotional, financial, and clinical costs of false positives, DBT has the potential to reduce the risks associated with callbacks.

Table 1 summarizes the clinical performance of DBT compared with conventional 2D mammography.

BENEFITS OF SCREENING WITH DIGITAL BREAST TOMOSYNTHESIS

In the randomized European clinical trials of DBT the two demonstrated benefits of screening with DBT have been an increase in breast cancer detection and, more importantly, a decrease in callback rates. The callback rate is the number of women that are asked to return for diagnostic evaluation from a screening mammogram study. The national benchmark for callback rates is 10% or less.[27] Calling a patient back from screening mammogram is expensive and anxiety inducing; most callbacks result in a negative diagnostic evaluation, with the inciting finding deemed to be overlapping tissue. Additional retrospective trials are discussed next.

Cancer Detection Rates

The thin slices obtained through the breast during DBT allows for better lesion visualization and margin analysis and increased cancer detection rates, benefiting patients with all types of breast density. For example, in a study by Friedewald and colleagues,[28] the detection of invasive breast cancer increased from 2.9 to 4.1 per 1000 women screened. This is a relative increase of 41%. The detection of DCIS, however, was unchanged. A tissue density subanalysis of the Friedewald study by Rafferty and colleagues[29] showed that although the dense and the nondense groups benefited from DBT, the heterogeneously dense group of women had the largest benefit, even over the extremely dense group. In addition to showing increased cancer detection rates, the Friedewald study showed a statistically significant decrease in callback rates.

Callback Rates

Some studies have shown no significant increase in cancer detection rates but have demonstrated a significant decrease in callback rates. For example, Hass and colleagues[30] showed a 29.7% decrease in callback rates and no significant increase in cancer detection. Sharpe and colleagues,[31] however, showed an 18.8% decrease in callback rates while demonstrating a 54.3% increase in cancer detection rates. Sharpe's study also suggested that patients with dense breast tissue benefit more from DBT.

Fig. 2 is an example of a breast cancer detected only on DBT in a patient with dense breasts.

Table 1
Summary of clinical performance of digital breast tomosynthesis compared with full-field digital mammography 2D mammography

	Sensitivity (%)	Specificity (%)	Accuracy (%)	False Positives (%)	PPV (%)	NPV (%)
2D Mammo	63–87	58–95	86.9	4.5	43–96	69–92
Tomosynthesis	91	88	90	—	95.5	77
2D Mammo + Tomo	76–99	69–96	—	6.6	50–93	95
2D Mammo + Tomo + US	97.7	82.8	93.7	—	94.0	96.3
Synthetic 2D Mammo + Tomo	88	71	—	—	—	—

Abbreviations: Mammo, mammography; NPV, negative predictive value; PPV, positive predictive value; Tomo, tomosynthesis; US, ultrasound.

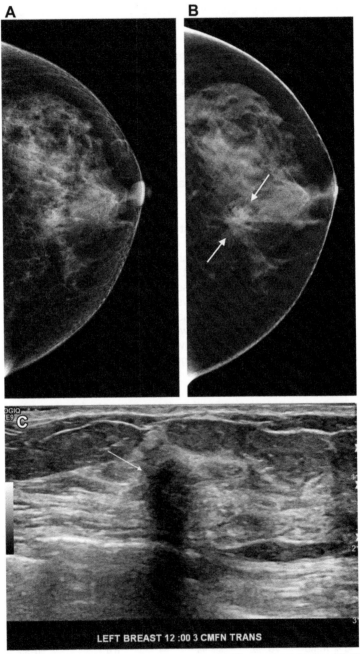

Fig. 2. 2D craniocaudal view (*A*) demonstrates no significant abnormality. (*B*) Single-slice DBT image demonstrates an irregular mass with spiculated margins in the posterior central left breast (*shown between the arrows*). A targeted ultrasound (*C*) of the lesion in question (*arrow*) demonstrates a nonparallel mass with angular margins and posterior shadowing, biopsy proven to be an invasive lobular breast cancer.

CALCIFICATIONS
Detection

Kopans and colleagues[32] had two radiologists compare the clarity of visualizing calcifications in mammograms of 119 women who underwent both 2D and DBT in a non-blinded study and concluded that DBT showed calcifications with superior clarity in 41.6% and with equal clarity in 50.4% when compared with 2D.

However, Tagliafico and colleagues[33] had six radiologists randomly, and in a blinded study, classify 109 microcalcifications on DBT and 2D and concluded that the 2D imaging provided higher sensitivity as compared with DBT (100% vs 91.1%), whereas the specificity of DBT was better than 2D (100% vs 94.6%).

Another nonblinded study compared the visibility of 179 microcalcifications on 2D with that of DBT and concluded that in 92.2% of cases, DBT provided equivalent or superior visualization of microcalcifications.[34]

Fig. 3 shows a case of DBT screen detected DCIS in a patient with dense breasts.

Extent of Ductal Carcinoma In Situ by Digital Breast Tomosynthesis

Berger and colleagues[35] determined the size of DCIS in 33 known cases of DCIS reviewed by three radiologists using FFDM and DBT and compared them with the final size on the pathology report of the surgical specimen. The results indicated that the estimated size of DCIS was more accurate when DBT was used. Another study evaluated the size estimation of 173 malignant breast lesions using DBT and 2D and concluded that "mis-sizing" was significantly less when DBT was used.[36]

EXTENT OF DISEASE

Imaging assessment of newly diagnosed breast cancer is integral to staging disease and can dictate the treatment course. Therefore, it is paramount that preoperative evaluation reflects the extent of disease before surgical intervention.

Assessment

Mun and colleagues[36] showed DBT to be more accurate than the current standard of 2D mammography in determining the local extent of breast cancer in the preoperative planning stage, especially in women with dense breasts. The study population was comprised of 169 women with one or more BI-RADS 4, 5, or 6 lesions. The lesions were then characterized as "mis-sized" if the predicted size differed by more than 1 cm than the size at the time of surgery. The results of the study showed that lesion size was more often overestimated with 2D compared with DBT. Furthermore, 2D mammography more commonly mis-sized lesions in women with dense breasts compared with size estimates using DBT.

A study by Mariscotti and coworkers[37] showed that DBT performs as well as MRI when added to conventional imaging (2D mammography and ultrasound) for preoperative assessment in women with breast cancer. The study examined 200 women with histologically proven breast cancer who had undergone DBT, MRI, 2D mammography, and ultrasound imaging. The addition of DBT to 2D mammography increased sensitivity of detecting breast cancer to 97.7%, which is close to the 98.8% sensitivity of MRI. Furthermore, when ultrasound was added to DBT and 2D mammography, sensitivity was nearly equal when compared with MRI (93.7% vs 92.3%). In another study comparing these modalities, Kim and colleagues[38] showed that the addition of DBT to 2D mammography also increased the positive predictive value and lowered false-positive rates when compared with digital mammography with MRI. Although these small, single institutions studies suggest that DBT may be equivalent to preoperative

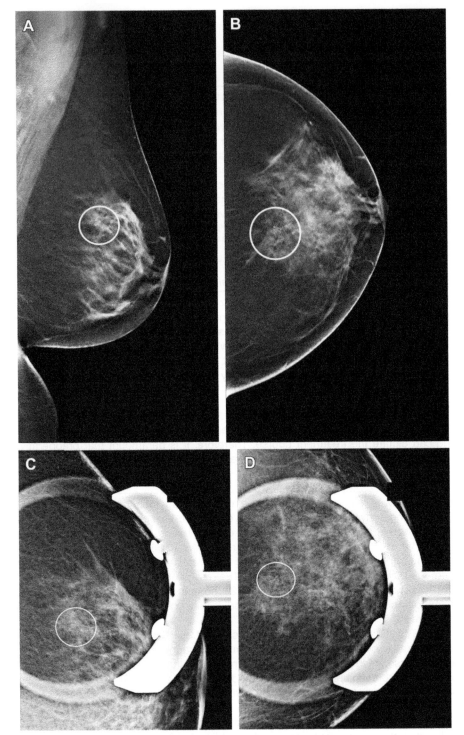

Fig. 3. Mediolateral oblique (*A*) and craniocaudal (*B*) slices in a 65 year old undergoing DBT screening mammogram demonstrates a group of faint calcifications (*circle*) in the 12:00 position of the left breast. For comparison, magnification mammogram [(*C*) lateral, (*D*) craniocaudal] demonstrates a group of fine pleomorphic calcifications (*circles* in (*C*) and (*D*)) with biopsy under stereotactic guidance and shown to be low-grade ductal carcinoma in situ.

breast MRI, DBT is limited in evaluation of the chest wall and has not been thoroughly studied to change the current standard of preoperative MRI.

Clinical Example of Extent of Disease

Fig. 4 demonstrates a case of multifocal breast cancer identified on DBT screening evaluation.

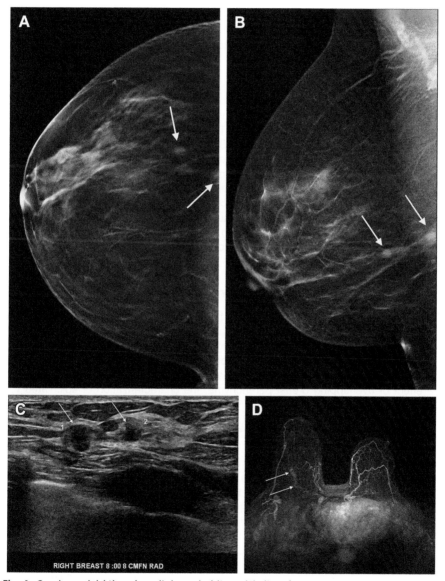

Fig. 4. Craniocaudal (A) and mediolateral oblique (B) slices from a DBT screening study in a 72-year-old woman demonstrates two focal asymmetries (*arrows*) in the lower outer right breast. (C) Targeted diagnostic ultrasound of the lesion demonstrates two masses (*arrows*), which were biopsy-proven invasive ductal carcinoma. (D) Preoperative breast MRI also demonstrates the multifocal breast cancer (*arrows*) and no additional findings.

INVASIVE LOBULAR CANCER

Detection of the extent of invasive lobular carcinoma (ILC) is a challenge on FFDM because ILC cells grow in files in between glandular structures with minimal distortion of architecture.[39] Because of this, it is common for FFDM to underestimate the extent of ILC. DBT enhances margin assessment on mammograms and according to Mariscotti and colleagues,[40] it provides a more accurate measurement of the size of all invasive tumors including ILC. A recent article by Chamming's and co-workers[41] also demonstrated significant increase in conspicuity of visualizing ILC in 23 patients on DBT as compared with 2D; however, their data did not demonstrate any significant improvement in determining the size of ILC when DBT was used.

HIGH-RISK PATIENT EVALUATION

In a detailed search of the literature, there were no dedicated studies or manuscripts that specifically evaluated the effects of DBT in the high-risk patient. In a study by Margolies and colleagues[42] evaluating how DBT changed patient management in a tertiary care facility, a subgroup of high-risk patients was identified and included patients with BRCA gene mutations and high risk based on family history or previous atypical or malignant biopsies. In the screening group of 711 patients in this study, 185 or 26.1% were considered high risk. No incremental benefit was shown in the subset of high-risk patients undergoing DBT. The authors suggest that the subgroup analyzed was too small to demonstrate a benefit from screening high-risk populations with DBT. Large and long-term studies are needed to determine if high-risk women are better served by screening them with DBT.

RADIAL SCAR AND SCLEROSING PAPILLARY LESIONS

The addition of DBT to 2D mammography has been shown to increase the detection rate of invasive cancers. However, several studies have also shown an increased sensitivity to stellate distortions simulating malignancy, increasing the recall rate, which has its associated adverse effects including psychosocial distress and decreased willingness to participate in subsequent screening. Because DBT reduces the effect of overlapping breast parenchyma, the characterization of spiculated tumors has increased.

An analysis of findings leading to recall in the Malmo Breast Tomosynthesis Screening Trial by Lång and colleagues[43] showed that stellate distortion was the major cause of recall when using either DBT or 2D mammography. However, there was a higher proportion of stellate distortion leading to recall in the DBT group compared with 2D mammogram alone (40.5% vs 31.9%). The use of DBT was able to identify more radial scars, postoperative scar tissue, sclerosing papillary lesions, and other benign lesions compared with 2D mammography alone. However, there were significantly fewer callbacks of round lesions (fibroadenomas and cysts) using DBT compared with digital mammography. Thus, although DBT may increase the callback rate for benign lesions, such as radial scar or sclerosing papillary lesion, it may also reduce further assessment of benign cysts and fibroadenomas. A longitudinal analysis done by Lang and colleagues[43] showed a drop in the false-positive callback rate in DBT readers over time, indicating that specificity in identifying lesions with DBT is improved with increased experience.

Fig. 5 illustrates postoperative scar and radial scar, both of which are readily identified by the long straight lines and stellate distortion.

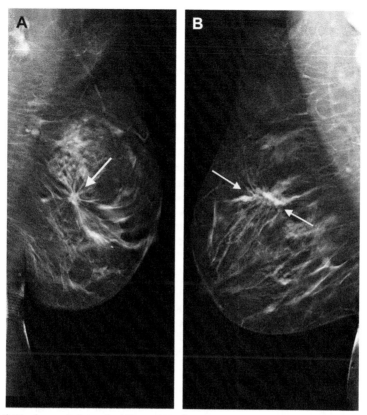

Fig. 5. (*A*) Single mediolateral oblique DBT slice in a 53 year old status post lumpectomy demonstrates architectural distortion (*arrow*) at the postsurgical scar. (*B*) Single mediolateral oblique DBT slice in another patient. Architectural distortion (Between *arrows*) was biopsy proven to be radial scar with atypia, which was surgically excised and showed no upgrade to malignancy.

DIGITAL BREAST TOMOSYNTHESIS–GUIDED BIOPSY AND SECOND-LOOK DIGITAL BREAST TOMOSYNTHESIS AFTER MRI

In addition to conventional stereotactic biopsy of asymmetries and calcifications, DBT has been used to perform image-guided biopsy of targets, such as architectural distortions that were not clearly seen on FFDM and demonstrated no ultrasound correlate.[44] Similarly, preoperative localization of tumors or areas of architectural distortion can be performed under DBT guidance. A special attachment and software localization package is available in most but not all of the currently available DBT units. In addition DBT has been used to evaluate surgical specimens. Urano and colleagues[45] demonstrated that DBT can provide a superior assessment of size of DCIS and extent of intraductal component on surgical specimens as compared with conventional 2D mammography in 65 surgical specimens.

Finally, DBT has been used to evaluate MRI-detected findings. A study by Clauser and colleagues[46] on 84 additional MRI findings in patients with breast cancer demonstrated that second-look ultrasound alone detected 52% of additional MRI findings, whereas adding second-look DBT to ultrasound resulted in identifying 75% of additional MRI findings. Very similar data were presented by Mariscotti and colleagues[47] where adding DBT to second-look ultrasound resulted in overall detection of 89% of MRI-detected additional lesions. A combination of MRI-directed ultrasound and DBT, with DBT biopsy and wire localization capability, could potentially avoid the need of costly and not readily available MRI-guided interventions.

SUMMARY

DBT has quickly emerged as a better mammogram for all types of breast densities, although patients with dense breasts seem to benefit the most. The radiation dose associated with DBT is well less than the FDA-allowed maximum from radiographic mammography studies and the use of synthetic views will lead to further minimizing radiation exposure. The evidence presented shows that patients undergoing DBT will have more breast cancers detected and fewer callbacks for additional imaging. There will be, however, an increase in the detection of spiculated lesions, such as radial scars. More studies are underway to evaluate the accuracy and benefits of DBT. Of particular interest is the effectiveness of DBT in high-risk patients and accuracy compared with MRI.

REFERENCES

1. Tabar L, Yen MF, Vitak B, et al. Mammography service screening and mortality in breast cancer patients: 20-year follow-up before and after introduction of screening. Lancet 2003;361(9367):1405–10.
2. Tabar L, Vitak B, Chen TH, et al. Swedish two-county trial: impact of mammographic screening on breast cancer mortality during 3 decades. Radiology 2011;260(3):658–63.
3. Frisell J, Lidbrink E, Hellström L, et al. Followup after 11 years–update of mortality results in the Stockholm mammographic screening trial. Breast Cancer Res Treat 1997;45(3):263–70.
4. Alexander FE, Anderson TJ, Brown HK, et al. 14 years of follow-up from the Edinburgh randomised trial of breast-cancer screening. Lancet 1999;353(9168):1903–8.
5. Andersson I, Aspegren K, Janzon L, et al. Mammographic screening and mortality from breast cancer: the Malmo mammographic screening trial. BMJ 1988;297(6654):943–8.
6. Bjurstam N, Björneld L, Duffy SW, et al. The Gothenburg breast screening trial: first results on mortality, incidence, and mode of detection for women ages 39-49 years at randomization. Cancer 1997;80(11):2091–9.
7. Pisano ED, Gatsonis C, Hendrick E, et al. Diagnostic performance of digital versus film mammography for breast-cancer screening. N Engl J Med 2005;353(17):1773–83.
8. Whitehead J, Carlile T, Kopecky KJ, et al. Wolfe mammographic parenchymal patterns. A study of the masking hypothesis of Egan and Mosteller. Cancer 1985;56(6):1280–6.
9. Niklason LT, Christian BT, Niklason LE, et al. Digital tomosynthesis in breast imaging. Radiology 1997;205(2):399–406.
10. Sechopoulos I. A review of breast tomosynthesis. Part I. The image acquisition process. Med Phys 2013;40(1):014301.
11. Sechopoulos I. A review of breast tomosynthesis. Part II. Image reconstruction, processing and analysis, and advanced applications. Med Phys 2013;40(1):014302.

12. Rodríguez-Ruiz A, Castillo M, Garayoa J, et al. Evaluation of the technical performance of three different commercial digital breast tomosynthesis systems in the clinical environment. Phys Med 2016;32(6):767–77.

13. Hu YH, Zhao B, Zhao W. Image artifacts in digital breast tomosynthesis: investigation of the effects of system geometry and reconstruction parameters using a linear system approach. Med Phys 2008;35(12):5242–52.

14. Wu T, Moore RH, Kopans DB. Voting strategy for artifact reduction in digital breast tomosynthesis. Med Phys 2006;33(7):2461–71.

15. Förnvik D, Andersson I, Svahn T, et al. The effect of reduced breast compression in breast tomosynthesis: human observer study using clinical cases. Radiat Prot Dosimetry 2010;139(1–3):118–23.

16. Sechopoulos I, Sabol JM, Berglund J, et al. Radiation dosimetry in digital breast tomosynthesis: report of AAPM Tomosynthesis Subcommittee Task Group 223. Med Phys 2014;41(9):091501.

17. Svahn TM, Houssami N, Sechopoulos I, et al. Review of radiation dose estimates in digital breast tomosynthesis relative to those in two-view full-field digital mammography. Breast 2015;24(2):93–9.

18. Paulis LE, Lobbes MB, Lalji UC, et al. Radiation exposure of digital breast tomosynthesis using an antiscatter grid compared with full-field digital mammography. Invest Radiol 2015;50(10):679–85.

19. Shin SU, Chang JM, Bae MS, et al. Comparative evaluation of average glandular dose and breast cancer detection between single-view digital breast tomosynthesis (DBT) plus single-view digital mammography (DM) and two-view DM: correlation with breast thickness and density. Eur Radiol 2015;25(1):1–8.

20. Houssami N, Turner RM. Rapid review: estimates of incremental breast cancer detection from tomosynthesis (3D-mammography) screening in women with dense breasts. Breast 2016;30:141–5.

21. Houssami N. Digital breast tomosynthesis (3D-mammography) for screening women with dense breasts. Expert Rev Med Devices 2016;13(6):515–7.

22. Destounis SV, Morgan R, Arieno A. Screening for dense breasts: digital breast tomosynthesis. AJR Am J Roentgenol 2015;204(2):261–4.

23. Daskalaki A, Bliznakova K, Pallikarakis N. Evaluation of the effect of silicone breast inserts on X-ray mammography and breast tomosynthesis images: a Monte Carlo simulation study. Phys Med 2016;32(2):353–61.

24. Ciatto S, Houssami N, Bernardi D, et al. Integration of 3D digital mammography with tomosynthesis for population breast-cancer screening (STORM): a prospective comparison study. Lancet Oncol 2013;14(7):583–9.

25. Gilbert FJ, Tucker L, Gillan MG, et al. The TOMMY trial: a comparison of TOMosynthesis with digital MammographY in the UK NHS Breast Screening Programme–a multicentre retrospective reading study comparing the diagnostic performance of digital breast tomosynthesis and digital mammography with digital mammography alone. Health Technol Assess 2015;19(4):i–xxv, 1–136.

26. Rafferty EA, Park JM, Philpotts LE, et al. Assessing radiologist performance using combined digital mammography and breast tomosynthesis compared with digital mammography alone: results of a multicenter, multireader trial. Radiology 2013;266(1):104–13.

27. Rosenberg RD, Yankaskas BC, Abraham LA, et al. Performance benchmarks for screening mammography. Radiology 2006;241(1):55–66.

28. Friedewald SM, Rafferty EA, Rose SL, et al. Breast cancer screening using tomosynthesis in combination with digital mammography. JAMA 2014;311(24):2499–507.

29. Rafferty EA, Durand MA, Conant EF, et al. Breast cancer screening using tomosynthesis and digital mammography in dense and nondense breasts. JAMA 2016;315(16):1784–6.

30. Haas BM, Kalra V, Geisel J, et al. Comparison of tomosynthesis plus digital mammography and digital mammography alone for breast cancer screening. Radiology 2013;269(3):694–700.

31. Sharpe RE Jr, Venkataraman S, Phillips J, et al. Increased cancer detection rate and variations in the recall rate resulting from implementation of 3D digital breast tomosynthesis into a population-based screening program. Radiology 2016; 278(3):698–706.

32. Kopans D, Gavenonis S, Halpern E, et al. Calcifications in the breast and digital breast tomosynthesis. Breast J 2011;17(6):638–44.

33. Tagliafico A, Mariscotti G, Durando M, et al. Characterisation of microcalcification clusters on 2D digital mammography (FFDM) and digital breast tomosynthesis (DBT): does DBT underestimate microcalcification clusters? Results of a multicentre study. Eur Radiol 2015;25(1):9–14.

34. Destounis SV, Arieno AL, Morgan RC. Preliminary clinical experience with digital breast tomosynthesis in the visualization of breast microcalcifications. J Clin Imaging Sci 2013;3:65.

35. Berger N, Schwizer SD, Varga Z, et al. Assessment of the extent of microcalcifications to predict the size of a ductal carcinoma in situ: comparison between tomosynthesis and conventional mammography. Clin Imaging 2016;40(6):1269–73.

36. Mun HS, Kim HH, Shin HJ, et al. Assessment of extent of breast cancer: comparison between digital breast tomosynthesis and full-field digital mammography. Clin Radiol 2013;68(12):1254–9.

37. Mariscotti G, Houssami N, Durando M, et al. Accuracy of mammography, digital breast tomosynthesis, ultrasound and MR imaging in preoperative assessment of breast cancer. Anticancer Res 2014;34(3):1219–25.

38. Kim WH, Chang JM, Moon HG, et al. Comparison of the diagnostic performance of digital breast tomosynthesis and magnetic resonance imaging added to digital mammography in women with known breast cancers. Eur Radiol 2016;26(6): 1556–64.

39. Mann RM, Veltman J, Barentsz JO, et al. The value of MRI compared to mammography in the assessment of tumour extent in invasive lobular carcinoma of the breast. Eur J Surg Oncol 2008;34(2):135–42.

40. Mariscotti G, Durando M, Houssami N, et al. Digital breast tomosynthesis as an adjunct to digital mammography for detecting and characterising invasive lobular cancers: a multi-reader study. Clin Radiol 2016;71(9):889–95.

41. Chamming's F, Kao E, Aldis A, et al. Imaging features and conspicuity of invasive lobular carcinomas on digital breast tomosynthesis. Br J Radiol 2017;90: 20170128.

42. Margolies L, Cohen A, Sonnenblick E, et al. Digital breast tomosynthesis changes management in patients seen at a tertiary care breast center. ISRN Radiol 2014; 2014:658929.

43. Lång K, Nergården M, Andersson I, et al. False positives in breast cancer screening with one-view breast tomosynthesis: an analysis of findings leading to recall, work-up and biopsy rates in the Malmö Breast Tomosynthesis screening trial. Eur Radiol 2016;26(11):3899–907.

44. Durand MA, Wang S, Hooley RJ, et al. Tomosynthesis-detected architectural distortion: management algorithm with radiologic-pathologic correlation. Radiographics 2016;36(2):311–21.

45. Urano M, Shiraki N, Kawai T, et al. Digital mammography versus digital breast tomosynthesis for detection of breast cancer in the intraoperative specimen during breast-conserving surgery. Breast Cancer 2016;23(5):706–11.
46. Clauser P, Carbonaro LA, Pancot M, et al. Additional findings at preoperative breast MRI: the value of second-look digital breast tomosynthesis. Eur Radiol 2015;25(10):2830–9.
47. Mariscotti G, Houssami N, Durando M, et al. Digital breast tomosynthesis (DBT) to characterize MRI-detected additional lesions unidentified at targeted ultrasound in newly diagnosed breast cancer patients. Eur Radiol 2015;25(9): 2673–81.

Anatomy and Breast Cancer Staging: Is It Still Relevant?

Jennifer K. Plichta, MD, MS[a], Brittany M. Campbell, BS[a],
Elizabeth A. Mittendorf, MD, PhD[b], E. Shelley Hwang, MD, MPH[a],*

KEYWORDS

- Breast cancer • Staging • Prognosis • Biomarkers

KEY POINTS

- Anatomic staging for breast cancer continues to provide prognostic information relevant to patients and clinicians.
- Prognostic staging for breast cancer now includes both anatomic factors and tumor-specific factors, such as receptor status and genomic profiles.
- By incorporating tumor biology, the new staging system will likely improve the future discrimination of prognosis between tumor stages.

WHY CLINICIANS STAGE PATIENTS

A patient's breast cancer stage provides a concise summary of the disease at the time of diagnosis and/or surgery. It conveys how much cancer is present, where it is located, and highlights important tumor characteristics. It also allows for efficient communication between clinicians and provides a framework for assessing and relaying prognostic information based on the sum of the tumor and disease features. By providing this prognostic framework, staging can be used to determine the best treatment approach for individual patients. In addition to its patient-specific purpose, it also forms the foundation on which changes in population-level cancer incidences can be more thoroughly and accurately evaluated, by allowing assessment of the overall impact of novel or changing breast cancer treatments. Staging information is also frequently used to define groups for inclusion in clinical trials, facilitating screening and evaluation of large groups of patients for research purposes.

To achieve these goals, the American Joint Committee on Cancer (AJCC) was organized in 1959 to develop a system of cancer staging using standardized language

Disclosure Statement: The authors have nothing to disclose.
[a] Department of Surgery, Duke University Medical Center, DUMC 3513, Durham, NC 27710, USA; [b] Department of Breast Surgical Oncology, University of Texas, MD Anderson Cancer Center, 1515 Holcombe Boulevard, Houston, TX 77030, USA
* Corresponding author.
E-mail address: shelley.hwang@duke.edu

Surg Oncol Clin N Am 27 (2018) 51–67
http://dx.doi.org/10.1016/j.soc.2017.07.010
1055-3207/18/© 2017 Elsevier Inc. All rights reserved.

surgonc.theclinics.com

acceptable to the American medical profession.[1] During this era, aggressive local treatments were standard (usually a radical mastectomy and postoperative radiation to the chest wall for most patients with breast cancer), and effective systemic therapies had not yet been established. Thus, the primary objective was to provide standard nomenclature for breast cancer prognostication to prevent futile care for those likely to die from the disease. The guiding philosophy was to develop a classification system that would convey the progression of the usual events that created the life history of a cancer, including tumor growth (size) and spread (to regional lymph nodes and/or distant organs).[1] The AJCC used the principles of the TNM system (T, tumor; N, nodes; M, metastasis), as described by the International Union Against Cancer (UICC)[2] to serve as the basis for categorizing the extent of disease. The aim was to create a staging system that would allow physicians to determine treatment more appropriately, to evaluate results of management more reliably, and to compare statistics from diverse institutions more confidently.[1]

Today, staging continues to be a critical tool used to communicate and understand a patient's breast cancer diagnosis, thus allowing for more accurate treatment discussions and decisions. In today's era of personalized medicine, breast cancer treatment is leading the charge to incorporate more patient-specific and tumor-specific data into determining a patient's prognosis and thus customizing treatment decisions. As treatments continue to evolve and improve, the staging system is also continuously being refined.

Despite significant changes in breast cancer treatment, traditional anatomic TNM staging remains relevant for several reasons. First, it allows investigators to continue to study historic groups of patients and relate them to contemporary patients. Second, it provides consistency in the way clinicians communicate with each other worldwide. Last, it is often the only source of staging classification available in low-income and middle-income countries and will likely remain the cornerstone on which evaluation and treatment decisions are made.[3] Moreover, early detection programs may be the most effective tools for improving outcomes in these countries and TNM staging directly reflects the success of such programs. However, in this modern era, many treatment decisions for patients with breast cancer are not based solely on the TNM stage. For example, local-regional treatments (eg, surgery and radiation) are often influenced by multicentricity and tumor margins, in addition to tumor size and nodal status. Similarly, endocrine therapy is routinely recommended for hormone receptor–positive disease and targeted therapies are frequently recommended for human epidermal growth factor receptor 2 (HER2)-positive tumors. Thus, modern staging systems have moved toward incorporating molecular markers into the staging classification system.

HOW CLINICIANS STAGE PATIENTS

Breast cancer staging is continually evolving, and it has been defined and updated by the AJCC for over 4 decades; the AJCC *Cancer Staging Manual*, 1st edition, was published in 1977.[1] Grouping cancer cases into stages was derived from survival rates being higher for localized disease compared with those in which the disease had spread beyond the original site, initially referred to as early and late cases. The AJCC *Cancer Staging Manual* was created to facilitate improved consistency in describing the extent of the neoplastic disease present, and thus allow clinicians to better determine appropriate treatments, more reliably evaluate the results of management strategies, and more accurately compare statistics or research outcomes.[1] Although it will not be fully adopted until January 2018, the most recent edition (8th) of the AJCC *Cancer Staging Manual,* was published in 2016 and includes 2 staging systems: the anatomic stage and the prognostic stage.[4] The anatomic stage includes the traditional anatomic factors, the primary tumor size (T), nodal status (N), and distant metastasis (M) based on clinical and/or pathologic assessments. However, additional tumor characteristics have recently been added to the AJCC prognostic staging system to more accurately determine the stage of a cancer, such as tumor grade, estrogen receptor (ER) status, progesterone receptor (PR) status, HER2 status, and (when available) tumor multigene panel testing (ie, Oncotype DX, Genomic Health, Redwood City, CA). Taken together, staging provides the most reliable source for accurately predicting a patient's outcome and, although anatomic staging may be predominantly used in some countries, prognostic staging is preferred for patients diagnosed and treated in the United States.

Determining a patient's breast cancer stage typically starts with a physical examination to provide an initial evaluation of the extent of the cancer, such as the tumor location, tumor size, and presence of regional and/or distant metastases. Imaging tests are then used to confirm physical examination findings. This may include a mammogram; breast or axillary ultrasound; breast MRI; computed tomography (CT) scan of the chest, abdomen, or pelvis; nuclear medicine bone scan; and/or PET scan. Depending on the examination and imaging findings, laboratory tests may be sent to make additional assessments, such as blood tests and/or tissue biopsies. When breast biopsies are performed, the pathologic assessment report routinely provides information on the tumor histology, grade, and receptor status (ER, PR, and HER2). If axillary lymph nodes or suspicious lesions of distant organs are biopsied, metastases may be identified.

The National Comprehensive Cancer Network guidelines for an invasive breast cancer staging workup include[5]

- History and physical examination
- Diagnostic bilateral mammogram
- Pathologic assessment review
- Determination of ER, PR, and HER2 status
- Breast MRI (optional).

Although many surgeons obtain a breast MRI with each new breast cancer diagnosis to more fully evaluate the extent of disease and rule out mammographically occult disease, wide variation in MRI use is observed and misconceptions about MRI benefits persist.[6] In general, breast MRIs have not been clearly shown to improve the surgeon's ability to obtain negative margins[7,8] or to improve recurrence or survival rates.[9,10] Similarly, routine axillary ultrasound to determine clinical nodal status is also frequently used but remains controversial.[11,12] The benefit of axillary staging by imaging is to avoid 2-stage axillary surgery; however, the main disadvantage is for those women who may have limited axillary disease managed via sentinel lymph node biopsy with or without axillary radiation. Thus, no consensus currently exists on routine use of breast MRI or staging axillary ultrasound.

For patients with early-stage breast cancer, consideration of additional studies is directed by signs or symptoms, and systemic imaging is not routinely indicated.[13] For patients with more advanced disease, additional studies to consider may include[14]

- Complete blood count
- Comprehensive metabolic panel, including liver function tests and alkaline phosphatase

- CT abdomen or pelvis with contrast or MRI with contrast
- CT chest with contrast
- Bone scan or sodium fluoride PET-CT
- Fluorodeoxyglucose (FDG) PET-CT (optional).

Depending on when staging is assessed, breast cancer staging can be divided into 4 types:

1. Clinical staging relies on the physical examination, imaging tests, and biopsies of affected areas. This designation is recorded with a lower case "c" before the TNM staging categories.
2. Pathologic staging can only be determined after a patient has had surgery to remove the primary tumor and regional lymph nodes. These results are then combined with the clinical stage to determine the final pathologic stage. This designation is recorded with a lower case "p" before the TNM staging categories.
3. Post-therapy or postneoadjuvant therapy staging determines how much cancer remains after a patient completes preoperative systemic therapy and/or radiation therapy before surgery. This is often assessed after surgery, but it may incorporate both clinical and pathologic staging information. This designation is recorded with a lower case "y" before the TNM staging categories.
4. Restaging is performed if a cancer returns after treatment and is used to determine the extent of disease recurrence. However, importantly, the formal stage of a cancer does not change over time, even if the cancer returns or progresses. Rarely, a cancer may be restaged after a significant disease-free interval, which would include the same assessments performed at the time of the initial diagnosis (ie, examinations, imaging, biopsies, and possibly surgery), and the new stage is recorded with a lower case "r" before the restaged TNM designation. A contralateral cancer is staged as a new episode of cancer, with the exception of direct tumor extension or dissemination via lymphatic spread.

When determining the anatomic stage, the categories for the primary tumor are the same for both clinical and pathologic assessments[4] (**Fig. 1**A; **Table 1**). The T stage should include the prefix "c" for clinical stage or "p" for pathologic stage, as appropriate. Tumor size should be rounded up to the nearest millimeter and, when multifocal, the largest tumor focus is used for T categorization (multiple foci are not added together). The additional suffix "m" can be used when the tumor is multifocal and the prefix "y" can be used when the patient has received preoperative (neoadjuvant) systemic therapy.

The categories for the regional lymph nodes vary between clinical and pathologic[4] assessments (see **Fig. 1**B; see **Table 1**). Similar to the T category, the N category should include the prefix "c" for clinical stage or "p" for pathologic stage, as appropriate. The additional suffix "sn" can be used when the lymph nodes have been evaluated by sentinel lymph node biopsy or "f" when the lymph nodes have been evaluated by fine-needle aspiration (FNA) or core needle biopsy without further resection of the nodes. Category cNX is considered invalid for most patients and, if a patient's clinical examination (and/or imaging) is negative, it should be more accurately listed as cN0; the exception to this being patients who have had prior axillary nodal clearance and cannot be evaluated by clinical examination or imaging.

To assess the M stage, clinical examination is used to classify patients as cM0 or cM1 (see **Table 1**), and the designation pM0 is considered invalid.[4] Patients who are microscopically confirmed to have metastatic disease can be categorized as pM1. Notably, M0 includes M0(i+). If a patient is deemed to have M1 disease before

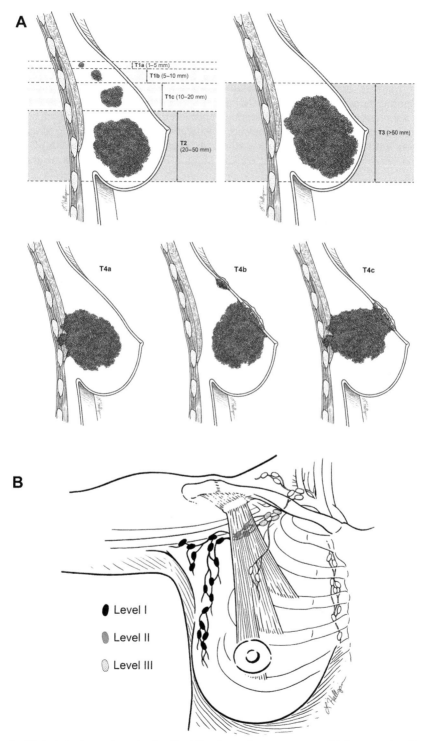

Fig. 1. Clinical staging categories for the (*A*) primary breast tumor and (*B*) regional axillary lymph nodes.[4] For the primary breast tumor (*A*), tumor size is used for delineating

preoperative systemic therapy, the patient is categorized as having stage IV disease and remains stage IV regardless of response to therapy. However, the stage designation should be updated if postsurgical imaging (within 4 months of diagnosis) reveals distant metastases, provided the patient has not received preoperative therapy.

For patients undergoing preoperative therapy, no pathologic stage group is assigned if there is a complete pathologic response (pCR), although these patients have been shown to have a significantly improved disease-free and overall survival, as confirmed in a recent meta-analysis.[15] However, when documenting staging for patients who received preoperative systemic therapy and experienced a pCR, one should continue to list the initial clinical staging information, as well as the pCR status.

Histopathologic tumor types include in situ carcinomas (ductal carcinoma in situ, Paget disease) and invasive carcinomas (ductal, inflammatory, medullary, medullary with lymphoid stroma, mucinous, papillary, tubular, lobular, Paget with infiltrating, undifferentiated, squamous cell, adenoid cystic, secretory, cribriform, and not otherwise specified). For histologic grading, all invasive breast cancers should be assigned a grade using the Nottingham modification of the Scarff-Bloom-Richardson grading system. Tumor grade is determined by scoring 3 morphologic features: tubule formation, nuclear pleomorphism, and mitotic count. Each feature is assigned a score from 1 (favorable) to 3 (unfavorable), and the summation of the 3 scores determines the category as follows:

- Grade 1 (low): 3 to 5 points
- Grade 2 (intermediate): 6 to 7 points
- Grade 3 (high): 8 to 9 points.

ANATOMIC STAGING, TUMOR GRADING, AND OUTCOMES

Although the anatomic extent of disease alone may not define the entire prognosis, it has remained a key prognostic factor in breast cancer (**Table 2**). In 1969, Fisher and colleagues[16] evaluated more than 2000 subjects with operative breast cancer entered into the National Breast Project by 45 institutions and reported that a larger tumor size was associated with a decreased survival, increased recurrence rates, and an increased likelihood of positive axillary lymph nodes. As such, tumor size was considered a key factor in breast cancer staging. Subsequently, a review of 24,136 female subjects with breast cancer from a Breast Cancer Survey was carried out by the American College of Surgeons in 1978.[17] Disease-free survival (cure rates) at 5 years were 60.5% for clinically localized disease and 33.9% for regional disease. Overall survival rates at 5 years were 72.8% for localized disease and 49.1% for regional disease. These findings confirmed that reduced cure and survival rates were associated with an increase in the number of positive nodes; a correlation with tumor size and

---

T categories 1 to 3; however, chest wall involvement results in categorization as T4a disease, whereas skin involvement via satellite nodules or ulceration is considered T4b disease and, when both are present, the tumor is categorized as T4c. Inflammatory breast cancer is categorized as T4d disease (not shown). For the regional axillary lymph nodes (*B*), patients are categorized as cN1 with metastases to movable ipsilateral level I to II nodes, whereas clinically fixed or matted nodes in the ipsilateral level I to II axilla are considered cN2. For cN3 disease, patients have metastases to ipsilateral infraclavicular (level III axillary) nodes, or to ipsilateral internal mammary nodes with level I to II axillary nodal metastases, or to ipsilateral supraclavicular nodes. (*Courtesy of* Duke University. Illustrated by Lauren Halligan, MSMI; copyright Duke University; with permission under a CC BY-ND 4.0 license.)

Table 1
The American Joint Committee *Cancer Staging Manual*, 8th edition, breast cancer definitions of anatomic and pathologic staging guidelines

T Category	T criteria (clinical and pathologic)
Tis	Only ductal carcinoma in situ identified (no invasive component)
T1	Tumor size ≤2 cm in greatest dimension (using the largest tumor foci, if multifocal) • T1mi: tumor size ≤1 mm • T1a: tumor size >1 mm but ≤5 mm • T1b: tumor size >5 mm but ≤10 mm • T1c: tumor size >10 mm but ≤20 mm
T2	Tumor size >2 cm but ≤5 cm in greatest dimension
T3	Tumor size >5 cm in greatest dimension
T4	Tumor of any size with direct extension to the chest wall and/or skin (ulceration or macroscopic nodules); invasion of the dermis alone does not qualify as T4 • T4a: tumor extension to the chest wall; invasion or adherence to the pectoralis muscle without chest wall invasion does not qualify as T4 • T4b: ulceration and/or ipsilateral macroscopic satellite nodules and/or skin edema (eg, peau d'orange) that does not meet criteria for inflammatory carcinoma • T4c: both T4a and T4b are present • T4d: inflammatory carcinoma
N Category	N criteria (clinical)
cN0	No regional lymph node metastases (by imaging or clinical examination)
cN1	Metastases to movable ipsilateral level I–II axillary lymph nodes
cN2	Metastases to ipsilateral level I–II axillary lymph nodes that are clinically fixed or matted, or to ipsilateral internal mammary nodes without axillary lymph node involvement • cN2a: metastases to ipsilateral level I–II axillary nodes that are clinically fixed or matted • cN2b: metastases to ipsilateral internal mammary nodes without axillary nodal involvement
cN3	Metastases to ipsilateral infraclavicular (level III axillary) lymph nodes, to ipsilateral internal mammary lymph nodes with level I–II axillary lymph node metastases, or to ipsilateral supraclavicular lymph nodes • cN3a: metastases to ipsilateral infraclavicular (level III axillary) nodes with or without level I–II axillary nodal involvement • cN3b: metastases to ipsilateral internal mammary nodes with level I–II axillary nodal metastases • cN3c: metastases to ipsilateral supraclavicular nodes with or without axillary or internal mammary nodal involvement
N Category	N criteria (pathologic)
pN0	No regional lymph node metastases identified or ITCs only • pN0(i+): regional lymph nodes with ITCs only (malignant cell clusters ≤0.2 mm)
pN1	Micrometastases, metastases to 1–3 axillary lymph nodes and/or clinically negative internal mammary nodes with micrometastases or macrometastases by sentinel lymph node biopsy • pN1mi: micrometastases (>0.2 mm but ≤2 mm) • pN1a: metastases to 1–3 axillary nodes, at least 1 metastasis > 2 mm • pN1b: metastases to ipsilateral internal mammary sentinel nodes, excluding ITCs • pN1c: pN1a and pN1b combined

(continued on next page)

Table 1 *(continued)*	
pN2	Metastases to 4–9 axillary lymph nodes or positive ipsilateral internal mammary lymph nodes by imaging in the absence of axillary lymph node metastases • pN2a: metastases to 4–9 axillary nodes, at least 1 metastasis > 2 mm • pN2b: metastases in clinically detected internal mammary nodes with or without microscopic confirmation; with pathologically negative axillary nodes
pN3	Metastases to ≥10 axillary lymph nodes, to infraclavicular level III axillary nodes, to positive ipsilateral internal mammary nodes by imaging in the presence of ≥1 positive level I–II axillary nodes, to >3 axillary nodes and micrometastases or macrometastases by sentinel lymph node biopsy in clinically negative ipsilateral internal mammary nodes, or to ipsilateral supraclavicular nodes • pN3a: metastases to ≥10 axillary nodes or to infraclavicular level III axillary nodes • pN3b: positive ipsilateral internal mammary nodes by imaging in the presence of ≥1 positive level I–II axillary nodes, or to >3 axillary nodes and micrometastases or macrometastases by sentinel lymph node biopsy in clinically negative ipsilateral internal mammary nodes • pN3c: metastases to ipsilateral supraclavicular nodes
M Category	M criteria (clinical and pathologic)
M0	No clinical or radiographic evidence of distant metastases (designated cM0, never pM0); imaging studies are not required to assign the cM0 category • cM0(i+): no clinical or radiographic evidence of distant metastases in the presence of tumor cells or deposits ≤ 0.2 mm detected microscopically or by molecular techniques in circulating blood, bone marrow, or other nonregional nodal tissue in a patient without symptoms or signs of metastases
M1	Distant metastases detected by clinical and/or radiographic means (cM1), or histologically proven metastases with at least 1 tumor deposit >0.2 mm (pM1)

Abbreviation: ITC, isolated tumor cells.

From AJCC Cancer Staging Manual. 8th edition. New York: Springer International Publishing; 2016.

prognosis was also noted.[17] Similarly, review of 24,740 cases in the Surveillance, Epidemiology, and End Results (SEER) program from 1977 to 1982 found that tumor diameter and lymph node status were independent but additive prognostic indicators: as tumor size increased, survival decreased regardless of nodal status; as nodal involvement increased, survival decreased regardless of tumor size.[18] Of note, the study also suggested that lymph node status indicates a tumor's ability to spread but that lymph node involvement was not mandatory for distant disease progression.[18]

Of 50,834 patients diagnosed between 1983 to 1987 in the SEER program, relative survival data clearly demonstrated separation of the stages with an expected progression from the best (stage I) to the worst (stage IV) using the AJCC *Cancer Staging Manual*, 4th edition, TNM staging system.[19] This separation of stages was again confirmed in the AJCC *Cancer Staging Manual*, 5th edition, in which survival rates for 50,383 patients with breast carcinoma were classified by the AJCC staging system. Clearly separate 5-year observed and relative survival rates were noted for each stage with an expected progression from the best (stage I: 5-year observed survival rate 87%, 5-year relative survival rate 98%) to the worst (stage IV: 5-year observed survival rate 13%, 5-year relative survival 16%).[20] At that time, numerous prognostic parameters for breast cancer had been postulated with well-supported literature for tumor size, regional lymph node involvement, metastasis, tumor

Table 2
Key references and findings in the history of breast cancer staging

Author, Y of Publication	Select Highlights
Fisher et al,[16] 1969	• Larger tumor size is associated with decreased survival, increased recurrence rates, and increased likelihood of positive axillary nodes
McGuire,[38] 1975	• Between 50%–60% of ER positive breast cancers will respond to endocrine therapy, whereas only 8%–16% of ER negative cancers will respond
Knight et al,[26] 1977	• ER absence is associated with earlier recurrence, independent of tumor size and lymph node status
AJCC guidelines, 1st edition,[1] 1977	• Lower stage cancers have higher recovery rates and greater survival time • Tumor size (T), spread to local lymph nodes (N) and distant metastases (M) are important staging factors; tumor grade was recorded but not included in the TNM classification
Nemoto et al,[17] 1980	• Expected survival decreases linearly with increasing number of histologically positive axillary nodes, up to 21 positive nodes
Clark et al,[27] 1983	• PR and ER positivity are both associated with increased time to recurrence and improved overall survival
AJCC guidelines, 2nd edition,[39] 1983	• Detection of cancers before direction extension or metastatic spread generally leads to improved survival
Slamon et al,[28] 1987	• HER2 gene amplification was a significant predictor of recurrence and overall survival, independent of other prognostic factors • For node positive disease, HER2 gene amplification had greater prognostic value than hormonal receptor status
AJCC guidelines, 3rd edition,[40] 1988	• T3N0M0 5-y survival (76%) most closely matches stage II (75%) rather than stage III (56%), thus reclassified as stage II
Carter et al,[18] 1989	• Both tumor size and number of positive lymph nodes are independent, additive prognostic indicators • Women with 1–3 positive lymph nodes have improved 5-y survival compared with those with 4 + positive nodes
Tandon et al,[41] 1989	• HER2 oncogene amplification is associated with significantly decreased DFS and 5-y OS • Axillary lymph node status is the most important prognostic indicator
Henson et al,[23] 1991	• Observed positive correlation between grade and stage • Both stage and grade are useful prognostic indicators, and provide the best prediction of outcome when used in combination
AJCC guidelines, 4th edition (SEER data),[19] 1992	• Relative survival is directly correlated with AJCC stage (best survival for stages 0-I and incrementally worse through stage IV)
Gusterson et al,[31] 1992	• Expression of c-erbB-2 is prognostically significant for node-positive breast cancer
Press et al,[30] 1993	• In node-negative women, HER2 overexpression is an independent risk factor for disease recurrence • Subgroup analysis confirmed a persistent increased risk in premenopausal and postmenopausal women, as well as ER negative and small (T1a) tumors

(continued on next page)

Table 2
(continued)

Author, Y of Publication	Select Highlights
Press et al,[29] 1997	• HER2 gene amplification is an independent predictor of poor clinical outcome (in the absence of adjuvant therapy) • HER2 gene amplification is a stronger discriminant than tumor size in this population
AJCC guidelines, 5th edition,[20] 1997	• 5-y observed survival decreases as stage increases (stage 0: 92%; stage I: 87%; stage IIA: 78%; stage IIB: 68%; stage IIIA: 51%; stage IIIB: 42%; stage IV: 13%) • 5-y relative survival decreases as stage increases (stage 0: 100%; stage I: 98%: stage IIA: 88%; stage IIB: 76%; stage IIIA: 56%; stage IIIB: 49%; stage IV: 16%) • Prognostic factors reviewed and literature support noted for: tumor size, regional lymph node involvement, metastasis, tumor histology, tumor grade, chromatin, tumor necrosis, mitotic counts, thymidine labeling index, S-phase flow cytometry, Ki-67, angiogenesis, and peritumoral LVI
Fitzgibbons et al,[32] 2000	• Axillary lymph node status is among the most important prognostic indicators for surviving breast cancer • Increasing tumor size, number of positive axillary lymph nodes, and grade are poor prognostic indicators in breast cancer
AJCC guidelines, 6th edition,[42] 2002	• Though data are not yet sufficient to incorporate histologic grade into TNM stage, it remains an important prognostic indicator
AJCC guidelines, 7th edition (NCDB data),[21] 2009	• Increasing tumor size and number of positive nodes demonstrate progressively worse 5-y survivals • 5-y observed survival decreases as stage increases (stage 0: 93%; stage I: 88%; stage IIA: 81%; stage IIB: 74%; stage IIIA: 67%; stage IIIB: 41%; stage IIIC: 49%; stage IV: 15%)
Elston & Ellis (in UICC 7th Edition),[43,44] 2010	• Revised grading criteria (Bloom-Richardson-Elston criteria) provided more objective and reproducible grading results • Using these criteria, grade was directly correlated with prognosis: grade I tumors had significantly better survival than grades II–III
Yi et al,[22] 2011	• Pathologic (anatomic) staging still associated with progressively worse 5-y disease-specific survival • Stage I: 98.8%, stage IIA: 96.3%, stage IIB: 94.5%, and stage IIIA: 88.6% • Staging that included pathologic stage, nuclear grade, and ER status was the most precise in predicting survival
Sparano et al. (TailorX Study),[34] 2015	• Women with T1-2, hormone receptor–positive, HER2 negative, axillary node-negative breast cancer that had a 21-gene recurrence score of 0–10 had a 98.7% DFS rate and 98% overall survival rate
Mittendorf et al,[33] 2016	• The Neo-Bioscore incorporates biomarkers and treatment response to determine prognosis in patients undergoing systemic chemotherapy before definitive surgery • Scoring included the previously defined CPS + EG staging system (clinical-pathologic stage, estrogen receptor status, tumor grade) and added ERBB2 status, which improved prognostic stratification

(continued on next page)

Table 2 (continued)	
Author, Y of Publication	**Select Highlights**
Harris et al,[35] 2016	• Of breast tumor biomarker assays, evidence supports use of Oncotype DX, EndoPredict, PAM50, Breast Cancer Index, and urokinase plasminogen activator and plasminogen activator inhibitor type 1 in select subgroups • Only ER, PR, and HER2 biomarkers should guide specific treatment regimen decisions, although disease stage, co-morbidities, and patient preference should also be considered
Cardoso et al,(MINDACT Study)[36] 2016	• Assessed clinical risk (using Adjuvant! Online) and genomic risk (using 70-gene signature) in women with early-stage breast cancer • Women with discordant disease (low clinical risk and high genomic risk, or high clinical risk and low genomic risk) had similar 5-y survival rates regardless of chemotherapy receipt
AJCC guidelines, 8th edition,[4] 2016	• Prognostic factors (nuclear grade, ER status, and HER2 status) create a risk profile (sum of scores = 0–3) combined with pathologic stage to create a new staging system • 5-y DSS and OS decreased as pathologic stage + risk profile score increased (ie, path stage IIA + risk profile 0 = 100% DSS and 96.8% OS vs path stage IIA = risk profile 3 = 91% DSS and 88.2% OS)

Abbreviations: DFS, disease-free survival; DSS, disease-specific survival; LVI, lymphovascular invasion; NCDB, National Cancer Database; OS, overall survival; SEER, Surveillance, Epidemiology, and End Results.

histology, tumor grade, chromatin, tumor necrosis, mitotic counts, thymidine labeling index, S-phase flow cytometry, Ki-67, angiogenesis, and peritumoral lymphatic vessel invasion.

Recent studies confirm the continued importance of anatomic staging. Review of 211,645 breast cancer cases diagnosed between 2001 and 2002, and reported in the National Cancer Database (NCDB), again demonstrated the significance of increasing tumor size and nodal burden because both correlated with progressively worse survival.[21] With regard to overall survival and disease stage (as classified by the AJCC *Cancer Staging Manual*, 7th edition), the 5-year observed survival rates were 93% for stage 0 disease and only 15% for stage IV disease.[21] Using a more contemporary database of 3728 patients with invasive breast cancer treated at MD Anderson from 1997 to 2006, pathologic (anatomic) staging was still associated with a progressively worse 5-year disease-specific survival on univariate and multivariate analyses: stage I, 98.8%; stage IIA, 96.3%; stage IIB, 94.5%; and stage IIIA, 88.6%.[22] Importantly, the combination of pathologic stage, nuclear grade, and ER status were the most precise in predicting survival, assuming proper multidisciplinary treatment with appropriate use of chemotherapy and endocrine therapy.[22]

Although tumor grade was not officially incorporated into the breast cancer staging system until the 8th edition, it has been recommended for reporting since the 1st edition in 1977.[1] In 1991, survival rates for 22,616 breast cancer cases in the SEER database were reviewed using both stage and tumor grade.[23] Survival rates for those with stage II, grade 1 disease were similar to those assigned stage I, grade 3 and were better than those assigned stage I, grade 4 (which would now be included with grade 3 tumors). These results suggested that combining histologic grade and breast cancer stage may improve the prediction of outcomes.[23] This was again confirmed in a more recent analysis of 161,708 patients in the SEER database.[24] Schwartz and colleagues[24] demonstrated that a higher histologic grade was associated with a progressive decrease in 10-year survival, independent of tumor size or nodal status, thus confirming grade as a prognostic factor. Although some investigators have questioned the reproducibility of histologic grading, specific methodology has been developed to address these concerns.[25]

EVIDENCE TO SUPPORT INCORPORATION OF BIOMARKERS AND IMPLEMENTATION

Tumor biomarkers have long been recognized as important prognostic factors in breast cancer and, for the first time, the AJCC *Cancer Staging Manual*, 8th edition, incorporates tumor biology. The first biomarkers to be recognized as having prognostic significance for breast cancer were the ERs and PRs. McGuire and colleagues[26] demonstrated as early as 1977 that the ER was an important prognostic factor in early-stage breast cancer, independent of anatomic staging factors. In 1983, both the ER and PR were examined in 189 subjects receiving adjuvant therapy for stage II breast cancer and it was found that the presence of either ER or PR was positively correlated with disease-free survival.[27] Studies such as these led to the recommendation that hormone receptor status should be routinely examined, to improve survival predictions. In 1987, the *HER-2/neu* oncogene was recognized to confer a worse prognosis in patients with early-stage breast cancer.[28] These findings were later confirmed in larger datasets of both node-negative[29,30] and as node-positive patients in the Ludwig Breast Cancer Study Group.[31]

In 2000, Fitzgibbons and colleagues[32] published the College of American Pathologists Consensus Statement 1999, which ranked factors as follows: category I, factors with prognostic value and useful in clinical patient management; category II, factors extensively studied biologically and clinically, but its value remained unvalidated; and category III, all other factors not sufficiently studied to demonstrate their prognostic value. Category I factors included TNM staging information, histologic grade, histologic type, mitotic figure counts, and hormone receptor status. Category II factors included HER2-neu, proliferation markers, lymphatic and vascular channel invasion, and p53. Following this publication, subsequent revisions of the AJCC guidelines continued to evaluate the potential incorporation of many of these category I and II factors. These efforts have resulted in the addition of new prognostic staging categories, which for the first time includes a select group of molecular markers.[4]

Evidence has now accumulated to support the combination of tumor biology and anatomic extent of disease demonstrating significant predictive synergy for breast cancer prognosis, beyond anatomic staging alone. Investigators at MD Anderson evaluated the performance of a risk profile, which included pathologic stage, tumor grade, lymphovascular invasion, hormone receptor status, and HER2 receptor status.[22] The incorporation of biomarkers yielded superior stratification of breast cancer specific survivals compared with TNM staging alone. These findings were confirmed by Winchester and colleagues,[4] who evaluated 238,265 women diagnosed with invasive breast cancer in 2010 to 2011 with a median follow-up of 37.6 months. Notably, patients with triple-negative cancer (all grades) had a worse survival, which was comparable to those at least 1 stage higher in the AJCC *Cancer Staging Manual*, 7th edition. Furthermore, several ER-positive or PR-positive subgroups (regardless of HER2 status) had a better survival than those with the same 7th edition stage group.[4] Recently, the MD Anderson group has built on their previous experience to develop the Neo-Bioscore, which incorporates biomarkers, as well as treatment response, to determine prognosis in patients who undergo systemic chemotherapy before definitive surgery.[33] Thus, there is evidence to propose that future staging systems should incorporate treatment response, as well as staging at diagnosis.

The breast cancer field has been replete with studies to support multigene panel testing for prediction of both prognosis and response to therapy. To date, the Oncotype DX assay has been tested in the largest prospective validation cohort. Among 10,253 women enrolled in a prospective study, 1626 women had a recurrence score of 0 to 10 and received endocrine therapy alone (without chemotherapy). At 5-year follow-up, this group had a distant disease-free survival of 99.3% (95% CI, 98.7–99.6), confirming the ability of this test to identify with high accuracy a group of patients who had an excellent outcome with endocrine therapy alone.[34]

More recently, an American Society of Clinical Oncology panel convened to provide guideline recommendations on the use of biomarkers for decision-making regarding systemic therapy for women with early-stage breast cancer.[35] After extensive review of published evidence, the panel concluded that in addition to ER, PR, and HER2 receptors, additional assays, including Oncotype DX, EndoPredict (Myriad Genetics, Salt Lake City, UT), PAM50 (Nanostring Technologies, Inc, Seattle, WA), Breast Cancer Index (Biotheranostics, San Diego, CA), and urokinase plasminogen activator and plasminogen activator inhibitor type 1, had clinical utility for making adjuvant treatment recommendations. Based on these and other recommendations, the AJCC *Cancer Staging Manual*, 8th edition, includes the Oncotype DX score (level I evidence) and the MammaPrint (Agendia Inc, Irvine, CA), EndoPredict, PAM50, and EndoPredict scores (level II evidence) as part of the staging for newly diagnosed breast cancers.

Following publication of the AJCC 8th edition guidelines, the MINDACT (Microarray in Node-Negative and 1–3 Positive Lymph Node Disease May Avoid Chemotherapy) trial reported that women with early-stage breast cancer and a low genomic risk (based on a 70-gene signature, MammaPrint) but high clinical risk (as determined by Adjuvant! Online) had similar 5-year survival rates regardless of chemotherapy receipt.[36] Survival rates were also similar for women with a high genomic risk and low clinical risk. These findings suggest that chemotherapy may not be significantly beneficial for women with discordant clinical and genomic risks (ie, high clinical risk and low genomic risk, or low clinical risk and high genomic risk).[36] Thus, in a summary of the changes to the AJCC *Cancer Staging Manual*, 8th edition, Giuliano and colleagues[37] reported that these findings are consistent with downstaging selected tumors with low-risk genomic profiling and would likely be incorporated in future updates to the manual.

For the of the AJCC *Cancer Staging Manual*, 8th edition, the new prognostic stage groups were determined based on breast cancer populations from the NCDB that were offered and mostly treated with appropriate endocrine and/or systemic therapy.[4] This highlights not only the importance of tumor and disease characteristics but also the critical need for appropriate multidisciplinary treatment. The authors recently performed an analysis comparing the 7th edition to the revised 8th edition AJCC staging system in 501,451 women in the NCDB diagnosed in 2004 to 2014, excluding patients undergoing neoadjuvant chemotherapy (**Table 3**). In this analysis, we found that 19.3% of women stages I to III will be upstaged and 23.8% will be downstaged, with the largest proportion of downstaged patients seen in the stage IB group becoming stage IA (9175, 76.7%). By providing a staging system that better reflects the current understanding of tumor biology and targeted therapy, this restaging is expected to provide a more accurate prediction of patient outcome. Work is ongoing to determine whether this expectation can be validated in large population-based datasets treated with contemporary systemic therapy regimens.

Table 3
Implications of the American Joint Committee on Cancer 8th edition staging guidelines, comparing 7th edition and 8th edition in patients in the National Cancer Database from 2004 to 2014

AJCC Guidelines, 7th Edition, Pathologic or Anatomic Stage	AJCC Guidelines 8th Edition Prognostic Stage									
	0 (%)	IA (%)	IB (%)	IIA (%)	IIB (%)	IIIA (%)	IIIB (%)	IIIC (%)	IV (%)	Total (N)
0	100	0	0	0	0	0	0	0	0	6955
IA	0	86.5	3.9	9.6	0	0	0	0	0	304279
IB	0	76.7	15.2	8.1	0	0	0	0	0	11,970
IIA	0	44.8	27.1	5.3	6.5	16.3	0	0	0	115819
IIB	0	0	27.8	0	1	25.7	14.4	31.2	0	16,982
IIIA	0	0	3.5	8.4	39.8	3.1	29.3	15.9	0	27,845
IIIB	0	0	0	0	0	5.8	35	59.2	0	3360
IIIC	0	0	0	0	0	6.1	39.7	54.2	0	11,458
IV	0	0	0	0	0	0	0	0	100	2783
Total (N)	6955	324249	50,885	38,628	18,739	24,967	16,328	17,917	2783	501451

Black shading represents patients with no change in their stage, light grey represents patients that were downstaged, and dark grey represents patients that were upstaged. Each percent is per row total for each stage using the AJCC 7th edition, then restaged based on the 8th edition (each cell contains row percent). Total from each column or row contains patient sample sizes for each stage. Overall N 5 501,451. Patients who did not have a corresponding prognostic stage in the 8th edition were excluded.

(Data from Plichta and colleagues, unpublished data, 2017.)

SUMMARY

The AJCC staging system continues to provide a universal, efficient, and consistent basis on which to communicate those factors that influence patient prognosis and treatment recommendations. The 8th edition of the AJCC staging system incorporates, for the first time, molecular biomarkers that have been validated to have critical prognostic significance. With these recent updates to the AJCC staging manual, clinicians are strongly encouraged to use the prognostic stage groups, including these additional variables whenever possible. These advancements in the understanding of the biology of breast cancer will undoubtedly continue to serve critical roles in the ongoing refinement of breast cancer staging and to advance both patient care and research.

ACKNOWLEDGMENTS

We would like to acknowledge and thank Lauren Halligan for her contributions in preparation of the figure for this article. We would also like to acknowledge and thank Samantha Thomas for her contributions in preparation of the data table summarizing the restaging of patients.

REFERENCES

1. Manual for staging of cancer. 1st edition. Philadelphia: Lippincott-Raven Publishers; 1977.
2. International Union Against Cancer (UICC): TNM Classification of malignant tumours. 2nd edition. Geneva, Switzerland; 1974.
3. Anderson BO, Yip CH, Smith RA, et al. Guideline implementation for breast healthcare in low-income and middle-income countries. Cancer 2008;113(S8):2221–43.
4. AJCC cancer staging manual. 8th edition. New York: Springer International Publishing; 2016.
5. National Comprehensive Cancer Network. Breast cancer screening and diagnosis (Version 1.2016). Available AT: https://www.nccn.org/professionals/physician_gls/pdf/breast-screening.pdf. Accessed April 11, 2017.
6. Morrow M, Hawley ST, McLeod MC, et al. Surgeon attitudes and use of MRI in patients newly diagnosed with breast cancer. Ann Surg Oncol 2017;24(7): 1889–96.
7. Turnbull L, Brown S, Harvey I, et al. Comparative effectiveness of MRI in breast cancer (COMICE) trial: a randomised controlled trial. Lancet 2010;375(9714):563–71.
8. Houssami N, Turner R, Morrow M. Preoperative magnetic resonance imaging in breast cancer: meta-analysis of surgical outcomes. Ann Surg 2013;257(2): 249–55.
9. Houssami N, Turner R, Macaskill P, et al. An individual person data meta-analysis of preoperative magnetic resonance imaging and breast cancer recurrence. J Clin Oncol 2014;32(5):392–401.
10. Yi A, Cho N, Yang KS, et al. Breast cancer recurrence in patients with newly diagnosed breast cancer without and with preoperative MR imaging: a matched cohort study. Radiology 2015;276(3):695–705.
11. Houssami N, Diepstraten SC, Cody HS 3rd, et al. Clinical utility of ultrasound-needle biopsy for preoperative staging of the axilla in invasive breast cancer. Anticancer Res 2014;34(3):1087–97.
12. Diepstraten SC, Sever AR, Buckens CF, et al. Value of preoperative ultrasound-guided axillary lymph node biopsy for preventing completion axillary lymph

node dissection in breast cancer: a systematic review and meta-analysis. Ann Surg Oncol 2014;21(1):51–9.

13. Moy L, Newell MS, Mahoney MC, et al. ACR appropriateness criteria stage I breast cancer: initial workup and surveillance for local recurrence and distant metastases in asymptomatic women. J Am Coll Radiol 2016;13(11S):e43–52.

14. National Comprehensive Cancer Network. Breast Cancer (Version 2.2017). Available at: https://www.nccn.org/professionals/physician_gls/pdf/breast.pdf. Accessed April 11, 2017.

15. Cortazar P, Zhang L, Untch M, et al. Pathological complete response and long-term clinical benefit in breast cancer: the CTNeoBC pooled analysis. Lancet 2014;384(9938):164–72.

16. Fisher B, Slack NH, Bross ID. Cancer of the breast: size of neoplasm and prognosis. Cancer 1969;24(5):1071–80.

17. Nemoto T, Vana J, Bedwani RN, et al. Management and survival of female breast cancer: results of a national survey by the American College of Surgeons. Cancer 1980;45(12):2917–24.

18. Carter CL, Allen C, Henson DE. Relation of tumor size, lymph node status, and survival in 24,740 breast cancer cases. Cancer 1989;63(1):181–7.

19. AJCC manual for staging of cancer. 4th edition. Philadelphia: Lippincott-Raven Publishers; 1992.

20. AJCC cancer staging manual. 5th edition. Philadelphia: Lippincott-Raven Publishers; 1997.

21. Edge S, Byrd DR, Compton CC, et al. AJCC cancer staging manual, Vol. 7. New York: Springer-Verlag; 2010.

22. Yi M, Mittendorf EA, Cormier JN, et al. Novel staging system for predicting disease-specific survival in patients with breast cancer treated with surgery as the first intervention: time to modify the current American Joint Committee on Cancer staging system. J Clin Oncol 2011;29(35):4654–61.

23. Henson DE, Ries L, Freedman LS, et al. Relationship among outcome, stage of disease, and histologic grade for 22,616 cases of breast cancer. The basis for a prognostic index. Cancer 1991;68(10):2142–9.

24. Schwartz AM, Henson DE, Chen D, et al. Histologic grade remains a prognostic factor for breast cancer regardless of the number of positive lymph nodes and tumor size: a study of 161 708 cases of breast cancer from the SEER Program. Arch Pathol Lab Med 2014;138(8):1048–52.

25. Elston E, Ellis I. Method for grading breast cancer. J Clin Pathol 1993;46(2):189.

26. Knight WA, Livingston RB, Gregory EJ, et al. Estrogen receptor as an independent prognostic factor for early recurrence in breast cancer. Cancer Res 1977;37(12):4669–71.

27. Clark GM, McGuire WL, Hubay CA, et al. Progesterone receptors as a prognostic factor in stage II breast cancer. N Engl J Med 1983;309(22):1343–7.

28. Slamon DJ, Clark GM, Wong SG, et al. Human breast cancer: correlation of relapse and survival with amplification of the HER-2/neu oncogene. Science 1987;235(4785):177–82.

29. Press MF, Bernstein L, Thomas PA, et al. HER-2/neu gene amplification characterized by fluorescence in situ hybridization: poor prognosis in node-negative breast carcinomas. J Clin Oncol 1997;15(8):2894–904.

30. Press MF, Pike MC, Chazin VR, et al. Her-2/neu expression in node-negative breast cancer: direct tissue quantitation by computerized image analysis and association of overexpression with increased risk of recurrent disease. Cancer Res 1993;53(20):4960–70.

31. Gusterson BA, Gelber RD, Goldhirsch A, et al. Prognostic importance of c-erbB-2 expression in breast cancer. International (Ludwig) Breast Cancer Study Group. J Clin Oncol 1992;10(7):1049–56.
32. Fitzgibbons PL, Page DL, Weaver D, et al. Prognostic factors in breast cancer. Arch Pathol Lab Med 2000;124(7):966–78.
33. Mittendorf EA, Vila J, Tucker SL, et al. The Neo-Bioscore update for staging breast cancer treated with neoadjuvant chemotherapy: incorporation of prognostic biologic factors into staging after treatment. JAMA Oncol 2016;2(7): 929–36.
34. Sparano JA, Gray RJ, Makower DF, et al. Prospective validation of a 21-gene expression assay in breast cancer. N Engl J Med 2015;373(21):2005–14.
35. Harris LN, Ismaila N, McShane LM, et al. Use of biomarkers to guide decisions on adjuvant systemic therapy for women with early-stage invasive breast cancer: American Society of Clinical Oncology Clinical Practice guideline. J Clin Oncol 2016;34(10):1134–50.
36. Cardoso F, van't Veer LJ, Bogaerts J, et al. 70-gene signature as an aid to treatment decisions in early-stage breast cancer. N Engl J Med 2016;375(8):717–29.
37. Giuliano AE, Connolly JL, Edge SB, et al. Breast Cancer—major changes in the American Joint Committee on Cancer eighth edition cancer staging manual. CA Cancer J Clin 2017;67:290–303.
38. McGuire WL. Current status of estrogen receptors in human breast cancer. Cancer 1975;36(S2):638–44.
39. AJCC manual for staging of cancer. 2nd edition. Philadelphia: Lippincott-Raven Publishers; 1983.
40. AJCC manual for staging of cancer. 3rd edition. Philadelphia: Lippincott-Raven Publishers; 1988.
41. Tandon AK, Clark GM, Chamness GC, et al. HER-2/neu oncogene protein and prognosis in breast cancer. J Clin Oncol 1989;7(8):1120–8.
42. Greene FL, American Joint Committee on Cancer, American Cancer Society. AJCC cancer staging manual. 6th edition. New York: Springer-Verlag; 2002.
43. International Union Against Cancer (UICC). TNM classification of malignant tumours. 7th edition. Chichester (United Kingdom): Wiley-Blackwell; 2010.
44. Elston CW, Ellis IO. Pathological prognostic factors in breast cancer. I. The value of histological grade in breast cancer: experience from a large study with long-term follow-up. Histopathology 1991;19(5):403–10.

Are There Alternative Strategies for the Local Management of Ductal Carcinoma in Situ?

Kelly J. Rosso, MD, Anna Weiss, MD, Alastair M. Thompson, BSc (Hons), MBChB, MD, FRCSEd (Gen)*

KEYWORDS

- Ductal carcinoma in situ (DCIS) • Active surveillance • Endocrine therapy

KEY POINTS

- Ductal carcinoma in situ (DCIS) is currently treated in similar ways to invasive breast cancer.
- Given the excellent breast cancer–specific survival for women with a diagnosis of DCIS, less invasive strategies than current therapy merit evaluation.
- Active surveillance of appropriately selected women with low-risk DCIS is the subject of several randomized clinical trials.
- Outcomes of invasive breast cancer and patient-reported outcome measures may change the way women with low-risk DCIS are managed in future.

INTRODUCTION

The management of ductal carcinoma in situ (DCIS) has largely shadowed the treatment of invasive breast cancer: surgical excision with adjuvant radiation and endocrine therapy for the prevention of further in situ or invasive events. As for invasive disease, patient selection for surgery, radiation therapy, choice of adjuvant endocrine therapy, and the potential role for neoadjuvant therapy have each become the subject of therapeutic trials in DCIS. Again as a parallel to invasive disease, locoregional control and event-free survival in the context of the morbidities of radiation therapy and drug therapies require consideration. There are now trials underway to address the question of overtreatment and determine whether nonsurgical management of low-risk (for progression) DCIS can be managed by medical therapy alone.

Disclosure: The authors have nothing to disclose.
Department of Breast Surgical Oncology, The University of Texas MD Anderson Cancer Center, FCT7.6092, Unit 1434, 1400 Pressler Street, Houston, Texas 77030-4008, USA
* Corresponding author.
E-mail address: AThompson1@mdanderson.org

SURGICAL MANAGEMENT

The current gold standard for surgical treatment of DCIS is excision to negative margins. Lumpectomy (segmental or partial mastectomy) with radiation or mastectomy represents guideline-concordant care for DCIS as outlined by the National Comprehensive Cancer Network (NCCN) treatment recommendations.[1] These guidelines are based on the findings of equivalent survival outcomes for patients with invasive breast cancer shown for both surgical approaches in randomized clinical trials.[2,3] The decision between breast conservation and mastectomy for DCIS is based on clinical, pathologic, and patient-related factors. DCIS is most commonly identified as a unifocal, nonpalpable lesion identified on mammography. Localization with a radioactive seed or wire is often necessary to facilitate breast conservation therapy (BCT). Multifocality, large-volume disease (with inability to obtain negative margins), or inability to obtain a favorable cosmetic outcome (even with oncoplastic techniques) may drive surgical decision making toward mastectomy. Although a nipple-sparing mastectomy may be appropriate for patients with early-stage, biologically favorable invasive cancers that are node negative and located in the periphery of the breast,[4] greater caution may be required for patients with DCIS. Extensive, centrally located, and subareolar DCIS less than 2 cm from the nipple areolar complex may be considered contraindications to a nipple-sparing approach. Contralateral prophylactic mastectomy incurs no survival benefit in patients who do not have a genetic predisposition for the development of invasive breast cancer[5] and thus should also be viewed with caution for individuals with DCIS.

When a mastectomy is planned for a diagnosis of DCIS, sentinel lymph node (SLN) biopsy should be considered, given the difficulty of axillary lymph node mapping if invasion is identified on final pathology after the breast has been removed. SLN biopsy alone carries a risk of wound infection, seroma, lymphedema, and pain/paresthesias, although lower than that associated with axillary lymph node dissection.[6] Hence, most clinicians caution that SLN biopsy for DCIS in BCT should not be routine[7–9] but considered at the time of completion mastectomy for positive/close margins following BCT (and attempted reexcision).[10]

RADIATION THERAPY

Women with DCIS who undergo breast-conserving surgery receive adjuvant radiotherapy in up to two-thirds of cases in published series. In contrast with invasive breast cancer, radiation therapy is rarely used following mastectomy for DCIS. Whole-breast radiotherapy following breast-conserving surgery reduces local recurrence (DCIS and invasive breast cancer) from 28.1% to 12.9% and reduces the incidence of invasive disease from 11.0% to 5.0% at 10 years as reported in a meta-analysis[11] based on key trials including the National Surgical Adjuvant Breast and Bowel Project (NSABP) B-17, NSABP B-24,[12] and the United Kingdom/Australia and New Zealand[13] (United Kingdom/ANZ) DCIS trials.

Although the extent of margin of clearance around DCIS has been hotly debated over the years, it is probable that at least a negative margin is required for the beneficial effects of breast radiotherapy to be realized. The dose and fractionation regimens for whole-breast radiotherapy for DCIS after breast-conserving surgery mirror practices for invasive disease, with a trend toward the use of hypofractionation and the potential added value of a boost to the tumor (DCIS) bed.[14] Whether alternative approaches to whole-breast irradiation to the DCIS resection bed (eg, using intracavity radiotherapy techniques) are equivalent to external beam radiation therapy is currently unclear and the subject of clinical trials. The side effects, such as skin toxicity and potential cardiac effects, as for invasive breast cancer, need to be considered with each approach. Although radiation therapy reduces in-breast recurrence by half (DCIS and invasive breast cancer), use of radiation therapy does not seem to alter long-term breast cancer–specific survival for patients diagnosed with pure DCIS.[11] There may be less benefit for radiation therapy following BCT for DCIS in the elderly population, similar to invasive disease. Although avoidance of radiation is associated with increased risk for locoregional recurrence, omission of radiation therapy may be a viable option for elderly patients with hormone receptor–positive disease receiving endocrine therapy, because such a strategy does not lead to decreased disease-free or overall survival.[15,16]

The Oncotype DX DCIS Score is a 12-gene assay that provides individualized 10-year risk of locoregional recurrence (in situ and invasive disease) following treatment with breast-conserving surgery alone.[17] The DCIS Score has been validated in different patient populations as an independent predictor of recurrence risk beyond clinical and pathologic variables and may support the omission of radiation therapy in some patients with low risk of recurrence.[18] The rigid eligibility criteria for the landmark validation study E5194 (25 mm maximum size for low-grade/intermediate-grade DCIS, 10 mm for high-grade DCIS, and 3-mm resection margins) and the historically high recurrence rates should be considered. Although clinical application of the DCIS score is not standard of care, it may inform clinicians and patients as to the likely benefits of adjuvant therapy.

ENDOCRINE THERAPY

The value of adjuvant endocrine therapy to prevent further DCIS or subsequent invasive breast cancer following resection of estrogen receptor (ER)–positive DCIS has followed the evidence in favor of such an approach for ER-positive invasive breast cancer but remains controversial. Not every DCIS is universally examined for ER (or HER2) status. There is a need not simply to show evidence of efficacy of endocrine therapy to reduce in-breast recurrence but also to recognize the potential to prevent contralateral and distant breast events balanced against the side effects of, and adherence to, endocrine therapy.

The NSABP B-24 trial found that in premenopausal and postmenopausal patients treated for DCIS with lumpectomy and adjuvant radiation therapy, tamoxifen reduced the risk of ipsilateral local recurrence by 30% and for contralateral breast cancer by 50%.[19] The absolute risk at 5 years of any (invasive or noninvasive) breast cancer event was small (tamoxifen arm 8% and placebo arm 13%) and survival was not influenced by treatment. A more complex trial design in the United Kingdom/ANZ DCIS trial (2 × 2 trial of tamoxifen vs radiation therapy) examined the use of tamoxifen versus no adjuvant therapy following complete local excision of DCIS in the presence or absence of radiation therapy.[13] The trial results suggested that, in the absence of radiation therapy, tamoxifen was associated with a 30% overall reduction in breast cancer events through reduction in DCIS recurrence, contralateral DCIS, and invasive disease events. However, tamoxifen was ineffective in preventing ipsilateral invasive recurrence and, in the presence of radiation therapy, tamoxifen had no added benefit. Survival was not affected by radiation therapy or tamoxifen in the United Kingdom/ANZ DCIS trial, with breast cancer accounting for only 20% of all deaths.[13] A meta-analysis including these 2 key trials suggests modest additional benefit of tamoxifen compared with a combination of breast-conserving surgery and radiation therapy for local recurrence, with a reduction from 14.1% to 9.7%.

Recently, the aromatase inhibitor anastrozole has been compared with tamoxifen in 2 large randomized trials enrolling postmenopausal women with DCIS. In NSABP B-35, which enrolled 3104 postmenopausal women who had undergone lumpectomy to clear margins and adjuvant radiation for DCIS, anastrozole treatment was associated with a small but statistically significant improvement in breast cancer–free interval compared with tamoxifen (hazard ratio [HR], 0.73; 95% confidence interval [CI], 0.56–0.96; $P = .023$), although disease-free survival was the same at 120 months (HR, 0.89; 95% CI, 0.75–1.07; $P = .21$).[20] Among postmenopausal women less than 60 years old (n = 1447), anastrozole was associated with significant improvements in breast cancer–free interval and disease-free survival compared with tamoxifen (HR, 0.53; 95% CI, 0.35–.080; and HR, 0.69; 95% CI, 0.51–0.93, respectively). However, the International Breast Intervention Study (IBIS) II trial, which enrolled 2980 postmenopausal women with DCIS who had undergone lumpectomy to clear margins with or without radiation, failed to show an improvement with anastrozole compared with tamoxifen (HR, 0.89; 95% CI, 0.64–1.23; $P = .49$).

The reduction in contralateral cancer and possibly local recurrence of DCIS with endocrine therapy needs to be weighed against the potential side effects of tamoxifen (hot flashes, deep vein thrombosis, or endometrial cancer) and aromatase inhibition (hot flashes, arthralgias, osteopenia, or osteoporosis). The impact on quality of life of endocrine therapy side effects and other diseases associated with these agents gives pause for thought. In addition, the issue of adherence is important with endocrine therapy, in which only 70% of women in the IBIS II[21] trial were still taking their endocrine agents at 5 years. If extrapolated to the wider community, this finding could diminish the value of adjuvant endocrine therapy for DCIS.

NEOADJUVANT THERAPY

Neoadjuvant therapy has become standard of care for advanced breast cancer and an option for reducing the size of the primary tumor in patients with early-stage invasive breast cancer (and hence facilitating breast conservation rather than mastectomy as a surgical option). However, there is currently little evidence in favor of the neoadjuvant approach for treatment of DCIS. For ER-positive DCIS, targeting the ER preoperatively has been the focus of the Cancer and Leukemia Group B (CALGB) 40903 trial. Patients receive 6 months of neoadjuvant letrozole before surgical intervention. There have been several trials targeting HER2-positive DCIS, with HER2 targeting agents including trastuzumab[22] and lapatinib.[23] The neoadjuvant approaches are largely used to further understand the biology of DCIS. If there is a clinical need to defer conventional surgical intervention for DCIS, such drug-based therapeutic approaches may be a useful option.

Thus, the standard approaches to managing DCIS have largely been derived and followed on from the treatment of invasive disease, despite the probability that most women diagnosed with DCIS will not die from breast cancer.[24] Hence, considered approaches to DCIS that reflect the concerns regarding overtreatment and the different outlook to invasive breast cancers have recently been developed.

MEDICAL THERAPY ALONE

Although surgical resection has been standard practice for DCIS, a small proportion of women in the United States ($\sim$1.5%) decline surgery and opt for medical intervention alone. Recent prospective, population-based data suggest that segmental mastectomy or modified radical mastectomy may be associated with surprisingly high levels of chronic pain, disability, and psychological distress, often resistant to management,

4 and 9 months after breast surgery.[25] Taken together with the exceptional long-term survival rates for women with DCIS, this has led some clinicians to question the need for surgical intervention.

However, DCIS (like invasive breast cancer) shows a spectrum of phenotypic behaviors ranging from indolence through progression to invasive disease. Thus, for nonsurgical management of DCIS, targeting low-risk (for progression) DCIS as the focus for medical management alone is most attractive, reflecting similar strategies implemented for selected patients with prostate and thyroid neoplasms. Internationally, there are 3 clinical trials (**Fig. 1**) designed to determine the effect of nonsurgical management of low-risk DCIS: the Comparison of Operative to Monitoring and Endocrine Therapy (COMET[26]) trial in the United States, the Low-risk DCIS (LORIS[27]) trial in the United Kingdom, and the Management of Low-grade DCIS (LORD[28]) trial in Europe. A fourth trial, the Low and Intermediate-risk Ductal Carcinoma Study, has been proposed in Australia and New Zealand. Although the LORIS trial has already shown the feasibility of randomizing patients between surgical and nonsurgical management, the US-based Comparison of Operative to Monitoring and Endocrine Therapy (COMET) trial merits particular attention. COMET, sponsored by the Alliance for Clinical Trials in Oncology, will not only randomize patients between guideline-concordant care (surgery, with or without radiation therapy and/or endocrine therapy) versus active surveillance (with the option of endocrine therapy) but will also monitor outcomes in those not participating in the trial. The identification of subsequent invasive breast cancer is the primary outcome; however, patient-reported outcomes and other breast and health outcome measures will also be captured. There are subtle differences between the 3 currently recruiting trials (COMET, LORIS, LORD) in terms of patient characteristics, imaging, and pathology features, and also some differences between the active surveillance arms (mammographic surveillance every 6 months in COMET but every 12 months in LORIS and LORD) (**Table 1**). However, the intent is for the 3 trials to ultimately allow for meta-analysis in order to provide high-level guidance regarding management options for patients with DCIS.

CONTROVERSIES FOR NONSURGICAL APPROACHES

Before guideline-concordant care or active surveillance, there is clearly a need to image and establish the diagnosis based on sufficient sampling of the lesion using core needle biopsies (**Fig. 2**). A legitimate concern for the conservative management of clinically low-risk DCIS (active surveillance, endocrine therapy, observation alone) is the failure to identify the presence of invasive carcinoma at the time of diagnosis. A meta-analysis examining 7350 cases of DCIS identified by core needle biopsy found invasive cancer at excision in 1736, thus underestimating the disease in 25.9% of cases.[29] More recent data from a national screening program with quality assurance measures in place for imaging and pathology suggest that the figure may still be around 20%.[30] Predictive variables associated with underestimating invasive disease include the presence of a palpable lesion, mammographic mass, the use of a smaller-gauge biopsy device (14 vs 11 gauge), and higher BIRADS (Breast Imaging Reporting and Data System) categorization. Subsequent studies evaluating upgrade rates further identified seemingly cumulative risk factors[31] and have led to the creation of predictive nomograms.[32,33]

To evaluate the safety of observation in DCIS, Pilewskie and colleagues[34] identified a cohort of 296 patients who met some of the eligibility criteria for the LORIS trial. Most patients (82%) had intermediate-grade DCIS on core biopsy, and more than half (62%) of the core biopsies in the study were performed with a vacuum-assisted 8-gauge or

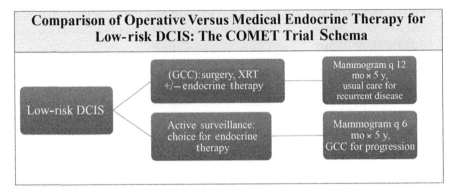

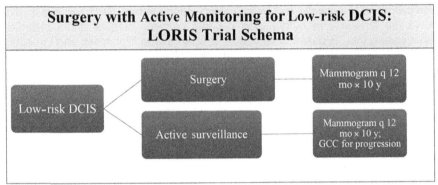

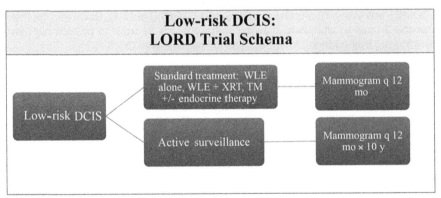

Fig. 1. Comparison of the COMET (Comparison of Operative to Monitoring and Endocrine Therapy), LORIS (Low-risk DCIS) and LORD (Management of Low-grade DCIS) trials. GCC, guideline-concordant care; q, every; TM, total mastectomy; WLE, wide local excision; XRT, external radiation therapy.

9-gauge core needle. Although this retrospective review did not mirror LORIS precisely, 20% of patients in this single-center retrospective review were found to have invasive carcinoma on final pathology. Intermediate-grade DCIS was a statistically significant factor; 23% of patients with intermediate-grade DCIS were upgraded based on final pathology compared with only 7% in those with low-grade DCIS. More recently, Grimm and colleagues[35] identified a contemporary cohort of patients diagnosed with DCIS by vacuum-assisted core biopsy (n = 307), some of whom

Table 1
Comparison of active surveillance trials in ductal carcinoma in situ

	COMET	LORIS	LORD
Patient characteristics			
Age (y)	$\geq$40	$\geq$46	$\geq$45
History of other cancer	NA	INCLUDE	EXCLUDE with exceptions[a]
History of breast cancer	EXCLUDE	EXCLUDE	NA
Synchronous ilnvasive cancer	EXCLUDE	EXCLUDE	EXCLUDE
Bilateral DCIS	INCLUDE	INCLUDE	EXCLUDE
Prior chemoprevention	EXCLUDE	NA	NA
High risk	INCLUDE	EXCLUDE[b]	EXCLUDE if BRCA mutation
Symptomatic	EXCLUDE	EXCLUDE	EXCLUDE
Imaging characteristics			
Morphology	Calcifications only	Calcifications only	Calcifications only
BIRADS	$\leq$3	NA	NA
Size	NA	NA	Any
Biopsy technique	VACB or surgical	VACB or surgical	VACB
Device Gauge, # of cores	NA, NA	$\leq$12 G, NA	8–9 G, 6 cores or 10–11G, 12 cores
Pathologic features			
Nuclear grade	Low and intermediate	Low and intermediate	Low
Hormone receptor	ER+ or PR+, HER2−	NA	NA
Comedonecrosis	EXCLUDE	EXCLUDE	NA
Key differences	Active surveillance arm: mammography q 6 mo × 5 y Two local pathologists to agree pathologic features	Active surveillance arm: mammography q 12 mo × 10 y Requires central pathology review before randomization	Active surveillance arm: mammography q 12 mo × 10 y
Outcome measures			
Primary	New ipsilateral invasive cancer in GCC and AS arms at 2 y	Ipsilateral invasive breast cancer–free survival time	Ipsilateral invasive breast cancer–free rate at 10 y
Secondary	QOL, psychological outcomes, rate of surgery, overall survival	Time to ipsilateral or contralateral invasive breast cancer, time to surgery, QOL, cost	Time to ipsilateral grade II–III DCIS, contralateral DCIS, contralateral invasive breast cancer, distant metastasis–free and overall survival

Abbreviations: AS, active surveillance; BIRADS, Breast Imaging Reporting and Data System; G, gauge; GCC, guideline-concordant care; NA, not applicable; q, every; QOL, quality of life; VACB, vacuum assisted core biopsy.
[a] Exceptions include in situ cancer of the cervix and basal carcinoma of the skin.
[b] If high risk per United Kingdom NICE (National Institute for Health and Care Excellence) guidelines.

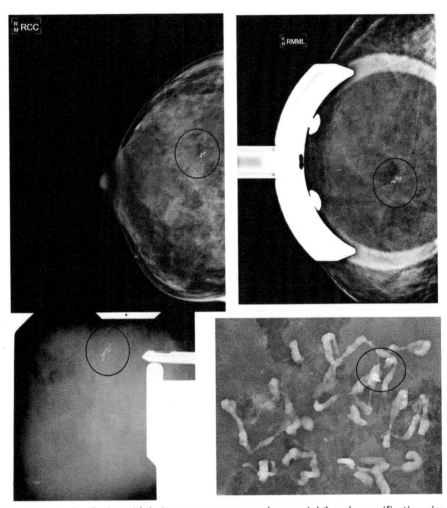

Fig. 2. Example of a low-risk lesion on mammogram (*upper right*) and magnification view (*upper left*) with stereotactic targeting (*lower left*) and multiple cores (*lower right*) containing microcalcifications (*circled*).

(n = 81) met the eligibility criteria for the active surveillance trials (COMET, LORIS, and LORD). The overall upgrade rate to invasive disease was 17% (53 of 307). However, upstage rates in patients who met trial inclusion criteria were more reassuringly 6% for COMET, 7% for LORIS, and 10% for LORD. All upstaged cases were node negative, hormone receptor positive (ER, PR), and HER2 nonamplified, indicating a traditionally very favorable subset in terms of long-term survival and provided strong reassurance that, using the current trials criteria, any potential for missed upgraded (invasive) lesions would likely not affect patient survival.

PATIENT-REPORTED OUTCOME MEASURES

A multitude of psychological, social, and physical stresses accompany the diagnosis and subsequent treatment of DCIS or invasive breast cancer. Anxiety, depression, fear of recurrence, pain, fatigue, body image issues, and sexual dysfunction have been found to affect quality of life and even long-term overall survival in patients with invasive breast cancer.[36–38] A recent meta-analysis of patient-reported outcomes identified that these treatment-associated physical, mental, and sexual health issues also pertain to women with a diagnosis of DCIS.[39]

In those women who undergo surgical management of DCIS, there is a risk of developing chronic pain at the surgical sites.[25] Persistent pain after lumpectomy may be as prevalent as pain after total mastectomy, leading to both physical and psychological disability, which is often resistant to management. One prospective study identified patient-specific and surgery-specific risk factors for postoperative pain, and showed remarkably high levels of chronic pain 4 and 9 months after breast surgery.[40] Prospective randomized trials designed to identify low-risk DCIS that can be safely managed with active surveillance may allow some women to safely avoid surgery and the associated complications.

SUMMARY

The contemporary understanding of the heterogeneous nature of DCIS has led to less invasive treatment in selected patients with low-risk disease and suggestions that the word carcinoma may not be appropriate in this diagnosis. A working group from the National Cancer Institute suggested that the word cancer to describe premalignant conditions such as DCIS should no longer be used, because this term almost mandates more aggressive treatment to halt otherwise definite progression to a lethal disease process.[41] Advocates of the name change call on studies linking patient anxiety and distress to overestimation of breast cancer risk.[42,43]

Treatment of DCIS, including surgery, radiation, and/or drug therapies, has largely followed the lead of invasive breast cancer. Although some benefit has been seen for the use of radiation therapy and/or endocrine agents in reducing locoregional events, without any impact on survival, the value of nonsurgical therapies (radiotherapy and endocrine therapy) for DCIS is less certain than for invasive breast cancer. However, trials around the world are seeking to determine whether DCIS at low risk for progression may be managed without surgical intervention, relying on medical therapy to control breast neoplasia reflecting the indolent process of DCIS in selected patients. In addition, alternative strategies, such as vaccinations and harnessing the immune system, are currently being investigated.[44,45] These strategies could offer promising insights and novel treatment approaches to appropriately selected women. A key to determining how best to manage DCIS in the future is the global activity of randomized clinical trials now underway, which are likely to take 5 to 10 years to produce clinically actionable data. In the meantime, appropriately selected patients should be offered entry into these trials to address this pressing question: are there alternative strategies to surgery for selected women in the management of DCIS?

REFERENCES

1. National Comprehensive Cancer Network, incorporated. Available at: https://www.nccn.org/patients/guidelines/stage_0_breast/. Accessed March 28, 2017.
2. Fisher B, Redmond C, Poisson R, et al. Eight-year results of a randomized clinical trial comparing total mastectomy and lumpectomy with or without irradiation in the treatment of breast cancer. N Engl J Med 1989;320(13):822–8.
3. Fisher B, Anderson S, Bryant J, et al. Twenty-year follow-up of a randomized trial comparing total mastectomy, lumpectomy, and lumpectomy plus irradiation for the treatment of invasive breast cancer. N Engl J Med 2002;347(16):1233–41.

4. Hieken TJ, Boolbol SK, Dietz JR. Nipple-sparing mastectomy: indications, contra-indications, risks, benefits, and techniques. Ann Surg Oncol 2016;23(10):3138–44.
5. Tuttle TM, Jarosek S, Habermann EB, et al. Increasing rates of contralateral pro-phylactic mastectomy among patients with ductal carcinoma in situ. J Clin Oncol 2009;27(9):1362–7.
6. Lucci A, McCall LM, Beitsch PD, et al. Surgical complications associated with sentinel lymph node dissection (SLND) plus axillary lymph node dissection compared with SLND alone in the American College of Surgeons Oncology Group Trial Z0011. J Clin Oncol 2007;25(24):3657–63.
7. Heymans C, van Bastelaar J, Visschers RG, et al. Sentinel node procedure obso-lete in lumpectomy for ductal carcinoma in situ. Clin Breast Cancer 2017;17(3):e87–93.
8. van Roozendaal LM, Goorts B, Klinkert M, et al. Sentinel lymph node biopsy can be omitted in DCIS patients treated with breast conserving therapy. Breast Can-cer Res Treat 2016;156(3):517–25.
9. Francis AM, Haugen CE, Grimes LM, et al. Is sentinel lymph node dissection war-ranted for patients with a diagnosis of ductal carcinoma in situ? Ann Surg Oncol 2015;22(13):4270–9.
10. Pilewskie M, Karsten M, Radosa J, et al. Is sentinel lymph node biopsy indicated at completion mastectomy for ductal carcinoma in situ? Ann Surg Oncol 2016;23(7):2229–34.
11. Correa C, McGale P, Taylor C, et al. Overview of the randomized trials of radio-therapy in ductal carcinoma in situ of the breast. J Natl Cancer Inst Monogr 2010;2010(41):162–77.
12. Wapnir IL, Dignam JJ, Fisher B, et al. Long-term outcomes of invasive ipsilateral breast tumor recurrences after lumpectomy in NSABP B-17 and B-24 randomized clinical trials for DCIS. J Natl Cancer Inst 2011;103(6):478–88.
13. Cuzick J, Sestak I, Pinder SE, et al. Effect of tamoxifen and radiotherapy in women with locally excised ductal carcinoma in situ: long-term results from the UK/ANZ DCIS trial. Lancet Oncol 2011;12(1):21–9.
14. Romestaing P, Lehingue Y, Carrie C, et al. Role of a 10-Gy boost in the conserva-tive treatment of early breast cancer: results of a randomized clinical trial in Lyon, France. J Clin Oncol 1997;15(3):963–8.
15. Kunkler IH, Williams LJ, Jack WJ, et al. Breast-conserving surgery with or without irradiation in women aged 65 years or older with early breast cancer (PRIME II): a randomised controlled trial. Lancet Oncol 2015;16(3):266–73.
16. Hughes KS, Schnaper LA, Bellon JR, et al. Lumpectomy plus tamoxifen with or without irradiation in women age 70 years or older with early breast cancer: long-term follow-up of CALGB 9343. J Clin Oncol 2013;31(19):2382–7.
17. Solin LJ, Gray R, Baehner FL, et al. A multigene expression assay to predict local recurrence risk for ductal carcinoma in situ of the breast. J Natl Cancer Inst 2013;105(10):701–10.
18. Rakovitch E, Nofech-Mozes S, Hanna W, et al. A population-based validation study of the DCIS Score predicting recurrence risk in individuals treated by breast-conserving surgery alone. Breast Cancer Res Treat 2015;152(2):389–98.
19. Fisher B, Land S, Mamounas E, et al. Prevention of invasive breast cancer in women with ductal carcinoma in situ: an update of the National Surgical Adjuvant Breast and Bowel Project experience. Semin Oncol 2001;28(4):400–18.
20. Margolese RG, Cecchini RS, Julian TB, et al. Anastrozole versus tamoxifen in postmenopausal women with ductal carcinoma in situ undergoing lumpectomy

plus radiotherapy (NSABP B-35): a randomised, double-blind, phase 3 clinical trial. Lancet 2016;387(10021):849–56.

21. Cuzick J, Sestak I, Forbes JF, et al. Anastrozole for prevention of breast cancer in high-risk postmenopausal women (IBIS-II): an international, double-blind, randomised placebo-controlled trial. Lancet 2014;383(9922):1041–8.

22. Neoadjuvant Herceptin for ductal carcinoma in situ of the breast. ClinicalTrials.gov. Identifier:NCT00496808.

23. Neoadjuvant trial of lapatinib for the treatment of women with DCIS breast cancer. ClinicalTrials.gov. Identifier:NCT00555152.

24. Narod SA, Iqbal J, Giannakeas V, et al. Breast cancer mortality after a diagnosis of ductal carcinoma in situ. JAMA Oncol 2015;1(7):888–96.

25. Bruce J, Thornton AJ, Scott NW, et al. Chronic preoperative pain and psychological robustness predict acute postoperative pain outcomes after surgery for breast cancer. Br J Cancer 2012;107(6):937–46.

26. COMET. Available at: http://www.pcori.org/research-results/2016/comparison-operative-versus-medical-endocrine-therapy-low-risk-dcis-comet. Accessed February 24, 2017.

27. LORIS. A phase III trial of surgery versus active monitoring for low risk ductal carcinoma in situ (DCIS). Available at: http://www.birmingham.ac.uk/research/activity/mds/trials/crctu/trials/loris/index.aspx. Accessed February 26, 2017.

28. EORTC LORD. Available at: http://www.eortc.org/research-groups/breast-cancer-group/ongoing-and-future-projects/. Accessed February 24, 2017.

29. Brennan ME, Turner RM, Ciatto S, et al. Ductal carcinoma in situ at core-needle biopsy: meta-analysis of underestimation and predictors of invasive breast cancer. Radiology 2011;260(1):119–28.

30. Nicholson S, Hanby A, Clements K, et al. Variations in the management of the axilla in screen-detected ductal carcinoma in situ: evidence from the UK NHS breast screening programme audit of screen detected DCIS. Eur J Surg Oncol 2015;41(1):86–93.

31. Doebar SC, de Monye C, Stoop H, et al. Ductal carcinoma in situ diagnosed by breast needle biopsy: predictors of invasion in the excision specimen. Breast 2016;27:15–21.

32. Park HS, Kim HY, Park S, et al. A nomogram for predicting underestimation of invasiveness in ductal carcinoma in situ diagnosed by preoperative needle biopsy. Breast 2013;22(5):869–73.

33. Lee SK, Yang JH, Woo SY, et al. Nomogram for predicting invasion in patients with a preoperative diagnosis of ductal carcinoma in situ of the breast. Br J Surg 2013;100(13):1756–63.

34. Pilewskie M, Stempel M, Rosenfeld H, et al. Do LORIS trial eligibility criteria identify a ductal carcinoma in situ patient population at low risk of upgrade to invasive carcinoma? Ann Surg Oncol 2016;23(11):3487–93.

35. Grimm LJ, Ryser MD, Partridge AH, et al. Surgical upstaging rates for vacuum assisted biopsy proven DCIS: implications for active surveillance trials. Ann Surg Oncol 2017. [Epub ahead of print].

36. Bower JE, Ganz PA, Desmond KA, et al. Fatigue in breast cancer survivors: occurrence, correlates, and impact on quality of life. J Clin Oncol 2000;18(4):743–53.

37. Hawley ST, Janz NK, Griffith KA, et al. Recurrence risk perception and quality of life following treatment of breast cancer. Breast Cancer Res Treat 2017;161(3):557–65.

38. Montazeri A. Health-related quality of life in breast cancer patients: a bibliographic review of the literature from 1974 to 2007. J Exp Clin Cancer Res 2008;27:32.
39. King MT, Winters ZE, Olivotto IA, et al. Patient-reported outcomes in ductal carcinoma in situ: a systematic review. Eur J Cancer 2017;71:95–108.
40. Bruce J, Thornton AJ, Powell R, et al. Psychological, surgical, and sociodemographic predictors of pain outcomes after breast cancer surgery: a population-based cohort study. Pain 2014;155(2):232–43.
41. Esserman LJ, Thompson IM Jr, Reid B. Overdiagnosis and overtreatment in cancer: an opportunity for improvement. JAMA 2013;310(8):797–8.
42. Partridge AH, Elmore JG, Saslow D, et al. Challenges in ductal carcinoma in situ risk communication and decision-making: report from an American Cancer Society and National Cancer Institute workshop. CA Cancer J Clin 2012;62(3):203–10.
43. Partridge A, Adloff K, Blood E, et al. Risk perceptions and psychosocial outcomes of women with ductal carcinoma in situ: longitudinal results from a cohort study. J Natl Cancer Inst 2008;100(4):243–51.
44. A HER-2/neu pulsed DC1 vaccine for patients with DCIS. ClinicalTrials.gov. Identifier:NCT00107211.
45. A randomized trial of HER-2/neu pulsed DC1 vaccine for patients with DCIS. ClinicalTrials.gov. Identifier:NCT02061332.

Lobular Breast Cancer
Different Disease, Different Algorithms?

Anita Mamtani, MD[a], Tari A. King, MD[b,c],*

KEYWORDS

- Invasive lobular carcinoma • E-cadherin • The Cancer Genome Analysis
- Breast conservation • Mastectomy • Chemotherapy • Aromatase inhibitors

KEY POINTS

- Invasive lobular breast cancer is a biologically unique entity, distinct from invasive ductal cancer.
- The characteristic molecular features of invasive lobular carcinoma (ILC) include its largely ER-positive and low-grade nature, and loss of E-cadherin protein expression.
- Tumor biology is of key importance in designing treatment approaches.
- Harnessing the growing knowledge of the molecular features inherent to lobular cancer holds promise for the next generation of tailored therapies.

INTRODUCTION

Invasive lobular carcinoma (ILC) is the second most common histologic form of breast cancer, comprising 10% to 15% of invasive tumors.[1] ILC is now recognized as a biologically distinct disease from the more common invasive ductal carcinoma (IDC), with a unique molecular pathogenesis and consequential implications on diagnosis and treatment. An understanding of these differences is of utmost importance to tailor management strategies. Ongoing investigations of the genomic basis of breast cancer are paving the road for novel approaches to treatment of ILC.

EPIDEMIOLOGY

The mean age of diagnosis of ILC is 57 years.[2] Risk factors include age at menarche, age at first birth, and use of hormone therapy, emphasizing the role of estrogen

The authors have nothing to disclose.
[a] Department of Surgery, Beth Israel Deaconess Medical Center, Harvard Medical School, Boston, MA, USA; [b] Department of Surgery, Brigham and Women's Hospital, 75 Francis Street, Boston MA 02215, USA; [c] Breast Oncology Program, Dana-Farber/Brigham and Women's Cancer Center, 450 Brookline Avenue, Boston, MA 02215, USA
* Corresponding author.
E-mail address: tking7@bwh.harvard.edu

Surg Oncol Clin N Am 27 (2018) 81–94
http://dx.doi.org/10.1016/j.soc.2017.07.005
1055-3207/18/© 2017 Elsevier Inc. All rights reserved.

exposure in pathogenesis. This relationship is also observed for most IDCs, but is more pronounced for ILC.[3] The incidence of ILC in the Western world has generally mirrored trends in use of hormone replacement therapy, with a steep increase between 1975 and 2000 and a decline between 2000 and 2004, but now increasing since 2005 with an unclear cause.[4]

Hereditary ILC is uncommon, but may be seen as a secondary tumor in families with hereditary diffuse gastric cancer syndrome, caused by a germline mutation in the tumor suppressor gene, CDH1. ILC otherwise accounts for a minority of cancers associated with known susceptibility genes, comprising less than 10% of cancers in patients with BRCA2 mutations, and less than 5% of cancers in patients with BRCA1 or TP53 mutations.[5]

HISTOLOGY

Classic ILC is histologically characterized by discohesive cells infiltrating the breast stroma in a single-file pattern[2] with a limited host inflammatory response (**Fig. 1**A).[6] Observed loss of membranous E-cadherin staining by immunohistochemistry may be a useful adjunct to confirm the diagnosis (see **Fig. 1**B). Several nonclassic forms of ILC have also been described, distinguished by morphology (alveolar, solid, dispersed, trabecular, and mixed) and cytology (apocrine, pleomorphic, signet ring, histiocytoid, and tubulolobular).[5] These variant forms show the typical cytologic

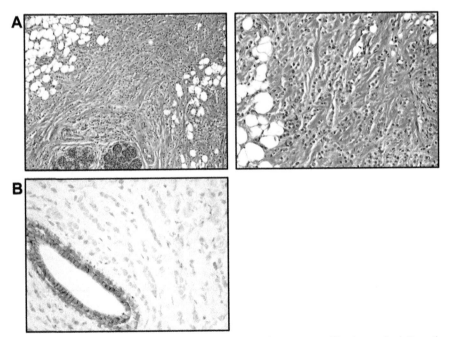

Fig. 1. (*A*) Hematoxylin and eosin staining, 10× and 20× magnifications, depicting the classic "single-file" morphology of ILC. (*B*) Immunohistochemistry of paraffin-embedded breast cancer tissue showing characteristic loss of membranous E-cadherin in lobular carcinoma. (*Courtesy of* Dr Stuart J. Schnitt, MD, Chief of Breast Oncologic Pathology, Dana-Farber/Brigham and Women's Cancer Center; Associate Director, Dana-Farber Cancer Institute/Brigham and Women's Hospital Breast Oncology Program; Professor of Pathology, Harvard Medical School.)

features of classic ILC, but display differing growth patterns. In the alveolar variant, cells are organized in globular arrangements, whereas the solid variant displays sheets of uniform cells with high frequency of mitoses. Conversely, the low-grade tubulolobular variant displays linear cells with tubular glands. The most aggressive pleomorphic variant of ILC exhibits greater atypia, nuclear pleomorphism, and frequent mitoses, with variable degrees of apocrine differentiation.[2]

Associated lobular neoplasia (LN), which refers to the noninvasive proliferative lobular lesions inclusive of atypical lobular hyperplasia and lobular carcinoma in situ (LCIS), is observed in more than 50% of classic ILCs.[2] The reported incidence of pure LN ranges from 0.5% to 4%,[2] and typically presents in younger women than does ILC. Histologically, LN displays pagetoid terminal duct involvement in more than 70% of cases. There exist 2 types of LN, type A (classic cellular features) and type B (larger, atypical cells with prominent nucleoli), with a small subgroup displaying pleomorphic cells with apocrine features and more aggressive biology, termed pleomorphic LCIS.[2]

LN is considered a risk factor for the subsequent development of invasive cancer of either the ductal or the lobular phenotype. The increased risk ranges from 1% to 2% per year and is conferred equally to both breasts.[7] Recent work demonstrating shared molecular alterations between LCIS and synchronous ILCs in a significant proportion of cases has also reopened the notion that some LCIS lesions may behave as nonobligate precursors of ILC.[2]

MOLECULAR BIOLOGY

More than 90% of ILCs are estrogen receptor (ER) positive and they are largely classified as luminal A at the level of the transcriptome, although this proportion is lower in more aggressive variants,[5] with highest rates of ER positivity observed in the classic form and alveolar variants, and lowest rates of ER positivity observed in pleomorphic ILCs (10%).[2] HER2 overexpression is rare, seen in only 3% to 5% of classic ILCs, but present in up to 80% of the more aggressive pleomorphic subgroup.[2,4]

Loss of E-cadherin expression is the most consistently reported hallmark feature of ILC (see **Fig. 1**B), demonstrated in up to 90% of cases, and thought to play a crucial role in pathogenesis.[2] E-cadherin is a calcium-dependent transmembrane protein involved in adherens-type junctions between epithelial cells, the loss of which predisposes to neoplastic proliferation. E-cadherin dysregulation results from somatic mutations in the CDH1 gene on chromosome 16q22.1, reported in 30% to 80% of ILCs, as well as by loss of heterozygosity at the CDH1 locus.[2,8] However, E-cadherin positivity does not, by itself, exclude a lobular neoplasm, and not all ILCs harbor CDH1 mutations. Other markers frequently expressed in ILC include GCDFP-15, seen in up to 90% of pleomorphic and signet ring subtypes,[2] cyclin D1 (80%), cathepsin D (86%), Bcl-2 (89%), and Ck 34BetaE12.[2]

In the Cancer Genome Analysis study, mutations in several key genes were found more frequently in ILC as compared with IDC, including CDH1 (63% in ILC vs 2% in IDC), P1K3CA (48% vs 33%), FOXA1 (7% vs 2%), RUNX1 (10% vs 3%), and TBX3 (9% vs 2%), respectively.[4] Conversely, GATA3 mutations were enriched in IDC (5% in ILC vs 13% in IDC). Importantly, when the analysis was limited to luminal A cancers, several alterations remained significantly more common among ILCs versus IDCs, as summarized in **Table 1**.[4] A later analysis of 417 ILCs by Desmedt and colleagues[9] reported that more than half of the cases contained a mutation in PIK3CA, PTEN, or AKT1, and there was also an increased frequency of HER2, HER3, FOXA1, and ESR1 alterations.

Table 1
Genomic alterations seen with increased frequency in luminal A lobular cancers (n = 106) versus luminal A ductal cancers (n = 201) in The Cancer Genome Analysis study

Gene	Q Value[a]
CDH1	1.4E−30
FOX1A	0.065
PIK3CA	Not stated
PTEN	0.035
RUNX1	Not stated
TBX3	0.05

[a] Depicted "q value" represents a P value that is adjusted for the proportion of expected false positives.

Data from Ciriello G, Gatza ML, Beck AH, et al. Comprehensive molecular portraits of invasive lobular breast cancer. Cell 2015;163:506–19.

CLINICAL PRESENTATION AND DIAGNOSIS

ILC may pose a diagnostic challenge because of its inherently insidious and infiltrative growth pattern. Although some patients present with an ill-defined palpable mass, others may display only vague skin thickening or diffuse nodularity, or disease may be clinically occult.[2] In keeping with their indolent phenotype, ILCs are not frequently associated with calcifications and have an innately discohesive growth pattern. As such, ILCs frequently display a scattered radiological appearance. Compared with IDCs, ILCs are more often mammographically occult, with sensitivity as low as 57% to 76%[2] and false negative rates as high as 25%.[10] These tumors also tend to be poorly circumscribed, which may limit the accuracy of both breast and axillary ultrasound. The sensitivity of ultrasound-guided fine-needle aspiration of lymph nodes in ILC is low, reported to be less than 40% in cases of pure ILC.[11,12] **Table 2** summarizes reported correlations between pathologic and radiologic tumor size as visualized by mammogram, ultrasound, and MRI.[13–17]

The utility of preoperative MRI in the workup and staging of lobular cancers remains controversial, with mixed data on resultant rates of mastectomy or reexcision after breast conservation. A recent large meta-analysis found that preoperative MRI increases rates of mastectomy for all cancer histologies, suggesting an unfavorable overestimation of the extent of disease.[18] On subset analysis of 766 ILC patients, although there was some reduction in the rate of reexcision after breast-conserving

Table 2
Correlation of pathologic and radiologic tumor size of lobular carcinomas

Study	Mammogram	Ultrasound	MRI
Boetes et al,[16] 2004 (n = 34)	0.34	0.24	0.81
Francis et al,[13] 2001 (n = 22)	0.79	0.56	0.87
Kepple et al,[17] 2005 (n = 29)	—	0.71	0.88
Kneeshaw et al,[15] 2003 (n = 21)	—	—	0.86
Munot et al,[14] 2002 (n = 20)	0.66	0.67	0.97

All values are reported as correlation coefficient.

Data from Mamtani A, King TA. Lobular breast cancer. Complex General Surgical Oncology, in press.

surgery (BCS) (odds ratio [OR] 0.56, P = .031), this observation was likely attributable to an increased likelihood of upfront mastectomy (adjusted OR 1.64, P = .034).[18]

American Joint Committee on Cancer TNM guidelines are used to stage all breast cancers, regardless of histology. The assessment of tumor size (T) category may be more complicated in ILCs, which often present in a multifocal or multicentric fashion.[2] In such cases, the T category is based on the size of the single largest mass, not an additive sum of multiple tumors. Many studies, including a large Surveillance, Epidemiology, and End Results (SEER) registry analysis of 263,408 patients with IDC or ILC, report that patients with ILC are more likely to present with tumors measuring greater than 2 cm at the time of diagnosis, as compared with IDC.[19] It is also well documented that the invasive lobular histology is an independent predictor for the likelihood of nodal micrometastases,[20–22] thought to be another demonstration of the underlying discohesive biology. Finally, although metastatic disease most commonly presents in the bones, lungs, and the central nervous system, ILCs display a fascinating predilection for gastrointestinal, peritoneal, and ovarian metastases.[2] The overwhelmingly ER-positive nature of ILCs also results in more frequent development of late metastases.

MANAGEMENT

The contemporary, multidisciplinary approach to the treatment of breast cancer includes individually tailored surgery, radiotherapy (RT), and systemic therapy. Although the overarching concepts of treatment are common among all breast cancer types, the largely ER-positive phenotype of ILC is central to the principles of management and the observed responses.

Surgery and RT provide locoregional control. The course of surgery, regardless of histology, is determined by the TNM stage at presentation. An operable cancer may be approached with upfront surgery if amenable, or undergo surgery after preoperative neoadjuvant therapy, if appropriate.

UPFRONT SURGERY

Patients with early-stage breast cancer are generally candidates for upfront surgery, either with BCT or mastectomy. BCT involves lumpectomy with negative margins followed by RT.

Factors that determine eligibility for BCT are shared between ILC and IDC. To be a candidate for BCT, patients must have tumors that can be removed with negative margins and acceptable cosmesis and must be able to receive RT thereafter. Accordingly, contraindications to BCT include cancers that are too large or diffuse for an acceptable oncologic and cosmetic result. In addition, any current or prior circumstances that preclude irradiation, such as a history of prior chest wall radiation, significant connective tissue or collagen vascular disease, and first trimester of pregnancy, are also contraindications. Determination of BCT candidacy can generally be made with greater than 95% accuracy by clinical examination and mammography alone.[23] Mastectomy is indicated for patients with contraindications to BCT, and those who prefer mastectomy.

Several randomized trials with long-term follow-up have demonstrated similar rates of locoregional recurrence (LRR) and survival with BCT and mastectomy for early-stage cancers.[24,25] Long-term survival is also shown to be equivalent with the use of BCT or mastectomy among a population of ILCs alone, but is dependent upon obtaining negative margins.[26] This is particularly true in the contemporary era of systemic therapies increasingly tailored to tumor biology, known to further reduce rates of LRR.[25,27,28]

The innately infiltrative growth pattern of ILC and difficult preoperative assessment of extent of disease have historically led surgeons to question the feasibility of BCT in ILC.[29] Mixed results have been reported; some studies demonstrate no significant increase in reexcisions to achieve negative margins,[30] whereas others have found an association with positive lumpectomy margins[29,31] and a higher likelihood of reoperation to obtain negative margins in ILC.[31,32] Despite these varying findings, when negative margins are obtained, patients with ILC are no more likely to experience LRR after BCT (**Table 3**), with contemporary rates ranging from 3.1% to 5.7%.[10,33–35] As defined by the recent consensus guidelines, "negative" margins are defined as no ink on tumor and include a subset analysis showing no benefit to a wider margin for ILC.[36] Based on these findings, the consensus panel concluded that these general recommendations should not be altered for lobular histology.[36]

The surgical approach to the axilla is similarly shared between ILC and IDC, although data on the patterns of nodal involvement in ILC vary, with some studies reporting no difference in the likelihood of axillary involvement when compared with IDC and others reporting an increased likelihood of nodal involvement.[19,37] Lobular histology has however been shown to independently predict for micrometastatic disease,[20–22] consistent with a discohesive biology.

Sentinel node biopsy (SLNB) is the standard method of axillary assessment for clinically node-negative patients and is equally feasible in both ILC and IDC.[38] Indications for axillary dissection (ALND) in clinically node-negative patients have been in evolution over the past decade, a decision related both to the nodal burden and to the breast surgery being performed.

Clinically node-negative (cN0) patients with a negative SLNB do not require ALND. Among women undergoing BCT, the ACOSOG Z0011 trial demonstrated low LRR rates and similar survival with SLNB alone as compared with ALND among early-stage, cN0 patients found to have 1 to 2 positive sentinel lymph nodes (SLNs).[39] The IBCSG 23-01 trial reported similar results for patients with micrometastatic disease in 1 to 2 SLNs, yet also included patients having mastectomy.[40] The AMAROS trial similarly showed noninferiority of SLNB and axillary irradiation compared with ALND in patients with 1 to 2 positive SLNs undergoing BCT or mastectomy.[41] These contemporary trials have allowed safe omission of ALND in select patients without a compromise in long-term outcomes.

Table 3
Local recurrence of lobular cancers after breast conservation therapy

Study	Stage	Received Adjuvant Therapy (%)	Follow-up (y)	Local Recurrence (%)
Braunstein et al,[33] 2015 (n = 79)	1–2	90	9.9	4.4
Galimberti et al,[35] 2011 (n = 382)	1–3	95	8.4	5.7
Molland et al,[10] 2004 (n = 76)	1–3	69	3.6	3.9
Sagara et al,[34] 2014 (n = 384)	1–3	96	6	3.1

Data from Mamtani A, King TA. Lobular breast cancer. Complex General Surgical Oncology, in press.

Patients who are clinically node positive should have the presence of axillary disease confirmed by fine-needle aspiration or core biopsy. In this setting, those having upfront surgery will require ALND. The management of the axilla in patients with nodal metastases who receive preoperative neoadjuvant therapy is discussed in the following section.

SURGERY FOLLOWING NEOADJUVANT THERAPY

Patients with locally advanced cancers should generally receive neoadjuvant therapy before proceeding to surgery. This approach affords an opportunity for downstaging of locally advanced disease without compromising survival and allows BCS in more patients who would otherwise need mastectomy. Neoadjuvant therapy also decreases the need for ALND[42] and provides insight into in vivo tumor chemosensitivity.

Patients with ILC are significantly less likely than those with IDC to experience a pathologic complete response (pCR) to neoadjuvant chemotherapy (NAC), ranging from 0% to 11% (Table 4).[43–51] In a meta-analysis including 1764 ILCs and 12,645 IDCs, IDCs had a significantly higher pCR rate (OR 3.1) and ability to undergo BCS (OR 2.1).[52] This is consistent with growing evidence that tumor biology is the principal determinant of response to NAC. The high ER-positivity and low proliferative rates in ILC predispose to a lesser response, a trend seen in most ER-positive breast cancers regardless of histology.[46,51] Expectedly, studies also show limited success in tumor downstaging to BCT in ILC.[48,53] Notably, despite having a reduced response to NAC, ILCs treated in this manner have very low LRR rates and no survival disadvantage when compared with all-comers undergoing BCT after NAC.[51,53] BCT rates in ILC after NAC are still increased from the otherwise anticipated baseline, supporting consideration of this approach for locally advanced ILCs.[48,54] Recent data suggest that although overall rates of pCR are low in ILC after NAC, lack of progesterone receptor expression and poor differentiation may identify those with the highest likelihood of benefit.[55]

An area of growing interest is the management of the axilla after NAC, with a recent prospective study demonstrating avoidance of ALND in 48% of biopsy-proven node-positive patients who downstaged to cN0 after NAC and had at least 3 negative SLNs

Table 4
Pathologic complete response to neoadjuvant chemotherapy among lobular versus other breast cancers

Study	N		pCR (%)		P
	ILC	Non-ILC	ILC	Non-ILC	
Cocquyt et al,[43] 2003	26	101	0	15	.007
Cristofanilli et al,[50] 2005	122	912	3	15	<.001
Delpech et al,[49] 2013	177	1718	3	14	<.001
Lips et al,[46] 2012	75	601	11	25	.01
Loibl et al,[47] 2014	1051	7969	6	17	<.001
Mathieu et al,[51] 2004	38	419	0	11	.04
Truin et al,[48] 2016	466	3622	5	20	<.0001
Tubiana-Hulin et al,[44] 2006	118	742	1	9	.002
Wenzel et al,[45] 2007	37	124	3	20	.009

Data from Mamtani A, King TA. Lobular breast cancer. Complex General Surgical Oncology, in press.

resected.[42] Several trials are underway to further investigate these approaches and to document long-term local-regional control. As ILCs will constitute small subsets of these studies, it is unlikely that recommendations for management of the axilla will differ between IDC and ILC.

Given the known ER-rich nature of most ILCs and favorable results in small retrospective studies, there is growing interest in neoadjuvant endocrine therapy (NET) for ILC. In one study, neoadjuvant letrozole was used for 3 or more months in 61 postmenopausal women with locally advanced cancers, after which they proceeded to surgery or continued on letrozole if tumors remained too large for BCS. At the time of publication, although there were no pCRs observed, the mean reduction in tumor volume was 66%, and the rate of successful BCS was 81% among 31 patients who had undergone surgery.[56] The PROACT trial demonstrated aromatase inhibitors to be as effective as tamoxifen for tumor downstaging in postmenopausal women with ER-positive disease.[57] The IMPACT trial showed similar results, randomizing patients to neoadjuvant tamoxifen, anastrozole, or both, showing equivalent tolerance and efficacy, but was unable to predict for outcome.[58] More recently, the ACOSOG Z1031 trial randomized stage II–III patients with ER-positive disease to 1 of 3 NET regimens and found marked improvements in surgical outcomes after NET, with the most favorable results in luminal A tumors.[59] Ongoing trials of relevance include the ALTERNATE trial, which randomizes women with ER-positive cancer to anastrozole or fulvestrant or a combination, and the PELOPS trial, which will assess response to preoperative endocrine therapy with or without the addition of palbociclib among patients with ILC.

RADIOTHERAPY

BCT by definition includes margin negative lumpectomy followed by adjuvant RT. Adjuvant whole-breast RT reduces the risk of both LRR and death from breast cancer after BCS.[24] Additional regional nodal irradiation may be indicated for those with involved lymph nodes or high-risk features. It is noteworthy that omission of RT may be considered in elderly women with early-stage ER-positive tumors, with small increases in absolute risk of LRR but no difference in mastectomy-free survival, disease-specific survival, or overall survival (OS).[60] Accelerated partial breast irradiation (APBI) is a newer technique involving more focused RT delivered in higher doses over a shorter time span. Notably, the recent American Society for Radiation Oncology guideline update categorizes lobular histology for "cautionary" use of APBI outside of a clinical trial.[61]

Selected patients may benefit from the use of RT after upfront mastectomy, determined by consideration of macrometastatic nodal deposits, large tumor size, and high-risk disease features. Similar to surgical trials, ILC patients comprise a minority in RT trials. A SEER study including 12,703 ILC patients treated from 2004 to 2009, of which 26% had a definite indication for post-mastectomy RT, found an improved 5-year breast cancer–specific survival from 80.9% to 84.7% (P = .0003) among ILC patients, a benefit to the same degree as IDC.[62] These data support continued consideration of RT using existing criteria, regardless of histology. The implications of margins at mastectomy remain controversial among radiation oncologists, with no data to support a definite benefit of RT after upfront mastectomy with close margins.

Considerations for RT in patients who undergo preoperative neoadjuvant therapy followed by surgery are similarly related to nodal burden, tumor size, and high-risk features, in addition to the response of disease to neoadjuvant therapy. Awaited data from ongoing trials including the NSABP B-51 trial will provide further insight.

ADJUVANT SYSTEMIC TREATMENT

Systemic adjuvant therapy is driven largely by tumor biology, rather than histology. Generally, patients with hormone receptor–positive cancers receive endocrine therapy, applicable to the vast majority of ILCs. Chemotherapy is offered for locally advanced cancers and considered for early-stage cancers with high-risk features such as large size, nodal involvement, high grade, high 21-gene recurrence scores, and more aggressive tumor biology, including triple-negative and HER2-positive receptor status. Although HER2 positivity is rare in most ILCs, this is overexpressed in up to 80% of pleomorphic ILCs, comprising a subset of patients who are more likely to benefit from targeted anti-HER2 therapy.[2]

Contemporary systemic therapies have a major impact on both locoregional and distant disease control,[25] and disease biology determines the efficacy of various therapies. Low rates of local recurrence (approximating 3%) are reported with 12-year follow-up among ER-positive patients who receive endocrine therapy, most relevant to ER-positive ILCs.[25] Randomized trials have demonstrated a measurable response in ILC to systemic hormonal and chemotherapy.[28,63,64] These studies include patients with ER-positive and ER-negative tumors, and hormone receptor status is evidently the chief determinant of response. Interestingly, studies of the utility of Oncotype Dx in ILC have shown that ILCs rarely (less than 2%) have a high recurrence score, as compared with rates approximating 20% in IDCs.[65]

Support for adjuvant endocrine therapy comes from trials demonstrating significant reduction in risk of recurrence at 15 years, summarized in a large Early Breast Cancer Trialists Collaborative Group meta-analysis.[27] Although studies specific to ILC remain limited, some data suggest a greater benefit with aromatase inhibitors compared with tamoxifen. In a retrospective analysis of the prospective BIG 1-98 trial, a greater benefit was observed with letrozole than tamoxifen among ILCs, with disease-free survival of 82% with letrozole versus 66% with tamoxifen at 8-year follow-up, and OS of 89% with letrozole versus 74% with tamoxifen.[63] One possible explanation for this differential response includes a paradoxic de novo resistance to tamoxifen and resultant proliferative response, which was observed in an in vitro study of ILC cell lines.[66] Conversely, the Tamoxifen and Exemestane Adjuvant Multinational trial, which randomized patients to exemestane alone, or an "early-switch" from tamoxifen for a total of 5 years, showed similar efficacy of both regimens for IDC and ILC. There was evidence of an effect of ER content, with benefit from monotherapy for ER-rich patients, as compared with a benefit from sequential treatment of ER-poor patients, regardless of histology.[64]

There are no randomized trials examining adjuvant chemotherapy regimens specifically in ILC. Although retrospective analyses do not show any definite reasons to deny adjuvant chemotherapy to ILC patients who otherwise meet indications for treatment, the limited response of classic ILCs to chemotherapy in the neoadjuvant setting suggests low chemosensitivity. In a retrospective study of 3685 postmenopausal patients with ILC and 19,609 postmenopausal patients with IDCs, treated either with adjuvant hormonal treatment alone or with hormonal treatment and chemotherapy, 10-year survival among ILC patients was 68% with hormonal treatment alone and 66% with combination therapy ($P = .45$), suggesting a limited benefit of chemotherapy in patients with ILC already receiving hormonal therapy.[67] However, chemotherapy may be more valuable for the minority of ILCs with ER-negative or HER2-positive subtype. In a retrospective subset analysis of the prospective phase III Herceptin Adjuvant trial of patients with HER2-positive tumors, there was a similar benefit after 1 year of adjuvant trastuzumab among ILCs and IDCs (disease-free survival hazard ratio [HR] 0.63

vs 0.77, $P = .49$) at 4 years of follow-up.[28] Presently, standard treatment with adjuvant trastuzumab is recommended for HER2-positive ILCs.

OUTCOMES

In keeping with the luminal A phenotype, outcomes and prognosis in ILC are generally favorable. In a large SEER study of 263,408 women (27,639 with ILC and 235,769 with IDC) treated between 1993 and 2003, a stage-matched analysis showed that the 5-year disease-free survival was significantly better for ILC than IDC, with an overall 14% survival benefit (HR 0.86) on multivariate analysis.[19] Although overall stage-corrected prognosis is favorable, some think that this may be offset by a higher stage at presentation,[68] and higher rates of late metastases in atypical locations. Pleomorphic ILCs are also a known exception, shown in retrospective series to present with larger tumor size, more nodal positivity, and frequently require mastectomy.[69]

SUMMARY AND FUTURE DIRECTIONS

Lobular breast cancer is increasingly recognized as a distinct disease from ductal cancer, with a unique molecular pathogenesis and differing genomic profile. Presently, locoregional and systemic treatment approaches remain shared among all breast cancer types. Continual discoveries of the molecular basis of this disease hold potential for advances in therapy and will pave the way for development of treatment algorithms tailored specifically to lobular disease.

ACKNOWLEDGMENTS

The authors thank Dr Stuart J. Schnitt for providing the histologic images for **Fig. 1**.

REFERENCES

1. Sledge GW, Chagpar A, Perou C. Collective wisdom: lobular carcinoma of the breast. Am Soc Clin Oncol Educ Book 2016;35:18–21.
2. Rakha EA, Ellis IO. Lobular breast carcinoma and its variants. Semin Diagn Pathol 2010;27:49–61.
3. Kotsopoulos J, Chen WY, Gates MA, et al. Risk factors for ductal and lobular breast cancer: results from the Nurses' Health Study. Breast Cancer Res 2010; 12:R106.
4. Ciriello G, Gatza ML, Beck AH, et al. Comprehensive molecular portraits of invasive lobular breast cancer. Cell 2015;163:506–19.
5. Christgen M, Steinemann D, Kuhnle E, et al. Lobular breast cancer: clinical, molecular and morphological characteristics. Pathol Res Pract 2016;212:583–97.
6. Mamtani A, King TA. Lobular breast cancer. Complex General Surgical Oncology, in press.
7. King TA, Reis-Filho JS. Lobular neoplasia. Surg Oncol Clin N Am 2014;23: 487–503.
8. Phipps AI, Li CI, Kerlikowske K, et al. Risk factors for ductal, lobular, and mixed ductal-lobular breast cancer in a screening population. Cancer Epidemiol Biomarkers Prev 2010;19:1643–54.
9. Desmedt C, Zoppoli G, Gundem G, et al. Genomic characterization of primary invasive lobular breast cancer. J Clin Oncol 2016;34:1872–81.
10. Molland JG, Donnellan M, Janu NC, et al. Infiltrating lobular carcinoma–a comparison of diagnosis, management and outcome with infiltrating duct carcinoma. Breast 2004;13:389–96.

11. Topps A, Clay V, Absar M, et al. The sensitivity of pre-operative axillary staging in breast cancer: comparison of invasive lobular and ductal carcinoma. Eur J Surg Oncol 2014;40:813–7.
12. Boughey JC, Middleton LP, Harker L, et al. Utility of ultrasound and fine-needle aspiration biopsy of the axilla in the assessment of invasive lobular carcinoma of the breast. Am J Surg 2007;194:450–5.
13. Francis A, England DW, Rowlands DC, et al. The diagnosis of invasive lobular breast carcinoma. Does MRI have a role? Breast 2001;10:38–40.
14. Munot K, Dall B, Achuthan R, et al. Role of magnetic resonance imaging in the diagnosis and single-stage surgical resection of invasive lobular carcinoma of the breast. Br J Surg 2002;89:1296–301.
15. Kneeshaw PJ, Turnbull LW, Smith A, et al. Dynamic contrast enhanced magnetic resonance imaging aids the surgical management of invasive lobular breast cancer. Eur J Surg Oncol 2003;29:32–7.
16. Boetes C, Veltman J, van Die L, et al. The role of MRI in invasive lobular carcinoma. Breast Cancer Res Treat 2004;86:31–7.
17. Kepple J, Layeeque R, Klimberg VS, et al. Correlation of magnetic resonance imaging and pathologic size of infiltrating lobular carcinoma of the breast. Am J Surg 2005;190:623–7.
18. Houssami N, Turner R, Morrow M. Preoperative magnetic resonance imaging in breast cancer: meta-analysis of surgical outcomes. Ann Surg 2013;257:249–55.
19. Wasif N, Maggard MA, Ko CY, et al. Invasive lobular vs. ductal breast cancer: a stage-matched comparison of outcomes. Ann Surg Oncol 2010;17:1862–9.
20. Gainer SM, Lodhi AK, Bhattacharyya A, et al. Invasive lobular carcinoma predicts micrometastasis in breast cancer. J Surg Res 2012;177:93–6.
21. Mittendorf EA, Sahin AA, Tucker SL, et al. Lymphovascular invasion and lobular histology are associated with increased incidence of isolated tumor cells in sentinel lymph nodes from early-stage breast cancer patients. Ann Surg Oncol 2008;15:3369–77.
22. Truin W, Roumen RM, Siesling S, et al. Sentinel lymph node biopsy and isolated tumor cells in invasive lobular versus ductal breast cancer. Clin Breast Cancer 2016;16:e75–82.
23. Morrow M, Schmidt R, Hassett C. Patient selection for breast conservation therapy with magnification mammography. Surgery 1995;118:621–6.
24. Darby S, McGale P, Correa C, et al. Effect of radiotherapy after breast-conserving surgery on 10-year recurrence and 15-year breast cancer death: meta-analysis of individual patient data for 10,801 women in 17 randomised trials. Lancet 2011;378:1707–16.
25. Anderson SJ, Wapnir I, Dignam JJ, et al. Prognosis after ipsilateral breast tumor recurrence and locoregional recurrences in patients treated by breast-conserving therapy in five National Surgical Adjuvant Breast and Bowel Project protocols of node-negative breast cancer. J Clin Oncol 2009;27:2466–73.
26. Fodor J, Major T, Tóth J, et al. Comparison of mastectomy with breast-conserving surgery in invasive lobular carcinoma: 15-year results. Rep Pract Oncol Radiother 2011;16:227–31.
27. Davies C, Godwin J, Gray R, et al. Relevance of breast cancer hormone receptors and other factors to the efficacy of adjuvant tamoxifen: patient-level meta-analysis of randomised trials. Lancet 2011;378:771–84.
28. Metzger-Filho O, Procter M, de Azambuja E, et al. Magnitude of trastuzumab benefit in patients with HER2-positive, invasive lobular breast carcinoma: results from the HERA trial. J Clin Oncol 2013;31:1954–60.

29. Moore MM, Borossa G, Imbrie JZ, et al. Association of infiltrating lobular carcinoma with positive surgical margins after breast-conservation therapy. Ann Surg 2000;231:877–82.

30. Morrow M, Keeney K, Scholtens D, et al. Selecting patients for breast-conserving therapy: the importance of lobular histology. Cancer 2006;106:2563–8.

31. Biglia N, Maggiorotto F, Liberale V, et al. Clinical-pathologic features, long term-outcome and surgical treatment in a large series of patients with invasive lobular carcinoma (ILC) and invasive ductal carcinoma (IDC). Eur J Surg Oncol 2013;39: 455–60.

32. Arps DP, Jorns JM, Zhao L, et al. Re-excision rates of invasive ductal carcinoma with lobular features compared with invasive ductal carcinomas and invasive lobular carcinomas of the breast. Ann Surg Oncol 2014;21:4152–8.

33. Braunstein LZ, Brock JE, Chen YH, et al. Invasive lobular carcinoma of the breast: local recurrence after breast-conserving therapy by subtype approximation and surgical margin. Breast Cancer Res Treat 2015;149:555–64.

34. Sagara Y, Barry WT, Mallory MA, et al. Surgical options and locoregional recurrence in patients diagnosed with invasive lobular carcinoma of the breast. Ann Surg Oncol 2015;22:4280–6.

35. Galimberti V, Maisonneuve P, Rotmensz N, et al. Influence of margin status on outcomes in lobular carcinoma: experience of the European Institute of Oncology. Ann Surg 2011;253:580–4.

36. Moran MS, Schnitt SJ, Giuliano AE, et al. Society of Surgical Oncology-American Society for Radiation Oncology consensus guideline on margins for breast-conserving surgery with whole-breast irradiation in stages I and II invasive breast cancer. Int J Radiat Oncol Biol Phys 2014;88:553–64.

37. Vandorpe T, Smeets A, Van Calster B, et al. Lobular and non-lobular breast cancers differ regarding axillary lymph node metastasis: a cross-sectional study on 4,292 consecutive patients. Breast Cancer Res Treat 2011;128:429–35.

38. Khakpour N, Hunt KK, Kuerer HM, et al. Sentinel lymph node dissection provides axillary control equal to complete axillary node dissection in breast cancer patients with lobular histology and a negative sentinel node. Am J Surg 2005;190: 598–601.

39. Giuliano AE, McCall L, Beitsch P, et al. Locoregional recurrence after sentinel lymph node dissection with or without axillary dissection in patients with sentinel lymph node metastases: the American College of Surgeons Oncology Group Z0011 randomized trial. Ann Surg 2010;252:426–32 [discussion: 432–3].

40. Galimberti V, Cole BF, Zurrida S, et al. Axillary dissection versus no axillary dissection in patients with sentinel-node micrometastases (IBCSG 23-01): a phase 3 randomised controlled trial. Lancet Oncol 2013;14:297–305.

41. Donker M, van Tienhoven G, Straver ME, et al. Radiotherapy or surgery of the axilla after a positive sentinel node in breast cancer (EORTC 10981-22023 AMAROS): a randomised, multicentre, open-label, phase 3 non-inferiority trial. Lancet Oncol 2014;15:1303–10.

42. Mamtani A, Barrio AV, King TA, et al. How often does neoadjuvant chemotherapy avoid axillary dissection in patients with histologically confirmed nodal metastases? Results of a prospective study. Ann Surg Oncol 2016;23:3467–74.

43. Cocquyt VF, Blondeel PN, Depypere HT, et al. Different responses to preoperative chemotherapy for invasive lobular and invasive ductal breast carcinoma. Eur J Surg Oncol 2003;29:361–7.

44. Tubiana-Hulin M, Stevens D, Lasry S, et al. Response to neoadjuvant chemotherapy in lobular and ductal breast carcinomas: a retrospective study on 860 patients from one institution. Ann Oncol 2006;17:1228–33.
45. Wenzel C, Bartsch R, Hussian D, et al. Invasive ductal carcinoma and invasive lobular carcinoma of breast differ in response following neoadjuvant therapy with epidoxorubicin and docetaxel + G-CSF. Breast Cancer Res Treat 2007; 104:109–14.
46. Lips EH, Mukhtar RA, Yau C, et al. Lobular histology and response to neoadjuvant chemotherapy in invasive breast cancer. Breast Cancer Res Treat 2012;136: 35–43.
47. Loibl S, Volz C, Mau C, et al. Response and prognosis after neoadjuvant chemotherapy in 1,051 patients with infiltrating lobular breast carcinoma. Breast Cancer Res Treat 2014;144:153–62.
48. Truin W, Vugts G, Roumen RM, et al. Differences in response and surgical management with neoadjuvant chemotherapy in invasive lobular versus ductal breast cancer. Ann Surg Oncol 2016;23:51–7.
49. Delpech Y, Coutant C, Hsu L, et al. Clinical benefit from neoadjuvant chemotherapy in oestrogen receptor-positive invasive ductal and lobular carcinomas. Br J Cancer 2013;108:285–91.
50. Cristofanilli M, Gonzalez-Angulo A, Sneige N, et al. Invasive lobular carcinoma classic type: response to primary chemotherapy and survival outcomes. J Clin Oncol 2005;23:41–8.
51. Mathieu MC, Rouzier R, Llombart-Cussac A, et al. The poor responsiveness of infiltrating lobular breast carcinomas to neoadjuvant chemotherapy can be explained by their biological profile. Eur J Cancer 2004;40:342–51.
52. Petrelli F, Barni S. Response to neoadjuvant chemotherapy in ductal compared to lobular carcinoma of the breast: a meta-analysis of published trials including 1,764 lobular breast cancer. Breast Cancer Res Treat 2013;142:227–35.
53. Boughey JC, Wagner J, Garrett BJ, et al. Neoadjuvant chemotherapy in invasive lobular carcinoma may not improve rates of breast conservation. Ann Surg Oncol 2009;16:1606–11.
54. Fitzal F, Mittlboeck M, Steger G, et al. Neoadjuvant chemotherapy increases the rate of breast conservation in lobular-type breast cancer patients. Ann Surg Oncol 2012;19:519–26.
55. Petruolo OA, Pilewskie M, Patil S, et al. Standard Pathologic Features Can Be Used to Identify a Subset of Estrogen Receptor-Positive, HER2 Negative Patients Likely to Benefit from Neoadjuvant Chemotherapy. Ann Surg Oncol 2017;24(9): 2556–62.
56. Dixon JM, Renshaw L, Dixon J, et al. Invasive lobular carcinoma: response to neoadjuvant letrozole therapy. Breast Cancer Res Treat 2011;130:871–7.
57. Cataliotti L, Buzdar AU, Noguchi S, et al. Comparison of anastrozole versus tamoxifen as preoperative therapy in postmenopausal women with hormone receptor-positive breast cancer: the pre-operative "Arimidex" compared to tamoxifen (PROACT) trial. Cancer 2006;106:2095–103.
58. Smith IE, Dowsett M, Ebbs SR, et al. Neoadjuvant treatment of postmenopausal breast cancer with anastrozole, tamoxifen, or both in combination: the immediate preoperative anastrozole, tamoxifen, or combined with tamoxifen (IMPACT) multicenter double-blind randomized trial. J Clin Oncol 2005;23:5108–16.
59. Ellis MJ, Suman VJ, Hoog J, et al. Randomized phase II neoadjuvant comparison between letrozole, anastrozole, and exemestane for postmenopausal women with estrogen receptor-rich stage 2 to 3 breast cancer: clinical and biomarker

outcomes and predictive value of the baseline PAM50-based intrinsic subtype–ACOSOG Z1031. J Clin Oncol 2011;29:2342–9.

60. Hughes KS, Schnaper LA, Bellon JR, et al. Lumpectomy plus tamoxifen with or without irradiation in women age 70 years or older with early breast cancer: long-term follow-up of CALGB 9343. J Clin Oncol 2013;31:2382–7.

61. Correa C, Harris EE, Leonardi MC, et al. Accelerated partial breast irradiation: executive summary for the update of an ASTRO evidence-based consensus statement. Pract Radiat Oncol 2017;7:73–9.

62. Stecklein SR, Shen X, Mitchell MP. Post-mastectomy radiation therapy for invasive lobular carcinoma: a comparative utilization and outcomes study. Clin Breast Cancer 2016;16:319–26.

63. Metzger Filho O, Giobbie-Hurder A, Mallon E, et al. Relative effectiveness of letrozole compared with tamoxifen for patients with lobular carcinoma in the BIG 1-98 trial. J Clin Oncol 2015;33:2772–9.

64. van de Water W, Fontein DB, van Nes JG, et al. Influence of semi-quantitative oestrogen receptor expression on adjuvant endocrine therapy efficacy in ductal and lobular breast cancer - a TEAM study analysis. Eur J Cancer 2013;49:297–304.

65. Barroso-Sousa R, Metzger-Filho O. Differences between invasive lobular and invasive ductal carcinoma of the breast: results and therapeutic implications. Ther Adv Med Oncol 2016;8:261–6.

66. Sikora MJ, Cooper KL, Bahreini A, et al. Invasive lobular carcinoma cell lines are characterized by unique estrogen-mediated gene expression patterns and altered tamoxifen response. Cancer Res 2014;74:1463–74.

67. Truin W, Voogd AC, Vreugdenhil G, et al. Effect of adjuvant chemotherapy in postmenopausal patients with invasive ductal versus lobular breast cancer. Ann Oncol 2012;23:2859–65.

68. Li CI, Uribe DJ, Daling JR. Clinical characteristics of different histologic types of breast cancer. Br J Cancer 2005;93:1046–52.

69. Buchanan CL, Flynn LW, Murray MP, et al. Is pleomorphic lobular carcinoma really a distinct clinical entity? J Surg Oncol 2008;98:314–7.

Molecular Subtypes and Local-Regional Control of Breast Cancer

Simona Maria Fragomeni, MD[a], Andrew Sciallis, MD[b],
Jacqueline S. Jeruss, MD, PhD[b,c],*

KEYWORDS

- Breast cancer • Molecular subtypes • Local-regional recurrence • Gene signatures
- Immunohistochemical surrogates

KEY POINTS

- The analysis of cancer gene expression patterns expands the understanding of breast cancer as a heterogeneous group of diseases.
- The presence or absence of estrogen, progesterone, and HER2/neu receptor (ER/PR/HER2) expression is key to molecular subtype stratification.
- Immunohistochemical techniques are widely applied to identify the markers of the different molecular subtypes.
- Gene expression profiling techniques, including commercially available tools such as Oncotype DX and MammaPrint, are considered complementary to the known prognostic factors.
- According to the currently available data, the different molecular subtypes are associated with different patterns of local-regional recurrence and response to treatment.

INTRODUCTION

Breast cancer is a heterogeneous disease that affects one anatomic site, yet is phenotypically variable.[1,2] The identification of different biological subtypes occurs primarily through the use of techniques including immunohistochemistry[3] and gene expression profiling.[1] To date, several studies have shown that the different biological subtypes are associated with variations in treatment response and disease-specific

Conflicts of Interest: The authors have nothing to disclose.
Funded by National Institutes of Health grant R01GM097220.
[a] Division of Gynecologic Oncology, Multidisciplinary Breast Center, Catholic University of the Sacred Heart of Rome, L.go Agostino Gemelli 8, 00168 Rome, Italy; [b] Division of Anatomic Pathology, Department of Pathology, University of Michigan, Ann Arbor, MI 48105, USA; [c] Division of Surgical Oncology, Department of Surgery, University of Michigan, 1500 East Medical Center Drive, Ann Arbor, MI 48105, USA
* Corresponding author. Department of Surgery, University of Michigan, 3303 Cancer Center, 1500 East Medical Center Drive, Ann Arbor, MI 48109-5932.
E-mail address: jjeruss@med.umich.edu

outcomes.[4–10] Currently, decision-making for individual patients is based on several factors, including tumor morphology and grade classification, tumor size, presence of lymph node metastases, and expression of estrogen receptor (ER), progesterone receptor (PR), and human epidermal growth factor receptor 2 (HER2)/neu (HER2). Although knowledge of these factors aids in treatment planning, there is a clear need to enhance the understanding of both prognostic and predictive markers that will facilitate customized treatment. The advent of novel technologies to aid in the identification of new markers also will be critical.

Through molecular analysis of breast cancers with gene expression profiling, both Perou and colleagues[1] and Sorlie and colleagues[2] showed that breast cancer could be subclassified into different subtypes. Broadly, these subtypes include luminal ER-positive (luminal A and luminal B), HER2 enriched, and basal-like (**Table 1**). Gene expression profiling can be costly, time-consuming, and, depending on the platform, may require a fresh tumor biopsy sample that has not been fixed in formalin.[11,12] Given these constraints, gene expression profiling can be difficult to implement on a broad scale. Nevertheless, several groups including the American Society of Clinical Oncology (ASCO), the National Comprehensive Cancer Network (NCCN), and the St Gallen Group have issued guidelines and recommendations supporting the implementation of molecular analysis as useful for risk stratification and for treatment planning.[13–15]

To facilitate the implementation of breast cancer subtype classification, efforts have been made to use immunohistochemical analysis to create approximated subtypes. Although taking this approach may enable stratification of breast cancers into subgroups that have outcomes comparable to those defined by gene expression profiling, there is not precise overlap.[16] Furthermore, in addition to the evaluation of standard biomarkers that can be assessed with immunohistochemistry (ER, PR, and HER2), the contribution of other factors, such as proliferative rate and expression of cytokeratins, also may be important. For example, the St Gallen 2013 classification included the evaluation of Ki67 (a marker of cell proliferation)[17] and a cutoff of PR of less than 20% as factors associated with the luminal B, HER2-negative subtype.[15]

The different molecular subtypes reflect the biological diversity of breast cancer. In a time in which medicine is moving toward a personalized approach, a critical goal is the correlation of the different disease subtypes with clinical outcomes and targeted therapeutics. Several studies have evaluated the variance in systemic disease recurrence and survival among the intrinsic subtypes.[18–21] To this end, additional work has pointed toward the growing significance of molecular subtypes in the risk of local-regional recurrence along with clinical and pathologic features.[5]

Table 1
Classification of molecular subtypes and correlation with biomarker staining on immunohistochemistry

Molecular Subtype	ER		PR	HER 2
Luminal A	Positive	and/or	Positive	Negative
Luminal B	Positive	and/or	Positive or negative[a]	Negative
Luminal B	Positive	and/or	Positive or negative [b]	Positive
HER2	Negative		Negative	Positive
Triple negative or basal-like	Negative		Negative	Negative

Abbreviations: ER, estrogen receptor; HER2, human epidermal growth factor receptor 2; PR, progesterone receptor.
[a] (PR <20% + Ki 67 >14%).
[b] (Any PR + any Ki 67).

Local-regional recurrence is described as ipsilateral, in-breast recurrence after lumpectomy, chest wall recurrence after mastectomy, or recurrence in the ipsilateral axillary, or supraclavicular lymph nodes (less commonly infraclavicular and/or internal mammary nodes).[22] Overall, among patients with stage I-II breast cancer, approximately 10% to 15% will develop a local recurrence after breast-conserving surgery (BCS) and radiation therapy, and 10% to 20% of patients with stage I-IIIA disease will experience a chest wall recurrence after mastectomy.[22] To date, several factors have been associated with aggressive cancer biology and the increased risk for local-regional recurrence. These factors include the following:

- Lymphovascular invasion[23]
- Young age[24]
- Increasing tumor size[25]
- Close or involved margin status[26,27]
- Positive nodal status[28,29]
- High tumor grade[23,30]
- Extensive intraductal component[31]
- Multifocal/multicentric disease[32]
- Negative hormone receptor status[33,34]
- Lack of adjuvant systemic therapy[35-37]

It follows that local-regional recurrence may be associated with a more aggressive tumor biology. The importance of adequate local disease control has been highlighted by findings from randomized studies showing the impact of local-regional recurrence on survival.[38-40] Data from the Early Breast Cancer Trialists' Collaborative Group overview analysis has demonstrated that for every 4 local recurrences prevented, approximately 1 death may be avoided.[41]

Defining the biological characteristics of breast cancer facilitates (1) characterization of different tumor histologic types, (2) understanding of disease prognosis, and (3) systemic treatment planning. Typically, immunohistochemistry is used to characterize intracellular or cell surface cancer-related protein expression. Among several factors, the most frequently evaluated immunohistochemical breast cancer prognostic and predictive markers include ER, PR, HER2, and Ki67.

ESTROGEN RECEPTOR/PROGESTERONE RECEPTOR

It has been known for some time that estrogen plays an important stimulatory role in the normal breast and in the development and progression of breast cancer. Moreover, ER is one of the most important prognostic biomarkers in breast cancer. ER belongs to a group of nuclear hormone receptors that act as transcription factors. There are 2 isoforms: ERα (the clinically measured isoform) and ERβ. Patients whose tumors are ER-positive benefit from endocrine therapy targeting ER (such as tamoxifen and aromatase inhibitors), and treatment can reduce local and distant recurrence and mortality.[42,43] However, ER-positive breast cancers do not respond as well to cytotoxic chemotherapy and are less likely to achieve a pathologic complete response (pCR) when compared with patients with ER-negative breast cancer who receive neoadjuvant chemotherapy.[44,45] PR also manifests as 2 major isoforms (PR-A and PR-B) and plays a role in downstream ER signaling.[46] It is likely that PR acts as a driver for the development of breast cancer that may be most impactful in postmenopausal women.[47] The ER is thought to regulate PR expression, and the presence of PR expression is considered indicative of a functional estrogen-ER axis.[48] In most cases, PR expression correlates with ER expression, and from a practical standpoint, robust

PR expression in the absence of ER may necessitate repeat testing. The presence of PR expression carries prognostic significance in early breast cancer with ER-positive and PR-positive cases having the best outcome.[49] Additionally, PR expression correlates with tumor responsiveness to endocrine therapy even when PR expression is low (ie, ≥1% of tumor cell nuclei).[50] However, in the setting of an ER-positive breast cancer, PR assessment may not add significant predictive information. That being said, breast cancers that are both ER-positive and PR-positive may derive greater benefit from endocrine therapy than ER-positive/PR-negative tumors.[51]

Currently, the evaluation of ER and PR receptor expression is standard practice and most often performed using immunohistochemistry. ER and PR immunoexpression manifests as nuclear staining, and heterogeneous ("physiologic") expression is typically observed in normal breast ductal epithelium. Up to 80% of breast cancers are ER-positive[52] and 55% to 65% are positive for PR expression.[53] ASCO and the College of American Pathologists (CAP) have provided recommendations regarding ER/PR measurement and reporting.[54] Per these recommendations, pathology reports for ER and PR results should include the following details: percentage and/or proportion of tumor cells staining positively in a tissue section or cytology preparation, the overall intensity of staining (weak, moderate, strong), and an interpretation as to hormone receptor status. As to the latter, ER and PR expression is considered positive when ≥1% of tumor cells stain positively, negative when less than 1%, and interpretable when preanalytic variables preclude an accurate assessment. These include the use of fixatives other than 10% neutral buffered formalin during tissue processing, duration of fixation less than 6 hours or more than 72 hours, delay in fixation/cold ischemic time more than 1 hour, decalcification of specimens using acids, and inappropriate intrinsic/extrinsic assay controls. Some institutions provide a composite score combining percentage and intensity of tumor cell hormone receptor expression.

Most pathology laboratories use immunohistochemical methods to determine ER and PR status. Testing is often performed on biopsy material before surgery, as there is excellent agreement in hormone receptor expression between biopsy and resection specimens.[55] This enables clinicians, oncologists, surgeons, and patients to possess vital prognostic and therapeutic information before establishing a treatment plan. However, there is institutional variability in the manner by which ER and PR immunoexpression is evaluated. At some centers, pathologists use digital image analysis (DIA) in which slides are scanned and converted into high-resolution computer images so that quantitative immunohistochemistry can be performed.[56] DIA is being used with greater frequency owing to established intraobserver and interobserver variability in scoring results by pathologists.[57] Finally, repeat testing of ER and PR on excision specimens in cases in which prior core biopsy showed weak or equivocal expression is also undertaken at some institutions.

ANDROGEN RECEPTOR

Another hormone receptor currently being studied in breast cancer research is the androgen receptor (AR). Like ER and PR, immunohistochemical AR expression is nuclear and usually strong and diffuse when present (ie, present in >80% of tumor cell nuclei). Expression is seen in most ER-positive breast cancers, as well as subsets of triple-negative breast cancer (TNBC) and HER2-positive carcinomas. In the spectrum of TNBCs, tumors with robust AR expression often manifest as apocrine carcinoma ("carcinoma with apocrine differentiation"), a ductal tumor in which the invasive cells exhibit extensive apocrine cell change (>90% of tumor cells exhibiting apocrine features).[58] Most pathologists view AR immunoexpression in 1% of tumor cell nuclei as AR-positive. Molecular studies using RNA expression profiling have revealed several potentially clinically relevant breast cancer subtypes. One of these is known as the molecular apocrine group, defined as tumors that are ER-negative but AR-positive.[59] These tumors often exhibit an expression profile that overlaps with luminal, basal-like, and occasionally HER2-positive groups. Interestingly, many of these tumors, but not all, show some degree of apocrine differentiation on histopathology.

From a clinical perspective, AR-positive breast cancers appear to behave favorably when compared with AR-negative tumors, regardless of ER status.[60] Among TNBCs, the significance of AR expression on prognosis and clinical course continues to be investigated. In some studies, AR-positive TNBC has a better prognosis when compared with AR-negative TNBC; however, others have found a decreased survival for patients with early-stage disease.[61] Further confounding the prognostic significance of AR expression is the presence of HER2 overexpression in molecular apocrine cases. The favorable clinical course of AR-positive TNBC may be related to the genetic overlap with luminal tumors. Because the AR can be targeted via aromatase inhibition, there has been considerable clinical interest in interrogating TNBC for AR expression; however, there are no guidelines regarding routine testing for AR for all patients with breast cancer.

HUMAN EPIDERMAL GROWTH FACTOR RECEPTOR 2

HER2 (erbB-2) is a transmembrane tyrosine kinase receptor that regulates cell growth, proliferation, and survival through several different signaling pathways, such as the mammalian target of rapamycin and RAS/RAF/MEK/extracellular signal-regulated kinase (ERK) pathways.[62] HER2 gene amplification is observed in 15% to 30% of breast cancers and is a strong prognostic biomarker for an aggressive clinical course.[63]

Importantly, HER2 gene overexpression is also a strong predictive marker of response to anti-HER2 therapy, which includes humanized monoclonal antibodies that bind to the extracellular domain of the HER2 receptor (trastuzumab and pertuzumab), small molecular receptor tyrosine kinase inhibitors (lapatinib), and an antibody drug conjugate of trastuzumab (ado-trastuzumab emtansine; T-DM1). Immunohistochemistry for HER2 protein overexpression has been developed, and testing for this protein is standard for invasive breast carcinomas whether primary or metastatic. Overexpression of the HER2 protein typically occurs secondary to HER2/neu gene amplification.[64] As per the most recent 2013 ASCO/CAP guideline recommendations[65] regarding HER2 testing in breast carcinoma, the threshold for a positive test on immunohistochemistry is strong circumferential staining in more than 10% of invasive tumor cells (score 3+), whereas criteria for a negative result includes (A) no staining observed or incomplete, faint/barely perceptible membrane staining in $\leq$10% of invasive tumor cells (score 0), or (B) incomplete, faint/barely perceptible membrane staining in greater than 10% of tumor cells (score 1+). An equivocal result (score 2+), is rendered when there is either incomplete and/or weak-to-moderate circumferential membrane staining in more than 10% of invasive tumor cells or there is complete, intense, circumferential membrane staining in $\leq$10% of invasive tumor cells. Breast cancers with an equivocal result for HER2 overexpression are reflexed to either fluorescence in situ hybridization (FISH), chromogenic in situ hybridization (CISH), or silver-enhanced in situ hybridization (SISH) assays to determine HER2 gene amplification. Immunohistochemistry and gene amplification assays usually yield similar results, as gene amplification induces immunohistochemically detected protein overexpression in 95% of cases. Most institutions use FISH, however CISH and SISH techniques are increasingly being used, as they may be implemented using light microscopy. Moreover, probes for *HER2* as well as centromere 17 (centromere enumeration probe, CEP17) are used so that the ratio of HER2 signals to CEP17 can be calculated. A positive (amplified) test result is rendered when the average HER2 copy number ≥6.0 signals per cell or HER2/CEP17 ratio ≥2.0, whereas a negative (not amplified) result is found when the average HER2 copy number is <4.0 and the HER2/CEP17 ratio is <2.0. As for HER2 immunohistochemistry, an equivocal result is observed with an HER2/CEP17 ratio less than 2.0 and the average HER2 copy number is ≥4.0 but less than 6.0.

KI67

Ki-67 is a nuclear proliferation marker expressed in all phases of the cell cycle except G_0.[66] In general, breast cancers expressing high levels of Ki67 correlate with worse outcomes.[67,68] Meta-analyses by de Azambuja and colleagues[68] in 2007 and Stuart-Harris and colleagues[69] in 2008, showed that Ki67 was associated with prognosis, disease-free survival, and overall survival. In 2009, the St Gallen Consensus stratified tumors according to the Ki67 value as low (less than 15%), intermediate (16%–30%), and highly proliferative (greater than 30%), to help identify patients who could potentially benefit from treatment with chemotherapy or endocrine therapy. Additional studies reported a Ki67 level higher than 10% to 14%[70,71] and 20%,[15] as characteristic of high risk for poor outcomes. The implementation of Ki67 has been complex, as some studies have used 10%, 14%, or 20% cutpoints for treatment recommendations.[72,73] Accordingly, Cheang and colleagues[74] defined a Ki67 cutoff to distinguish luminal A and B subtypes using immunohistochemistry. This work defined the luminal A subtype as ER-positive and/or PR-positive, HER2-negative, and Ki67 low (ie, a Ki67 index of <14%), and the luminal B subtype as ER-positive and/or PR-positive, HER2-negative, and Ki67 high (ie, a Ki67 index of ≥14%) and showed that stratification using the immunohistochemical panel of 4 biomarkers (ie, ER, PR, HER2, and Ki67) was statistically significant.[74] ASCO guidelines have not included Ki67 in the list of routinely assessed markers for breast cancer prognosis.[75] In Europe, the St Gallen International Expert Consensus recommended the use of proliferation markers, such as Ki67, in addition to standard parameters (stage, grade, hormone receptor status) when choosing systemic treatment regimens.[15] A role for Ki67 was also found in the neoadjuvant setting, in particular for patients undergoing preoperative endocrine therapy,[76] indicating how a variation in Ki67 expression may predict long-term outcomes. Nishimura and colleagues,[77] in 2010, investigated the role of Ki67 in neoadjuvant systemic treatment and found that marker values before starting treatment could help to predict response, whereas those measured after chemotherapy could help predict disease-free survival. Additionally, measurement of Ki67 is cost-effective when compared with multigene assays. At some centers, Ki67 is included in surgical pathology reports along with other standard markers, and can aid in the identification of luminal B tumors not identified by ER, PR, and HER2.

MOLECULAR SUBTYPES
Luminal A

Frequency: 30% to 40% of all invasive breast cancers. *Gene expression profiling (GEP):* PIK3CA mutations, MAP3KI mutations, ESR1 high expression, XBP1 high expression, GATA3 mutations, FOXA1 mutations; gain of 1q, 8q, loss of 8p, 16q. *Morphology:* Grading 1 or 2; most are well-differentiated carcinomas of no special type (NST), classic lobular carcinomas, tubular, mucinous, neuroendocrine and cribriform carcinomas.[78] *Immunohistochemical profile (IHC):* ER-positive, PR high expression ($\geq$20%), HER2-negative, and low Ki-67.[79,80] Several studies showed that a Ki-67 of 14% was the cutoff point to separate luminal A from luminal B subtypes.[74] More recently, this cutoff was changed to 20%.[81]

Luminal B (Human Epidermal Growth Factor Receptor 2–Negative)

Frequency: 20% to 30% of all invasive breast cancer. *GEP:* TP53 mutations, PIK3CA mutations, Cyclin D1 amplification, MDM2 amplification, ATM loss, enhanced genomic instability, focal amplifications (eg, 8p12, 11q13). *Morphology:* Grading 2 or 3; less well-differentiated cancers, mostly invasive ductal carcinomas NST and also some invasive micropapillary carcinomas.[78] *IHC profile:* ER-positive, lower PR expression (<20%),[15] HER2-negative and higher level of Ki67 labeling index (>14% or 20%).[52,74] *Correlation to oncotype results:* high recurrence score is suggestive of luminal B like subtype.[15] Furthermore, on a molecular basis, it seems that luminal A and luminal B breast cancers have specific gene profiles that lead to oncogenic proliferation.

Human Epidermal Growth Factor Receptor 2

Frequency: 12% to 20% of all invasive breast cancers. *GEP:* HER2 amplification, TP53 mutations, PIK3CA mutations, FGFR4 high expression, epidermal growth factor receptor (EGFR) high expression, APOBEC mutations, cyclin D1 amplification, high genomic instability.[1,2,82–85] *Morphology:* grading 2 or 3; infiltrating carcinoma NST, apocrine and pleomorphic lobular carcinomas. *Classification:* in the study from Fountzilas and colleagues,[86] hormone receptor status was shown to affect survival, metastatic spread, and treatment response. Therefore, on IHC, HER2-positive tumors can be divided into 2 subtypes: HER2-enriched subtype (ER-negative and/or PR-negative/HER2-positive)[86–88] and luminal HER2 subtype (ER-positive and/or PR-positive, HER2-positive); and further divided into 2 phenotypes based on PR expression: ER-positive, PR-positive, HER2-positive and ER-positive, PR-negative, HER2-positive. There is preclinical evidence for crosstalk between the HER2 and ER signaling pathways with a negative effect on the response to endocrine therapy.[89–93]

Triple-Negative Breast Cancer

Representing 15% to 20% of all invasive breast cancers, TNBC is defined by the absence of expression of ER, PR, and HER2. Despite its simple definition, it is a morphologically, genetically, and clinically heterogeneous category of breast cancer. Most TNBCs manifest as invasive ductal carcinoma NST; however, the category also includes variants such as metaplastic carcinoma, carcinoma with medullary features (formerly known as medullary carcinoma), carcinoma with apocrine features (formerly known as apocrine carcinoma), secretory carcinoma (formerly known as juvenile breast cancer), and adenoid cystic carcinoma.[58] Gene expression profiling has enabled the subdivision of these cancers into different, prognostically significant subtypes that, in some cases, correlate with a particular pathologic variant. The most common, and best-characterized, molecular subtypes of TNBC are basal-like 1 (BL1), basal-like 2 (BL2), immunomodulatory (IM), mesenchymal (M), mesenchymal stemlike (MSL), and luminal androgen receptor (LAR).[94] BL1 breast cancers usually manifest clinically and pathologically as invasive ductal carcinoma NST and have high Ki67 proliferative indices, and their expression profile is enriched in genes associated with basal cytokeratin genes (including *KRT5*), cell cycle and DNA replication, and DNA damage response pathways. BL2 tumors also manifest as invasive ductal carcinoma NST and also show increased basal cytokeratin gene expression, *TP63*, and growth factor signaling (eg, EGF and insulinlike growth factor 1 receptor pathways). In general, the immunomodulatory subtype of TNBC overlaps with carcinoma with medullary features, as both often contain a brisk lymphocytic infiltrate. Mesenchymal and MSL subtypes may present clinically as metaplastic carcinoma, defined as breast cancer with epithelial and mesenchymal differentiation, sometimes taking the form of heterologous elements like bone and cartilage. These tumors are enriched in genes important for cell differentiation and growth factor signaling pathways. Finally, the LAR subtype often presents as carcinoma with apocrine differentiation and correlates with the molecular apocrine type. As expected, LAR shows increased expression of luminal cytokeratin genes (including *KRT7* and *KRT1*) and enriched in AR mRNA and protein expression, possibly explaining their responsiveness to hormone therapies.

Gene Expression Testing

The information obtained from microarray-based gene expression profiling has revealed further information about breast cancer as a group of different diseases with different biological characteristics and behaviors.[95,96] A key finding, in addition to the validation of ER-positive and ER-negative cancers as different diseases from a molecular point of view, was that the expression of proliferation-related genes was also associated with prognosis of ER-positive tumors.[12,97] Through the advent of methods for gene expression testing, a prognostic multigene assessment has also been developed and validated in clinical trials, and integrated into clinical practice.[98] Through the work of Perou and colleagues[1] and Sorlie and colleagues,[2] a group of "intrinsic genes" was identified, revealing 4 molecular subtypes of breast cancer[1]: luminal A and B, HER2-enriched, and basal-like. The groups of genes primarily responsible for the segregation of molecular subtypes are genes related to expression of ER, regulation of proliferation, HER2, and genes mapping to chromosome 17.[1,2] The prognostic signatures currently available provide clinicians with data complementary to factors with known prognostic significance, including tumor size and nodal status (**Table 2**). To date, these gene signatures are more informative for patients with ER-positive disease, but have a more limited role for patients with ER-negative tumors. One of the main objectives of molecular subtyping was the ability to identify factors to aid in the discrimination between patients a with favorable versus an unfavorable prognosis to guide therapeutic decision-making.[96] In recent years, several prognostic signatures have been identified[96] that revealed overlapping groups of patients with a poor prognosis,[99] primarily characterized by cancers with high expression of proliferation-related genes.[95,99] Given the significance of proliferation-related gene expression for prognosis for both ER-positive and ER-negative disease, these factors are active targets for cytotoxic chemotherapies.[95,100] In terms of outcome prediction generated from molecular subtyping, the insights obtained appear to extend beyond the short-term time frame (eg, 10 years instead of 5),[101,102] serving as complementary to the parameters routinely used in clinical practice.[96,99]

70 Gene Signature

MammaPrint (Agendia, Amsterdam, Netherlands) is a microarray-based test, primarily implemented in Europe, that can be used for risk stratification (ie, low or high) for patients with ER-positive or ER-negative breast cancer. It was based on data derived from stage I and II patients younger than 55 years, with node-negative tumors smaller than 5 cm. The test can be performed with fresh or formalin-fixed tumor samples. Much of the data related to this test were obtained from retrospective studies, and the findings were then confirmed prospectively by the RASTER study.[103] The results

Table 2
Gene signatures

Test	Method	Result	Clinical Application	Level of Evidence
MammaPrint	• Microarray • 70 gene • Fresh tissue, frozen material and alternatively formalin fixed and paraffin embedded (FFPE)	Distant metastasis at 5 y (without adjuvant treatment): • Low risk 13% • High risk 56%	Prognosis of N0, <5 cm diameter, stage I/II disease, age <61 y	II
Oncotype DX	• qRT – PCR • 21-gene • Fresh frozen tissue and/or FFPE	Risk of 10 y distant recurrence: • Low (<18) • Intermediate (18–30) • High (≥31)	Prediction of recurrence risk in ER+ and N0 disease treated with tamoxifen	I
Prosigna/PAM50	• qRT – PCR • 50-gene • Routinely processed tissue (e.g. FFPE)	Risk of distant recurrence from 5 to 10 y after diagnosis: • Node-negative cancers Low (0–40) Intermediate (41–60) High (61–100) • Node-positive cancers Low (0–40) High (41–100)	Prediction of recurrence risk in hormone receptor positive breast cancer after 5 y of hormonal therapy in postmenopausal women	I

of the prospective MINDACT trial recently published showed survival rates of approximately 95% at 5 years for low-risk patients who did not receive chemotherapy.[104]

21 Gene Recurrence Score Assay

In the United States, implementation of the Oncotype DX assay has been widespread for patients with node-negative hormone receptor–positive breast cancer.[105] It is performed using a reverse-transcription polymerase chain reaction on RNA isolated from paraffin-embedded breast cancer tissue, measuring the expression of 21 genes (16 cancer-related genes and 5 reference genes). The Oncotype DX 21 gene recurrence score (RS) assay has been defined as a continuous variable (ranging from 0 to 100). This assay can be considered as an independent prognostic factor in node-negative, ER-positive breast cancer, measuring the risk of distant relapse at 10 years. With values ranging from 0 to 100, patients are stratified into 3 groups: (1) low risk (RS <18), (2) intermediate risk (RS 18–31), and (3) high risk (RS ≥31). These groups are associated with 10-year relapse rates of 7%, 14%, and 30%, respectively. For patients with ER-positive tumors, those who fall into the high-risk group may have greater benefits from the use of chemotherapy.[105] Appropriate management of patients in the intermediate-risk group will be revealed through results of the TAILORx study (NCT00310180). Patients (ER-positive and node-negative) enrolled in TAILORx were assigned to low-risk (RS <11), intermediate-risk (RS 11–25), and high-risk groups (RS >25). The main aim of the study was to evaluate the risk of relapse after surgery for the intermediate-risk group. Patients in this risk category were randomly assigned to hormone treatment alone or in combination with chemotherapy. The trial completed enrollment and results are pending. Emerging data from several studies highlight how Oncotype DX may also play a role in different patient scenarios, including those with positive lymph nodes, ER-positive and HER2-positive disease, and patients treated with aromatase inhibitors instead of tamoxifen.[106,107]

Based on the available evidence, guidelines have been developed for the use of for Oncotype DX clinically. NCCN guidelines suggest that Oncotype DX can be used as a predictor of recurrence and can be used as a guide for treatment decision-making in ER-positive, node-negative breast cancer based on level I evidence.[14]

ASCO guidelines suggest it can be used as a tumor marker for risk of recurrence.[108]

In Europe, the latest St Gallen International Expert Consensus recommended that the validated assay should be used to clarify the indication for chemotherapy and added to other known prognostic and predictive factors.[15] Along with the ability of the RS to aid in predicting the response to adjuvant chemotherapy,[107,109] additional studies have shown how the RS can be predictive of local-regional and distant recurrence.[105,110] Although evidence suggests that the RS obtained with the Oncotype DX correlates with traditional clinicopathologic data, the information obtained regarding prognosis from tumor size, lymph node status, and histologic grade remain as independent variables.[109,111]

Clinical Outcomes: Local-Regional Recurrence

Significant progress has been made in terms of systemic therapy and targeted treatments, improving outcomes for patients with breast cancer. Optimal local-regional control continues to be relevant in terms of clinical outcomes. The risk of a local-regional recurrence (LRR) has been correlated to different parameters (both pathologic and clinical) with the aim to guide treatment decisions.

RISK FACTORS FOR LOCAL-REGIONAL RECURRENCE
Breast-Conserving Therapy

Age
Studies have found that age is a risk factor for LRR after breast-conserving therapy, with 10-year local recurrence rates reportedly higher for younger patients.[112,113] One relevant study showing the impact of age was the EORTC 22881 to 10882 trial.[114] A tumor bed boost used in addition to standard whole breast irradiation resulted in a reduction in local recurrence from 23.9% to 13.5% in patients aged 40 years or younger when compared with a decrease from 7.3% to 3.8% in patients older than 60 years.[114] Accordingly, clinicians should consider patient age when considering treatment planning in patients undergoing BCS.

Margins
Positive margins (defined as ink on invasive carcinoma or ductal carcinoma in situ) are associated with a twofold increase in the risk of local recurrence when compared with negative margins (>2 mm). This was an independent risk factor, not mitigated by radiation boost or other characteristics. There is no evidence that more widely free margins reduced this risk even in cases with other risk factors, including young age, unfavorable biology, lobular cancers, or cancers with an extensive intraductal component (EIC).[115]

Extensive intraductal component
EIC is defined as an infiltrating ductal cancer in which more than 25% of the tumor volume is ductal cancer in situ (DCIS) and DCIS extends beyond the invasive cancer into

surrounding normal breast parenchyma. Invasive breast carcinoma is accompanied by EIC in 15% to 30% of patients.[14] It can be considered as a risk factor for local recurrence.[114,116,117]

Mastectomy

Several studies have identified risk factors for local recurrence after mastectomy (Jagsi and colleagues[118] and the Breast Cancer Cooperative Group (DBCG82) b and c studies).[119] Jagsi and colleagues[118] demonstrated how tumor size larger than 2 cm, margins less than 2 mm, premenopausal status, and lymphovascular invasion can be considered as independent prognostic factors for LRR. Ten-year LRR was 1.2% for those patients with no risk factors, and as high as 40.6% for those with 3 risk factors. This retrospective analysis suggested the benefit of postmastectomy radiation therapy (PMRT) to reduce the risk of recurrence for patients with node-negative disease and high-risk factors. In the Breast Cancer Cooperative Group (DBCG82) b and c studies, tumor size, histology positive for ductal carcinoma, high tumor grade, invasion of the pectoralis major fascia, several positive nodes, and extracapsular spread were identified as risk factors for LRR.[119,120] Abdulkarim and colleagues[121] reported an increased risk of local-regional recurrence in women with node-negative, TNBC with tumors ≤5 cm when mastectomy was performed without radiation. This prospective study further identified that risk factors for LRR include node-positive disease, tumors larger than 2 cm, and lymphovascular invasion.

Additional Risk Factors

Large tumor size, poor tumor differentiation, nodal status, multifocal/multicentric disease, and adjuvant treatment have all been found to be relevant to the assessment of the risk for LRR.[122]

Lymphovascular invasion
Lymphovascular invasion is a factor associated with a higher risk of recurrence. In patients treated with mastectomy, this parameter is one of the risk factors to be considered when offering postmastectomy radiation therapy.[14,123]

Receptor status
ER, PR, and HER2 status, known as predictors of response to targeted treatment, also have a prognostic role after breast-conserving therapy and mastectomy.[42] As described in the analysis of the Danish 82 b and c trials, triple-negative disease was associated with higher local recurrence rates after mastectomy.[6]

BRCA1 and 2 mutation carriers
Patients with sporadic breast cancer treated with BCS have an approximate 10% risk of ipsilateral breast tumor recurrence. Although some studies have reported a risk reduction of contralateral breast cancers in BRCA mutation carriers who take tamoxifen or undergo oophorectomy, contralateral prophylactic mastectomy can decrease the risk to less than 10%.[124] Risk reduction strategies in BRCA1/2 mutation carriers, including bilateral prophylactic mastectomy, oophorectomy, and/or the use of tamoxifen are being implemented in many countries.[124,125] BRCA1 mutation cancers are more likely to have ER-negative breast cancer and are also more likely to develop tumors with a higher histologic grade.

There are several studies showing that the different intrinsic subtypes have differences in overall prognosis[2] and different rates of local-regional disease recurrence (**Table 3**).

Table 3
Local-regional recurrence by molecular subtype

Molecular Subtype	Frequency, %
Luminal A	0.8–8
Luminal B	1.5–8.7
HER2[a]	1.7–9.4
Triple negative	3–17

Abbreviation: HER2, human epidermal growth factor receptor 2.
  Patients treated with upfront surgery.
  [a] Luminal HER2-positive and HER2-enriched.

INTRINSIC SUBTYPES, WHAT ROLE?
Luminal A

The luminal A molecular subtype is generally associated with a highly favorable prognosis[126] and typically shows less frequent and less extensive lymph nodal involvement.[127,128] This subtype also tends to have a more indolent course with a slower evolution over time when compared with the other molecular subtypes.[129] Additionally, a positive hormone receptor status is both a favorable prognostic factor and also predictive of response to endocrine therapy.[42,130,131] In terms of LRR, several retrospective studies have shown similar outcomes with percentages ranging between 0.8% and 8.0%.[4,5,9,132,133]

Luminal B

The luminal B molecular subtype is associated with a more intermediate prognosis when compared with the luminal A molecular subtype.[126] The risk of LRR for luminal B tumors, as described in literature, ranges from 1.5% and 8.7% with a peak of incidence in the first 5 years after diagnosis.[4,5,9,132,133]

Luminal Tumor Considerations

The luminal molecular subtypes have lower local-regional recurrence rates, with both conservative surgery and mastectomy.[134] In the study by Lowery and colleagues,[134] it was estimated that the rate of LRR for both luminal A and B subtypes after BCS and radiation was approximately 5%, even in the setting of noncompliance with endocrine therapy. It is important for clinicians to reinforce that endocrine therapy reduces the LRR and mortality rates by more than 50% in patients with ER-positive breast cancer between 5 and 10 years from diagnosis.[42]

HER2-Positive Disease

Historically, HER2 overexpression has been associated with a higher frequency of LRR based on studies in which patients were not treated with HER2-targeted therapy, ranging between 4% and 15%.[4,5,9,132,133] In the meta-analysis from Lowery and colleagues,[134] 12,592 patients were evaluated for LRR after BCS with radiation therapy and mastectomy. The results showed increased rates of LRR for patients with HER2-positive tumors, with higher rates of recurrence observed after BCS versus mastectomy. In this study, fewer than 6% of the HER2-positive patients were treated with trastuzumab. A subgroup analysis of 9306 patients from 9 studies showed a lower rate of LRR after mastectomy for luminal HER2-negative tumors, when compared with luminal HER2-positive cancers (7.5% vs 9.4%), although in this analysis the use of trastuzumab was also low. In this subgroup analysis, no difference was observed in the risk of LRR after BCS for luminal HER2-negative tumors compared with luminal HER2-positive (Relative Risk (RR) 0.8%–95% confidence interval) tumors. Overall, both luminal HER2-negative and luminal HER2-positive cancers showed a positive trend toward lower LRR rates when compared with ER-negative/HER2-positive and TNBC subtypes.[134] More recently, patients with HER2-positive tumors receive targeted therapies, including trastuzumab and pertuzumab, and this has modified the natural course of this disease subtype, resulting in improved outcomes.[126] HER2-positivity is a predictive factor for response to trastuzumab[135] and also a prognostic factor for LRR.[131,136–138] In a study by Panoff and colleagues,[139] patients with HER2-positive tumors who underwent mastectomy and received trastuzumab, had an LRR of 1.7%. This finding was supported by an analysis of 6 studies from Yin and colleagues,[140] who also showed trastuzumab treatment resulted in a decrease in LRR by 50%. It has been suggested that breast cancer cells with radiation damage could be more vulnerable to injury when deprived of the mitogenic cell signaling provided by the HER2 pathway activation.[141] Further to this point, a study conducted in patients with T1 (a or b) HER2-positive breast cancer showed a risk of LRR of 2.0% to 5.7% for those who did not receive trastuzumab, and 0% for those patients treated with trastuzumab ± chemotherapy at 5 years after diagnosis.[142]

Triple-Negative Breast Cancer

TNBC is associated with an unfavorable prognosis when compared with the other breast cancer subtypes secondary to a higher risk of disease recurrence.[126,143,144] For TNBC, the involvement of regional lymph nodes is associated with a poor prognosis, without a direct relationship to the number of involved nodes.[135] The TNBC subtype has been associated with a higher risk of local-regional relapse[10] and contralateral disease, as shown by Bessonova and colleagues[145] and Malone and colleagues,[143] and also systemic relapse.[126] Peak incidence for recurrence in TNBC has been reported in the first 1 to 3 years, as reported in studies by Jatoi and colleagues[129] and Kumar and Aggarwal.[146] In the meta-analysis by Lowery and colleagues,[134] the TNBC subtype was associated with increased LRR rates, after BCS and mastectomy, ranging from 3% to 17%. Other studies have reported that TNBC is not associated with higher LRR risk.[147,148] Abdulkarim and colleagues[121] reported no difference in local recurrence events, whereas Wang and colleagues[147] found patients with TNBC undergoing mastectomy to have inferior outcomes. Several other studies have described the TNBC subtype as having the highest risk for LRR.[4,5,9,10,22,132,133] Moreover, after the diagnosis of a local-regional recurrence, this molecular subtype is associated with a high incidence of distant metastases and cancer-related mortality.[146]

Another topic of debate is the apparent radiation resistance of this molecular subtype, which may be impacted by ER negativity, shorter cell cycle duration, and less time for DNA damage repair. Kyndi and colleagues[6] reported a smaller reduction in LRR rates after PMRT in TNBC, and no overall survival benefit, thought to be secondary to radio-resistance–associated hormone receptor negativity.[146] Some studies are evaluating ways to improve radio-sensitivity through use of cisplatin-based chemoradiation in the setting of TNBC.[126]

LOCAL-REGIONAL RECURRENCE AND MOLECULAR SUBTYPES IN THE NEOADJUVANT SETTING

Huang and colleagues[149] reported in the neoadjuvant setting that multifocal/multicentric disease, number of positive axillary nodes, axillary dissection with fewer than 10 nodes, lymphovascular invasion, extracapsular extension, skin or nipple involvement, and ER-negative disease were significantly associated with LRR. Patients who achieved a pCR had a lower rate of LRR (2% vs 12%). The study by Levy and colleagues[150] evaluated the long-term local-regional control rates after breast-conserving therapy for patients undergoing surgery before or after chemotherapy. In this study, ER-negative and/or PR-negative disease were associated with higher rates of LRR, and the 10-year LRR rate was not related to surgical treatment approach.[150] Mamounas and colleagues[151] also reported that after neoadjuvant treatment, surgical approach was not related to a different incidence in LRR. Thus, for patients treated with neoadjuvant therapy, as for patients treated with surgery first, clinical stage, nodal involvement, and histology can be considered prognostic factors for LRR. Two large trials, NSABP B-18 and B-27, have also shown that a pCR (defined in these studies as the absence of invasive tumor in the breast), after Neoadjuvant Chemotherapy can be considered as a prognostic factor for LRR.[151] von Minckwitz and colleagues[152] studied 6377 patients after neoadjuvant treatment, and found pCR was associated with better outcomes in luminal B/HER2-negative, HER2-positive (nonluminal), and TNBC subtypes, but not for patients with luminal B/HER2-positive or luminal A cancers. Liedtke and colleagues[153] found that patients experiencing a pCR had excellent outcomes regardless of receptor status, but, when comparing patients with TNBC who did not achieve a pCR with other subtypes, TNBC was associated with a lower overall and postrecurrence survival rate, with a risk of relapse and death found to be higher in the first 3 years after diagnosis. Despite this, when patients with TNBC achieve a pCR, they have improved survival. In a series published by Swisher and colleagues[154] at the MD Anderson Cancer Center, the LRR-free survival rate for patients with TNBC with residual disease posttreatment was estimated at approximately 89.9% versus 98.6% for patients with a pCR. This study concluded that TNBC was an independent predictive factor for LRR.[154] The role of pCR on LRR was not observed for patients with HER2-positive subtypes.[154] Similar findings were reported in the studies of Peterson and colleagues[155] and Kiess and colleagues.[156] Taken together, these findings point toward the role of molecular subtypes in the locoregional recurrence and could help to facilitate patient selection for optimal treatment planning.

LOCAL-REGIONAL RECURRENCE AND AXILLARY DISEASE

Many changes have occurred in the management of the axilla over the past several years. Two trials that have proposed treatment changes include the AMAROS trial and ACOSOG Z0011. The AMAROS trial was a multicenter phase 3 trial in which patients were enrolled with T1 and T2 breast cancers (both unifocal and multifocal), a clinically negative axilla, and positive sentinel nodes. Patients were treated with BCS or mastectomy and were assigned to axillary node dissection versus radiation treatment (breast tangential fields, axillary and supraclavicular nodes). The study endpoints were to evaluate the axillary recurrence, disease-free survival (DFS), overall survival, and quality of life in terms of arm lymphedema and motility. The investigators showed additional metastases were found in 33% of cases and no differences were identified in terms of DFS and overall survival between the 2 treatment groups, with less morbidity reported in the axillary radiation therapy group (lymphedema 11% vs 23%).[157]

The American College of Surgeons (ACOSOG) Z0011 trial enrolled clinically node-negative women with T1 and T2 breast cancer with 1 to 2 positive sentinel nodes who underwent BCS and breast irradiation (breast tangential fields). This study showed that 27% of patients in the axillary dissection arm had additional positive non-sentinel nodes. There was no difference in regional recurrence and no difference in overall survival and DFS between those who had completion axillary dissection versus those undergoing sentinel node dissection alone. Nodal recurrences were reported in 1% of patients.[158,159] These results suggest that regional control can be achieved by radiation and systemic therapy, regardless of cancer subtypes.[160]

ONGOING TRIALS AND FUTURE PERSPECTIVES

Currently, PMRT is not recommended for patients at low risk for LRR (<10%).[161] The St Gallen recommendations indicate PMRT should be considered in cases in which the 10-year LRR rate is 20% or higher.[162,163] Therefore, the need to quantify the LRR rate is essential, and molecular subtyping could be a key part of this evaluation.

Currently there are several trials examining the need for radiation therapy based on disease subtype.

IDEA Study (Individualized Decisions for Endocrine Therapy Alone)

In this prospective multicenter study, after the confirmation of a stage 1 invasive breast cancer, after BCS, hormone receptor–positive, HER2-negative patients with an Oncotype DX RS ≤18 could be included. The enrolled patients receive endocrine therapy alone without radiotherapy.[164]

PRECISION Trial (Profiling Early Breast Cancer for Radiotherapy Omission)

This trial is a prospective study performed on unifocal T1 (≤2 CM), ER-positive (≥10%), PR-positive, HER2-negative, grade 1 or 2, pN0 or pN0(i+) associated with a PAM 50 (Prosigna, Seattle, WA) low-risk score. All the participants undergo omission of radiation therapy and will receive adjuvant endocrine treatment.[165]

LUMINA

This prospective single-arm study aims to evaluate the risk of ipsilateral breast cancer recurrence after breast-conserving therapy without radiation. Patients included in the study are 55 years of age; tumors ≤2 cm; ductal, tubular, or mucinous disease; ER-positive and PR-positive; HER2-negative; node-negative; with negative margins.[166]

SUPREMO Trial

A randomized phase III trial assessing the role of chest wall irradiation in women with intermediate-risk breast cancer following mastectomy. This is a trial from the Medical Research Council/European Organization for Research and Treatment of Cancer not yet recruiting.[167]

SUMMARY

Luminal A cancers are associated with a better prognosis and an LRR that occurs more frequently after 5 or 10 years from diagnosis. Although the expression of ER and PR receptors overlaps between luminal A and luminal B cancers, it is critical to identify luminal B breast cancers because this subgroup is associated with a worse prognosis and could benefit from additional local and systemic treatment. HER2-positive cancers have improved outcomes in both local and systemic control with targeted therapies. TNBC remains a clinical challenge, and several clinical trials are ongoing in attempts to identify mechanisms to help improve outcomes for this patient subgroup. The increasing prognostic and predictive information obtained from both prospective and retrospective studies on molecular subtypes will allow clinicians to customize treatment in terms of surgery, regional and systemic therapy, and follow-up. Implementing knowledge about tumor biology allows clinicians to distinguish high-risk versus favorable, low-risk disease subtypes through several different criteria. Further investigations will be necessary to potentially change guidelines regarding treatments offered for the local-regional control of breast cancer.

REFERENCES

1. Perou CM, Sorlie T, Eisen MB, et al. Molecular portraits of human breast tumours. Nature 2000;406(6797):747–52.
2. Sorlie T, Perou CM, Tibshirani R, et al. Gene expression patterns of breast carcinomas distinguish tumor subclasses with clinical implications. Proc Natl Acad Sci 2001;98(19):10869–74.
3. Nielsen TO, Hsu FD, Jensen K, et al. Immunohistochemical and clinical characterization of the basal-like subtype of invasive breast carcinoma. Clin Cancer Res 2004;10(16):5367–74.
4. Millar EKA, Graham PH, O'Toole SA, et al. Prediction of local recurrence, distant metastases, and death after breast-conserving therapy in early-stage invasive breast cancer using a five-biomarker panel. J Clin Oncol 2009;27(28):4701–8.
5. Voduc KD, Cheang MCU, Tyldesley S, et al. Breast cancer subtypes and the risk of local and regional relapse. J Clin Oncol 2010;28(10):1684–91.
6. Kyndi M, Sørensen FB, Knudsen H, et al. Estrogen receptor, progesterone receptor, HER-2, and response to postmastectomy radiotherapy in high-risk breast cancer: the Danish Breast Cancer Cooperative Group. J Clin Oncol 2008;26(9):1419–26.
7. Gabos Z, Thoms J, Ghosh S, et al. The association between biological subtype and locoregional recurrence in newly diagnosed breast cancer. Breast Cancer Res Treat 2010;124(1):187–94.
8. Metzger-Filho O, Sun Z, Viale G, et al. Patterns of recurrence and outcome according to breast cancer subtypes in lymph node-negative disease: results from international breast cancer study group trials VIII and IX. J Clin Oncol 2013;31(25):3083–90.
9. Arvold ND, Taghian AG, Niemierko A, et al. Age, breast cancer subtype approximation, and local recurrence after breast-conserving therapy. J Clin Oncol 2011;29(29):3885–91.
10. Haffty BG, Yang Q, Reiss M, et al. Locoregional relapse and distant metastasis in conservatively managed triple negative early-stage breast cancer. J Clin Oncol 2006;24(36):5652–7.
11. Arpino G, Generali D, Sapino A, et al. Corrigendum to "Gene expression profiling in breast cancer: a clinical perspective" [The Breast 22 (2013) 109–120]. Breast 2016;25(2):86.
12. Reis-Filho JS, Pusztai L. Gene expression profiling in breast cancer: Classification, prognostication, and prediction. Lancet 2011;378(9805):1812–23.
13. ASCO guidelines on breast cancer. Available at: https://www.asco.org/practice-guidelines/quality-guidelines/guidelines/breast-cancer. Accessed January 17, 2017.
14. Gradishar WJ, Robert CH, Anderson BO, et al. NCCN Guidelines Version 1.2016 Breast Cancer Panel Members. Natl Compr Cancer Netw 2016. Available at: https://www.nccn.org. Accessed September 10, 2017.

15. Goldhirsch A, Winer EP, Coates AS, et al. Personalizing the treatment of women with early breast cancer: highlights of the St Gallen international expert consensus on the primary therapy of early breast Cancer 2013. Ann Oncol 2013;24(9):2206–23.

16. Cheang MC, Martin M, Nielsen TO, et al. Defining breast cancer intrinsic subtypes by quantitative receptor expression. Oncologist 2015;20(5):474–82.

17. Gerdes J, Schwab U, Lemke H, et al. Production of a mouse monoclonal antibody reactive with a human nuclear antigen associated with cell proliferation. Int J Cancer 1983;31(1):13–20.

18. Hennigs A, Riedel F, Gondos A, et al. Prognosis of breast cancer molecular subtypes in routine clinical care: a large prospective cohort study. BMC Cancer 2016;16(1):734.

19. Li Z, Hu P, Tu J, et al. Luminal B breast cancer: patterns of recurrence and clinical outcome. Oncotarget 2016;7(40):1–10.

20. Ehinger A, Malmström P, Bendahl P-O, et al. Histological grade provides significant prognostic information in addition to breast cancer subtypes defined according to St Gallen 2013. Acta Oncol 2017;56(1):68–74.

21. García Fernández A, Chabrera C, García Font M, et al. Differential patterns of recurrence and specific survival between luminal A and luminal B breast cancer according to recent changes in the 2013 St Gallen immunohistochemical classification. Clin Transl Oncol 2015;17(3):238–46.

22. Freedman GM, Fowble BL. Local recurrence after mastectomy or breast-conserving surgery and radiation. Oncology (Williston Park) 2000;14(11): 1561–81 [discussion: 1582–4].

23. Magee B, Swindell R, Harris M, et al. Prognostic factors for breast recurrence after conservative breast surgery and radiotherapy: results from a randomised trial. Radiother Oncol 1996;39(3):223–7.

24. Bouvet M, Babiera GV, Tucker SL, et al. Does breast conservation therapy in young women with breast cancer adversely affect local disease control and survival rate? The M. D. Anderson Cancer Center Experience. Breast J 1997;3(4): 169–75.

25. Van Dongen JA, Voogd AC, Fentiman IS, et al. Long-term results of a randomized trial comparing breast-conserving therapy with mastectomy: European organization for research and treatment of cancer 10801 trial. J Natl Cancer Inst 2000;92(14):1143–50.

26. Jager JJ, Volovics L, Schouten LJ, et al. Loco-regional recurrences after mastectomy in breast cancer: prognostic factors and implications for postoperative irradiation. Radiother Oncol 1999;50(3):267–75.

27. Obedian E, Haffty BG. Negative margin status improves local control in conservatively managed breast cancer patients. Cancer J Sci Am 2000;6(1):28–33.

28. Touboul E, Buffat L, Belkacémi Y, et al. Local recurrences and distant metastases after breast-conserving surgery and radiation therapy for early breast cancer. Int J Radiat Oncol Biol Phys 1999;43(1):25–38.

29. Pisansky TM, Ingle JN, Schaid DJ, et al. Patterns of tumor relapse following mastectomy and adjuvant systemic therapy in patients with axillary lymph node-positive breast cancer. Impact of clinical, histopathologic, and flow cytometric factors. Cancer 1993;72(4):1247–60.

30. O'Rourke S, Galea MH, Morgan D, et al. Local recurrence after simple mastectomy. Br J Surg 1994;81(3):386–9.

31. Voogd AC, Peterse JL, Crommelin MA, et al. Histological determinants for different types of local recurrence after breast-conserving therapy of invasive breast cancer. Eur J Cancer 1999;35(13):1828–37.

32. Wilson LD, Beinfield M, McKhann CF, et al. Conservative surgery and radiation in the treatment of synchronous ipsilateral breast cancers. Cancer 1993;72(1): 137–42.

33. Borger J, Kemperman H, Hart A, et al. Risk factors in breast-conservation therapy. J Clin Oncol 1994;12:653–60.

34. Recht A, Gray R, Davidson NE, et al. Locoregional failure 10 years after mastectomy and adjuvant chemotherapy with or without tamoxifen without irradiation: experience of the Eastern Cooperative Oncology Group. J Clin Oncol 1999; 17(6):1689–700.

35. Harris JR, Schnitt SJ, Park CC, et al. Outcome at 8 years after breast-conserving surgery and radiation therapy for invasive breast cancer: influence of margin status and systemic therapy on local recurrence. J Clin Oncol 2000;18(8): 1668–75.

36. Fisher B, Dignam J, Bryant J, et al. Five versus more than five years of tamoxifen therapy for breast cancer patients with negative lymph nodes and estrogen receptor-positive tumors. J Natl Cancer Inst 1996;88(21):1529–42.

37. Fisher B, Anderson S, Redmond CK, et al. Reanalysis and results after 12 years of follow-up in a randomized clinical trial comparing total mastectomy with lumpectomy with or without irradiation in the treatment of breast cancer. N Engl J Med 1995;333(22):1456–61.

38. Fisher B, Anderson S, Bryant J, et al. Twenty-year follow-up of a randomized trial comparing total mastectomy, lumpectomy, and lumpectomy plus irradiation for the treatment of invasive breast cancer. N Engl J Med 2002;347(16):1233–41.

39. Overgaard M, Jensen M-B, Overgaard J, et al. Postoperative radiotherapy in high-risk postmenopausal breast-cancer patients given adjuvant tamoxifen: Danish Breast Cancer Cooperative Group DBCG 82c randomised trial. Lancet 1999;353(9165):1641–8.

40. Ragaz J, Olivotto IA, Spinelli JJ, et al. Locoregional radiation therapy in patients with high-risk breast cancer receiving adjuvant chemotherapy: 20-year results of the British Columbia Randomized Trial. JNCI J Natl Cancer Inst 2005;97(2): 116–26.

41. Abe O, Abe R, Enomoto K, et al. Effects of radiotherapy and of differences in the extent of surgery for early breast cancer on local recurrence and 15-year survival: an overview of the randomised trials. Lancet 2005;366(9503):2087–106.

42. Early Breast Cancer Trialists' Collaborative Group (EBCTCG). Effects of chemotherapy and hormonal therapy for early breast cancer on recurrence and 15-year survival: an overview of the randomised trials. Lancet 2005;365(9472): 1687–717.

43. Early Breast Cancer Trialists' Collaborative Group (EBCTCG) EBCTCG, Davies C, Godwin J, Gray R, et al. Relevance of breast cancer hormone receptors and other factors to the efficacy of adjuvant tamoxifen: patient-level meta-analysis of randomised trials. Lancet 2011;378(9793):771–84.

44. Colleoni M, Viale G, Zahrieh D, et al. Chemotherapy is more effective in patients with breast cancer not expressing steroid hormone receptors: a study of preoperative treatment. Clin Cancer Res 2004;10(19):6622–8.

45. Ring A, Smith I, Ashley S, et al. Oestrogen receptor status, pathological complete response and prognosis in patients receiving neoadjuvant chemotherapy for early breast cancer. Br J Cancer 2004;91(12):2012–7.

46. Lange CA. Challenges to defining a role for progesterone in breast cancer. Steroids 2008;73(9–10):914–21.
47. Chlebowski RT, Hendrix SL, Langer RD, et al. Influence of estrogen plus progestin on breast cancer and mammography in healthy postmenopausal women: The women's health initiative randomized trial. JAMA 2003;289(24):3243–53.
48. Clarke RB. Steroid receptors and proliferation in the human breast. Steroids 2003;68:789–94.
49. Pichon M-F, Pallud C, Brunet M, et al. Relationship of presence of progesterone receptors to prognosis in early breast cancer. Cancer Res 1980;40(SEPTEMBER): 3357–60.
50. Mohsin SK, Weiss H, Havighurst T, et al. Progesterone receptor by immunohistochemistry and clinical outcome in breast cancer: a validation study. Mod Pathol 2004;17(12):1545–54.
51. Bardou VJ, Arpino G, Elledge RM, et al. Progesterone receptor status significantly improves outcome prediction over estrogen receptor status alone for adjuvant endocrine therapy in two large breast cancer databases. J Clin Oncol 2003;21(10):1973–9.
52. Harvey JM, Clark GM, Osborne CK, et al. Estrogen receptor status by immunohistochemistry is superior to the ligand-binding assay for predicting response to adjuvant endocrine therapy in breast cancer. J Clin Oncol 1999;17(5):1474–81.
53. Schiff R, Osborn CK, FS. Clinical aspects of estrogen and progesterone receptors. In: Harris JR, Lippman ME, Morrow M, Osbourne CK, editors. Diseases of the Breast, 4th edition. Philadelphia: Wolters Kluwer Lippincott Williams and Wilkins; 2012. p. 408–30.
54. Hammond MEH, Hayes DF, Dowsett M, et al. American Society of Clinical Oncology/College of American Pathologists guideline recommendations for immunohistochemical testing of estrogen and progesterone receptors in breast cancer. Arch Pathol Lab Med 2010;134(7):e48–72.
55. Harris GC, Denley HE, Pinder SE, et al. Correlation of histologic prognostic factors in core biopsies and therapeutic excisions of invasive breast carcinoma. Am J Surg Pathol 2003;27(1):11–5.
56. Hamilton PW, Bankhead P, Wang Y, et al. Digital pathology and image analysis in tissue biomarker research. Methods 2014;70(1):59–73.
57. Stålhammar G, Fuentes Martinez N, Lippert M, et al. Digital image analysis outperforms manual biomarker assessment in breast cancer. Mod Pathol 2016;2(4):1–12.
58. Lakhani SR, Ellis IO, Schnitt SJ, et al. World Health Organization (WHO) Classification of Breast Tumours, 4th edition, IARC WHO Classification of Tumours. Geneva (Switzerland): WHO Press; 2012.
59. Farmer P, Bonnefoi H, Becette V, et al. Identification of molecular apocrine breast tumours by microarray analysis. Oncogene 2005;24(29):4660–71.
60. Vera-Badillo FE, Templeton AJ, De Gouveia P, et al. Androgen receptor expression and outcomes in early breast cancer: a systematic review and meta-analysis. J Natl Cancer Inst 2014;106(1):djt319.
61. Lehmann-Che J, Hamy A-S, Porcher R, et al. Molecular apocrine breast cancers are aggressive estrogen receptor negative tumors overexpressing either HER2 or GCDFP15. Breast Cancer Res 2013;15(3):R37.
62. Wieduwilt MJ, Moasser MM. The epidermal growth factor receptor family: biology driving targeted therapeutics. Cell Mol Life Sci 2008;65(10):1566–84.
63. Slamon DJ, Clark GM, Wong SG, et al. Human breast cancer: correlation of relapse and survival with amplification of the HER-2/neu oncogene. Science 1987;235(4785):177–82.

64. Pegram MD, Konecny G, Slamon DJ. The molecular and cellular biology of HER2/neu gene amplification/overexpression and the clinical development of herceptin (trastuzumab) therapy for breast cancer. Cancer Treat Res 2000;103:57–75.

65. Wolff A, Hammond M, Hicks D, et al. Recommendations for human epidermal growth factor receptor 2 testing in breast cancer: American Society of Clinical Oncology/College of American Pathologists clinical practice guideline update. J Clin Oncol 2013;31(31):3997–4013.

66. Gerdes J, Li L, Schlueter C, et al. Immunobiochemical and molecular biologic characterization of the cell proliferation-associated nuclear antigen that is defined by monoclonal antibody Ki-67. Am J Pathol 1991;138(4):867–73.

67. Trihia H, Murray S, Price K, et al. Ki-67 expression in breast carcinoma: its association with grading systems, clinical parameters, and other prognostic factors–a surrogate marker? Cancer 2003;97(5):1321–31.

68. de Azambuja E, Cardoso F, de Castro G, et al. Ki-67 as prognostic marker in early breast cancer: a meta-analysis of published studies involving 12,155 patients. Br J Cancer 2007;96(10):1504–13.

69. Stuart-Harris R, Caldas C, Pinder SE, et al. Proliferation markers and survival in early breast cancer: a systematic review and meta-analysis of 85 studies in 32,825 patients. Breast 2008;17(4):323–34.

70. Jonat W, Arnold N. Is the Ki-67 labelling index ready for clinical use? Ann Oncol 2011;22(3):500–2.

71. DeCensi A, Guerrieri-Gonzaga A, Gandini S, et al. Prognostic significance of Ki-67 labeling index after short-term presurgical tamoxifen in women with ER-positive breast cancer. Ann Oncol 2011;22(3):582–7.

72. Keshgegian AA, Cnaan A. Proliferation markers in breast carcinoma. Mitotic figure count, S-phase fraction, proliferating cell nuclear antigen, Ki-67 and MIB-1. Am J Clin Pathol 1995;104(1):42–9.

73. Clahsen PC, van de Velde CJ, Duval C, et al. The utility of mitotic index, oestrogen receptor and Ki-67 measurements in the creation of novel prognostic indices for node-negative breast cancer. Eur J Surg Oncol 1999;25(4):356–63.

74. Cheang MCU, Chia SK, Voduc D, et al. Ki67 index, HER2 status, and prognosis of patients with luminal B breast cancer. J Natl Cancer Inst 2009;101(10): 736–50.

75. Inwald EC, Klinkhammer-Schalke M, Hofstädter F, et al. Ki-67 is a prognostic parameter in breast cancer patients: results of a large population-based cohort of a cancer registry. Breast Cancer Res Treat 2013;139(2):539–52.

76. Dowsett M, Smith IE, Ebbs SR, et al. Prognostic value of Ki67 expression after short-term presurgical endocrine therapy for primary breast cancer. JNCI J Natl Cancer Inst 2007;99(2):167–70.

77. Nishimura R, Osako T, Okumura Y, et al. Clinical significance of Ki-67 in neoadjuvant chemotherapy for primary breast cancer as a predictor for chemosensitivity and for prognosis. Breast Cancer 2010;17(4):269–75.

78. Vuong D, Simpson PT, Green B, et al. Molecular classification of breast cancer. Virchows Arch 2014;465(1):1–14.

79. Carey LA, Perou CM, Livasy CA, et al. Race, breast cancer subtypes, and survival in the Carolina Breast Cancer Study. JAMA 2006;295(21):2492–502.

80. Subik K, Lee JF, Baxter L, et al. The expression patterns of ER, PR, HER2, CK5/6, EGFR, KI-67 and AR by immunohistochemical analysis in breast cancer cell lines. Breast Cancer (Auckl) 2010;4(1):35–41.

81. Prat A, Cheang MCU, Martín M, et al. Prognostic significance of progesterone receptor-positive tumor cells within immunohistochemically defined luminal A breast cancer. J Clin Oncol 2013;31(2):203–9.

82. Sorlie T, Tibshirani R, Parker J, et al. Repeated observation of breast tumor subtypes in independent gene expression data sets. Proc Natl Acad Sci U S A 2003;100(14):8418–23.

83. Koboldt DC, Fulton RS, McLellan MD, et al. Comprehensive molecular portraits of human breast tumours. Nature 2012;490(7418):61–70.

84. Prat A, Carey LA, Adamo B, et al. Molecular features and survival outcomes of the intrinsic subtypes within HER2-positive breast cancer. JNCI J Natl Cancer Inst 2014;106(8):dju152.

85. Staaf J, Ringnér M, Vallon-Christersson J, et al. Identification of subtypes in human epidermal growth factor receptor 2–positive breast cancer reveals a gene signature prognostic of outcome. J Clin Oncol 2010;28(11):1813–20.

86. Fountzilas G, Dafni U, Bobos M, et al. Differential response of immunohistochemically defined breast cancer subtypes to anthracycline-based adjuvant chemotherapy with or without paclitaxel. PLoS One 2012;7(6):e37946. Aziz SA, ed.

87. Kneubil MC, Brollo J, Botteri E, et al. Breast cancer subtype approximations and loco-regional recurrence after immediate breast reconstruction. Eur J Surg Oncol 2013;39(3):260–5.

88. Vici P, Pizzuti L, Natoli C, et al. Triple positive breast cancer: a distinct subtype? Cancer Treat Rev 2015;41(2):69–76.

89. De Laurentiis M, Arpino G, Massarelli E, et al. A meta-analysis on the interaction between HER-2 expression and response to endocrine treatment in advanced breast cancer. Clin Cancer Res 2005;11(13):4741–8.

90. Dowsett M, Allred C, Knox J, et al. Relationship between quantitative estrogen and progesterone receptor expression and human epidermal growth factor receptor 2 (HER-2) status with recurrence in the arimidex, tamoxifen, alone or in combination trial. J Clin Oncol 2008;26(7):1059–65.

91. Osborne CK, Schiff R. Mechanisms of endocrine resistance in breast cancer. Annu Rev Med 2011;62(1):233–47.

92. Shou J, Massarweh S, Osborne CK, et al. Mechanisms of tamoxifen resistance: increased estrogen receptor-HER2/neu cross-talk in ER/HER2-positive breast cancer. J Natl Cancer Inst 2004;96(12):926–35.

93. Alqaisi A, Chen L, Romond E, et al. Impact of estrogen receptor (ER) and human epidermal growth factor receptor-2 (HER2) co-expression on breast cancer disease characteristics: implications for tumor biology and research. Breast Cancer Res Treat 2014;148(2):437–44.

94. Lehmann BD, Bauer JA, Chen X, et al. Identification of human triple-negative breast cancer subtypes and preclinical models for selection of targeted therapies. J Clin Invest 2011;121(7):2750–67.

95. Reis-Filho JS, Weigelt B, Fumagalli D, et al. Molecular profiling: moving away from tumor philately. Sci Transl Med 2010;2(47):47ps43.

96. Weigelt B, Baehner FL, Reis-Filho JS. The contribution of gene expression profiling to breast cancer classification, prognostication and prediction: a retrospective of the last decade. J Pathol 2010;220(2):263–80.

97. Desmedt C, Sotiriou C. Proliferation: the most prominent predictor of clinical outcome in breast cancer. Cell Cycle 2006;5(19):2198–202.

98. Pusztai L, Broglio K, Andre F, et al. Effect of molecular disease subsets on disease-free survival in randomized adjuvant chemotherapy trials for estrogen receptor-positive breast cancer. J Clin Oncol 2008;26(28):4679–83.

99. Wirapati P, Sotiriou C, Kunkel S, et al. Meta-analysis of gene expression profiles in breast cancer: toward a unified understanding of breast cancer subtyping and prognosis signatures. Breast Cancer Res 2008;10(4):R65.

100. Iwamoto T, Bianchini G, Booser D, et al. Gene pathways associated with prognosis and chemotherapy sensitivity in molecular subtypes of breast cancer. JNCI J Natl Cancer Inst 2011;103(3):264–72.

101. Buyse M, Loi S, van't Veer L, et al. Validation and clinical utility of a 70-gene prognostic signature for women with node-negative breast cancer. JNCI J Natl Cancer Inst 2006;98(17):1183–92.

102. Desmedt C, Piette F, Loi S, et al. Strong time dependence of the 76-gene prognostic signature for node-negative breast cancer patients in the TRANSBIG multicenter independent validation series. Clin Cancer Res 2007;13(11): 3207–14.

103. Drukker CA, Bueno-de-Mesquita JM, Retèl VP, et al. A prospective evaluation of a breast cancer prognosis signature in the observational RASTER study. Int J Cancer 2013;133(4):929–36.

104. Cardoso F, van't Veer LJ, Bogaerts J, et al. 70-Gene signature as an aid to treatment decisions in early-stage breast cancer. N Engl J Med 2016;375(8):717–29.

105. Paik S, Shak S, Tang G, et al. A multigene assay to predict recurrence of tamoxifen-treated, node-negative breast cancer. N Engl J Med 2004;351(27): 2817–26.

106. Dowsett M, Cuzick J, Wale C, et al. Prediction of risk of distant recurrence using the 21-gene recurrence score in node-negative and node-positive postmenopausal patients with breast cancer treated with anastrozole or tamoxifen: a TransATAC Study. J Clin Oncol 2010;28(11):1829–34.

107. Albain KS, Barlow WE, Shak S, et al. Prognostic and predictive value of the 21-gene recurrence score assay in postmenopausal women with node-positive, oestrogen-receptor-positive breast cancer on chemotherapy: a retrospective analysis of a randomised trial. Lancet Oncol 2010;11(1):55–65.

108. Harris LN, Ismaila N, McShane LM, et al. Use of biomarkers to guide decisions on adjuvant systemic therapy for women with early-stage invasive breast cancer: American Society of Clinical Oncology Clinical Practice Guideline. J Clin Oncol 2016;34(10):1134–50.

109. Tang G, Shak S, Paik S, et al. Comparison of the prognostic and predictive utilities of the 21-gene Recurrence Score assay and Adjuvant! for women with node-negative, ER-positive breast cancer: results from NSABP B-14 and NSABP B-20. Breast Cancer Res Treat 2011;127(1):133–42.

110. Mamounas EP, Tang G, Fisher B, et al. Association between the 21-gene recurrence score assay and risk of locoregional recurrence in node-negative, estrogen receptor-positive breast cancer: results from NSABP B-14 and NSABP B-20. J Clin Oncol 2010;28(10):1677–83.

111. Habel LA, Shak S, Jacobs MK, et al. A population-based study of tumor gene expression and risk of breast cancer death among lymph node-negative patients. Breast Cancer Res 2006;8(3):R25.

112. Elkhuizen PH, van de Vijver MJ, Hermans J, et al. Local recurrence after breast-conserving therapy for invasive breast cancer: high incidence in young patients and association with poor survival. Int J Radiat Oncol 1998;40(4):859–67.

113. Fowble BL, Schultz DJ, Overmoyer B, et al. The influence of young age on outcome in early stage breast cancer. Int J Radiat Oncol Biol Phys 1994; 30(1):23–33.

114. van Werkhoven E, Hart G, Tinteren HV, et al. Nomogram to predict ipsilateral breast relapse based on pathology review from the EORTC 22881-10882 boost versus no boost trial. Radiother Oncol 2011;100(1):101–7.

115. Moran MS, Schnitt SJ, Giuliano AE, et al. Society of Surgical Oncology–American Society for Radiation Oncology consensus guideline on margins for breast-conserving surgery with whole-breast irradiation in stages I and II invasive breast cancer. Int J Radiat Oncol 2014;88(3):553–64.

116. Jones HA, Antonini N, Hart AAM, et al. Impact of pathological characteristics on local relapse after breast-conserving therapy: a subgroup analysis of the EORTC boost versus no boost trial. J Clin Oncol 2009;27(30):4939–47.

117. Gage I, Schnitt SJ, Nixon AJ, et al. Pathologic margin involvement and the risk of recurrence in patients treated with breast-conserving therapy. Cancer 1996; 78(9):1921–8.

118. Jagsi R, Raad RA, Goldberg S, et al. Locoregional recurrence rates and prognostic factors for failure in node-negative patients treated with mastectomy: implications for postmastectomy radiation. Int J Radiat Oncol Biol Phys 2005; 62(4):1035–9.

119. Nielsen HM, Overgaard M, Grau C, et al. Loco-regional recurrence after mastectomy in high-risk breast cancer–risk and prognosis. An analysis of patients from the DBCG 82 b&c randomization trials. Radiother Oncol 2006;79(2):147–55.

120. Recht A, Comen EA, Fine RE, et al. Postmastectomy radiotherapy: an American Society of Clinical Oncology, American Society for Radiation Oncology, and Society of Surgical Oncology focused guideline update. Pract Radiat Oncol 2016; 6(6):e219–34.

121. Abdulkarim BS, Cuartero J, Hanson J, et al. Increased risk of locoregional recurrence for women with T1-2N0 triple-negative breast cancer treated with modified radical mastectomy without adjuvant radiation therapy compared with breast-conserving therapy. J Clin Oncol 2011;29(21):2852–8.

122. Clarke M, Collins R, Darby S, et al. Effects of radiotherapy and of differences in the extent of surgery for early breast cancer on local recurrence and 15-year survival: an overview of the randomised trials. Lancet 2005;366(9503): 2087–106.

123. Su Y-L, Li S-H, Chen Y-Y, et al. Post-mastectomy radiotherapy benefits subgroups of breast cancer patients with T1-2 tumor and 1-3 axillary lymph node(s) metastasis. Radiol Oncol 2014;48(3):314–22.

124. Metcalfe K, Lynch HT, Ghadirian P, et al. Contralateral breast cancer in *BRCA1* and *BRCA2* mutation carriers. J Clin Oncol 2004;22(12):2328–35.

125. Garcia-Etienne CA, Barile M, Gentilini OD, et al. Breast-conserving surgery in BRCA1/2 mutation carriers: are we approaching an answer? Ann Surg Oncol 2009;16(12):3380–7.

126. Tsoutsou PG, Vozenin M-C, Durham A-D, et al. How could breast cancer molecular features contribute to locoregional treatment decision making? Crit Rev Oncol Hematol 2017;110:43–8.

127. Sanpaolo P, Barbieri V, Genovesi D. Prognostic value of breast cancer subtypes on breast cancer specific survival, distant metastases and local relapse rates in conservatively managed early stage breast cancer: a retrospective clinical study. Eur J Surg Oncol 2011;37(10):876–82.

128. García Fernández A, Chabrera C, García Font M, et al. Mortality and recurrence patterns of breast cancer patients diagnosed under a screening programme versus comparable non-screened breast cancer patients from the same population: analytical survey from 2002 to 2012. Tumor Biol 2014;35(3):1945–53.

129. Jatoi I, Anderson WF, Jeong J-H, et al. Breast cancer adjuvant therapy: time to consider its time-dependent effects. J Clin Oncol 2011;29(17):2301–4.

130. van der Leij F, Elkhuizen PHM, Bartelink H, et al. Predictive factors for local recurrence in breast cancer. Semin Radiat Oncol 2012;22(2):100–7.

131. Haffty BG. Molecular and genetic markers in the local-regional management of breast cancer. Semin Radiat Oncol 2002;12(4):329–40.

132. Albert JM, Gonzalez-Angulo AM, Guray M, et al. Estrogen/progesterone receptor negativity and HER2 positivity predict locoregional recurrence in patients with T1a,bN0 breast cancer. Int J Radiat Oncol 2010;77(5):1296–302.

133. Nguyen PL, Taghian AG, Katz MS, et al. Breast cancer subtype approximated by estrogen receptor, progesterone receptor, and HER-2 is associated with local and distant recurrence after breast-conserving therapy. J Clin Oncol 2008; 26(14):2373–8.

134. Lowery AJ, Kell MR, Glynn RW, et al. Locoregional recurrence after breast cancer surgery: a systematic review by receptor phenotype. Breast Cancer Res Treat 2012;133(3):831–41.

135. Romond EH, Perez EA, Bryant J, et al. Trastuzumab plus adjuvant chemotherapy for operable HER2-positive breast cancer. N Engl J Med 2005; 353(16):1673–84.

136. Haffty BG, Brown F, Carter D, et al. Evaluation of HER-2 neu oncoprotein expression as a prognostic indicator of local recurrence in conservatively treated breast cancer: a case-control study. Int J Radiat Oncol Biol Phys 1996;35(4): 751–7.

137. Elkhuizen PH, Voogd AC, van den Broek LC, et al. Risk factors for local recurrence after breast-conserving therapy for invasive carcinomas: a case-control study of histological factors and alterations in oncogene expression. Int J Radiat Oncol Biol Phys 1999;45(1):73–83.

138. Pierce LJ, Merino MJ, D'Angelo T, et al. Is c-erb B-2 a predictor for recurrent disease in early stage breast cancer? Int J Radiat Oncol Biol Phys 1994;28(2): 395–403.

139. Panoff JE, Hurley J, Takita C, et al. Risk of locoregional recurrence by receptor status in breast cancer patients receiving modern systemic therapy and post-mastectomy radiation. Breast Cancer Res Treat 2011;128(3):899–906.

140. Yin W, Jiang Y, Shen Z, et al. Trastuzumab in the adjuvant treatment of HER2-positive early breast cancer patients: a meta-analysis of published randomized controlled trials. PLoS One 2011;6(6):e21030.

141. Pietras RJ, Poen JC, Gallardo D, et al. Monoclonal antibody to HER-2/neu receptor modulates repair of radiation- induced DNA damage and enhances radiosensitivity of human breast cancer cells overexpressing this oncogene. Cancer Res 1999;59:1347–55.

142. Fehrenbacher L, Capra AM, Quesenberry CP, et al. Distant invasive breast cancer recurrence risk in human epidermal growth factor receptor 2-positive T1a and T1b node-negative localized breast cancer diagnosed from 2000 to 2006: a cohort from an integrated health care delivery system. J Clin Oncol 2014;32(20):2151–8.

143. Malone KE, Begg CB, Haile RW, et al. Population-based study of the risk of second primary contralateral breast cancer associated with carrying a mutation in BRCA1 or BRCA2. J Clin Oncol 2010;28(14):2404–10.

144. Tun N, Villani G, Ong K, et al. Risk of having BRCA1 mutation in high-risk women with triple-negative breast cancer: a meta-analysis. Clin Genet 2014;85(1):43–8.

145. Bessonova L, Taylor TH, Mehta RS, et al. Risk of a second breast cancer associated with hormone-receptor and HER2/neu status of the first breast cancer. Cancer Epidemiol Biomarkers Prev 2011;20(2):389–96.

146. Kumar P, Aggarwal R. An overview of triple-negative breast cancer. Arch Gynecol Obstet 2016;293(2):247–69.

147. Wang J, Xie X, Wang X, et al. Locoregional and distant recurrences after breast conserving therapy in patients with triple-negative breast cancer: a meta-analysis. Surg Oncol 2013;22(4):247–55.

148. Moran MS. Radiation therapy in the locoregional treatment of triple-negative breast cancer. Lancet Oncol 2015;16(3):e113–22.

149. Huang EH, Tucker SL, Strom EA, et al. Predictors of locoregional recurrence in patients with locally advanced breast cancer treated with neoadjuvant chemotherapy, mastectomy, and radiotherapy. Int J Radiat Oncol 2005;62(2):351–7.

150. Levy A, Borget I, Bahri M, et al. Loco-regional control after neo-adjuvant chemotherapy and conservative treatment for locally advanced breast cancer patients. Breast J 2014;20(4):381–7.

151. Mamounas EP, Anderson SJ, Dignam JJ, et al. Predictors of locoregional recurrence after neoadjuvant chemotherapy: results from combined analysis of National Surgical Adjuvant Breast and Bowel Project B-18 and B-27. J Clin Oncol 2012;30(32):3960–6.

152. von Minckwitz G, Untch M, Blohmer J-U, et al. Definition and impact of pathologic complete response on prognosis after neoadjuvant chemotherapy in various intrinsic breast cancer subtypes. J Clin Oncol 2012;30:1796–804.

153. Liedtke C, Mazouni C, Hess KR, et al. Response to neoadjuvant therapy and long-term survival in patients with triple-negative breast cancer. J Clin Oncol 2008;26(8):1275–81.

154. Swisher SK, Vila J, Tucker SL, et al. Locoregional control according to breast cancer subtype and response to neoadjuvant chemotherapy in breast cancer patients undergoing breast-conserving therapy. Ann Surg Oncol 2016;23(3):749–56.

155. Peterson DJ, Truong PT, Sadek BT, et al. Locoregional recurrence and survival outcomes by type of local therapy and trastuzumab use among women with node-negative, HER2-positive breast cancer. Ann Surg Oncol 2014;21(11):3490–6.

156. Kiess AP, McArthur HL, Mahoney K, et al. Adjuvant trastuzumab reduces locoregional recurrence in women who receive breast-conservation therapy for lymph node-negative, human epidermal growth factor receptor 2-positive breast cancer. Cancer 2012;118(8):1982–8.

157. Donker M, van Tienhoven G, Straver ME, et al. Radiotherapy or surgery of the axilla after a positive sentinel node in breast cancer (EORTC 10981-22023 AMAROS): a randomised, multicentre, open-label, phase 3 non-inferiority trial. Lancet Oncol 2014;15(12):1303–10.

158. Giuliano AE, McCall L, Beitsch P, et al. Locoregional recurrence after sentinel lymph node dissection with or without axillary dissection in patients with sentinel lymph node metastases. Ann Surg 2010;252(3):423–6.

159. Giuliano AE, Ballman K, McCall L, et al. Locoregional recurrence after sentinel lymph node dissection with or without axillary dissection in patients with sentinel lymph node metastases. Ann Surg 2016;264(3):413–20.
160. Morrow M. Rethinking the local therapy of breast cancer: integration of biology and anatomy. Ann Surg Oncol 2015;22(10):3168–73.
161. Olivotto IA, Truong PT, Chua B. Postmastectomy radiation therapy: who needs it? J Clin Oncol 2004;22(21):4237–9.
162. Goldhirsch A, Glick JH, Gelber RD, et al. Meeting highlights: international consensus panel on the treatment of primary breast cancer. J Natl Cancer Inst 1998;90(21):1601–8.
163. Jwa E, Shin KH, Lim HW, et al. Identification of risk factors for locoregional recurrence in breast cancer patients with nodal stage N0 and N1: who could benefit from post-mastectomy radiotherapy? PLoS One 2015;10(12):e0145463. St-Pierre Y, ed.
164. The IDEA Study (Individualized Decisions for Endocrine Therapy Alone). Available at: https://clinicaltrials.gov/show/NCT02400190.
165. The PRECISION Trial (Profiling Early Breast Cancer for Radiotherapy Omission): A Phase II study of breast-conserving surgery without adjuvant radiotherapy for favorable-risk breast cancer. Available at: https://clinicaltrials.gov/ct2/show/NCT02653755.
166. A Prospective Cohort Study evaluating risk of local recurrence following breast conserving surgery and endocrine therapy in low risk luminal a breast cancer - Full Text View - ClinicalTrials.gov. Available at: https://clinicaltrials.gov/ct2/show/NCT01791829.
167. Radiation therapy or standard therapy in treating women with stage II breast cancer who have undergone mastectomy. Available at: https://clinicaltrials.gov/ct2/show/NCT00966888.

Neoadjuvant Endocrine Therapy: Who Benefits Most?

Julie Grossman, MD[a], Cynthia Ma, MD, PhD[a], Rebecca Aft, MD, PhD[b],*

KEYWORDS

- Neoadjuvant endocrine therapy • Estrogen receptor–positive breast cancer
- Neoadjuvant chemotherapy • Aromatase inhibitors

KEY POINTS

- Neoadjuvant endocrine therapy (NET) can be used to downstage breast cancers in postmenopausal women with estrogen receptor–positive tumors.
- NET can be used in selected premenopausal women and is often combined with ovarian suppression.
- Complete pathologic responses are infrequent with NET; however, residual disease does not imply poor prognosis.
- NET as a single agent is less effective than in combination with trastuzumab in patients with human epidermal growth factor receptor 2 (HER2)-overexpressing tumors.
- Aromatase inhibitors are more effective than tamoxifen for downstaging with NET.

OVERVIEW

Neoadjuvant treatment of breast cancer has been established as an important strategy for understanding prognosis, biomarker evaluation, and targeted therapeutics development. Neoadjuvant treatment allows for real-time evaluation of drug efficacy by assessment of in vivo sensitivity as well as insight into the molecular alterations associated with tumor response through analysis of serial tumor biopsies. Neoadjuvant chemotherapy (NCT) has been incorporated into clinical practice for downstaging tumors for less extensive surgery and for assessing tumor response, which is associated with prognosis.[1] Similar to NCT, neoadjuvant endocrine therapy (NET) can downstage tumors and provide information on the tumor endocrine responsiveness. NET, however, has been less frequently incorporated into practice due to the slow tumor response requiring prolonged therapy as well as the less defined prognostic information that is obtained after treatment.[2] NET was initially limited to elderly

The authors have nothing to disclose.

[a] Department of Medicine, Washington University, 660 South Euclid Avenue, St Louis, MO 63110, USA; [b] Department of Surgery, Washington University, 660 South Euclid Avenue, St Louis, MO 63110, USA
* Corresponding author.
E-mail address: Aftr@wudosis.wustl.edu

postmenopausal women with large tumors who were poor candidates for NCT or surgery.[3–6] More recently, the ability to identify early endocrine responsiveness and the development of highly effective aromatase inhibitors (AIs) has resulted in a broader use of NET. The National Comprehensive Cancer Network guidelines suggests that appropriate candidates for NET are patients with estrogen receptor (ER)-rich tumors (Allred score of 7–8),[7] which correspond to luminal A or luminal B breast cancers.[8] Intensity of ER positivity, however, does not always parallel responsiveness to endocrine therapy.[9] Current research is directed toward identifying those patients who receive the greatest benefit from endocrine-directed therapy who could avoid cytotoxic chemotherapy. The most common class of drugs used for NET are the AIs (**Table 1**).

NEOADJUVANT ENDOCRINE THERAPY VERSUS NEOADJUVANT CHEMOTHERAPY

NET is as efficacious as NCT in downsizing tumors in patients with ER-positive disease, although the latter has more pathologic complete responses (pCRs).

Three randomized clinical trials have been conducted evaluating tumor response with NET versus NCT, all of which have shown similar response rates (**Table 2**).[10] In all 3 studies, toxicities were significantly higher with NCT versus NET. Although these studies demonstrate that downstaging is similar with both treatments, long-term outcome data are not readily available nor are defined biomarkers for patient selection for each therapy.

Semiglazov and colleagues[11] evaluated 239 postmenopausal women with ER-positive and/or progesterone receptor (PR)-positive breast cancer comparing anastrozole or exemestane for 3 months versus 4 cycles of doxorubicin plus paclitaxel every 21 days. Study endpoints included overall objective response determined by palpation, mammography, or ultrasound and the number of patients who qualified for breast-conserving surgery (BCS). The clinical objective response (determined by palpation) was similar in the endocrine group (64%) compared with chemotherapy (64%). Rates of pCR (3% vs 6%) and disease progression (9% vs 9%) did not differ significantly between the endocrine therapy or chemotherapy arms, respectively ($P>.05$). Rates of BCS were slightly higher in the endocrine group (33% vs 24%; $P = .058$). Overall, NET with AIs was better tolerated and resulted in rates similar to chemotherapy in overall objective response and BCS in postmenopausal women with ER-positive and/or PR-positive tumors.

The Grupo Español de Investigación en Cáncer de Mama (GEICAM) trial enrolled patients with operable breast cancer (T2/T3) and immunophenotypically defined luminal disease (ER-positive, PR-positive, HER2-negative, and cytokeratin 8/18-positive)[12]; 95 patients were randomized to either NCT (epirubicin plus cyclophosphamide [EC] × 4 cycles followed by docetaxel × 4 cycles) or NET (exemestane × 24 weeks, combined with goserelin in premenopausal patients). The primary endpoint was clinical response measured by MRI. The clinical response rate did not differ significantly between the arms. The clinical response was 66% for NCT (13% complete response and 53% partial response) and 48% for NET (6% complete response and 42% partial response) ($P = .07$). Three patients with NCT and 0 with NET achieved a pCR ($P =$ not significant). Mastectomy rates were similar in both arms (NCT, 47%, and NET, 56%; $P = .18$).

The Neoadjuvant Chemotherapy Versus Endocrine Therapy (NEOCENT) trial was a multicenter trial that enrolled 44 postmenopausal women, ages less than 70, with strongly ER-positive tumors, greater than 2 cm on mammogram or ultrasound, or nodal disease greater than 2 cm.[13] Patients were randomized to NCT with 6 cycles

Table 1
Neoadjuvant endocrine therapies

Drug Class	Mechanism	Method of Administration	Generic Name	Trade Name	Comments
Selective ER modulators	Binds to ER	Oral	Tamoxifen Torimefene	Nolvadex Fareston	
Antiestrogens	Selective ER down-regulator	Intramuscular injection	Fulvestrant[a]	Faslodex	Used in postmenopausal women only
AIs	Inhibits peripheral conversion of androgen to estrogen	Oral	Letrozole Anastrozole Exemestane	Femara Arimdex Aromasin	Reversible inhibitor — Steroidal inhibitor irreversibly binds to enzyme
Luteinizing hormone-releasing hormone agonists	Activates GnRH receptor, leads to paradoxic decrease in follicle-stimulating hormone/luteinizing hormone	Subcutaneous injection	Goserelin Leuprolide	Zolodex Lupron	Suppresses ovarian function in premenopausal women

[a] Fulvestrant is not approved for NET and for this use is investigational.

Table 2
Neoadjuvante endocrine therapy versus neoadjuvant chemotherapy trials

Source (Trial Name)	No.	Patient Characteristics at Baseline	Chemotherapy	Endocrine Therapy	Primary Endpoint	Response (per Primary Endpoint)	Rate of Breast Cancer Surgery
Semiglazov et al,[11] 2007	239	Postmenopausal ER+ and/or PR+, stages IIA to IIIB	Doxorubicin + paclitaxel × 4 cycles	Anastrozole or exemestane ×12 wk	CR by palpation	64% CT vs 64% ET	24% CT vs 33% ET
Alba et al,[12] 2012 (GEICAM/2006–03)	95	51% premenopausal ER+/PR+/HER2−/cytokeratin 8/18+	EC × 4 cycles, followed by docetaxel × 4 cycles	Exemestane (+ goserelin if premenopausal) × 24 wk	OR by RECIST criteria, MRI	66% CT vs 48% ET	47% CT vs 56% ET
Palmieri et al,[13] 2014 (NEOCENT)	44	Postmenopausal ER+	5-fluorouracil + EC ×6 cycles, switched to docetaxel after 3 cycles if stable disease or progressive disease	Letrozole ×18 wk	OR by ultrasound, mammography	55% CT vs 59% ET	55%CT Vs 68% ET

Abbreviations: CR, clinical response; CT, chemotherapy; EC, epirubicin + cyclophosphamide; ET, endocrine therapy; OR, objective response.

of fluorouracil with EC or letrozole NET daily for 18 weeks to 23 weeks. Radiological objective response was similar in both groups, 12/22 (55%) in the chemotherapy arm and 13/22 (59%) in the letrozole arm.

In all 3 studies, toxicity was significantly increased in patients treated with NCT. The GEICAM trial found grade III–IV toxicity was more frequent with NCT (47% NCT vs 9% NET; P = .0001). The most frequent toxicities observed from chemotherapy were alopecia (79%), grade 3/4 neutropenia (33%), and grade 2 neuropathy (30%). Findings were similar in the NEOCENT trial.[11–13]

PATIENT SELECTION: PREMENOPAUSAL WOMEN WITH ESTROGEN RECEPTOR–POSITIVE, HER2-POSITIVE TUMORS

Most NET trials have been conducted in postmenopausal women, which have demonstrated downsizing of tumors. The main NET trials often limit accrual to postmenopausal women with ER-positive breast cancers. These studies are discussed in more detail later. NET can be used to downstage ER-positive, HER2-positive tumors; however, the proliferation rate remains high. Data is limited for use of NET in premenopausal women and women with ER-positive, HER2-positive tumors.

Neoadjuvant Endocrine Therapy in Premenopausal Women

Premenopausal women have been excluded from most of the NET trials. Treatment of premenopausal women with AIs combined with ovarian suppression or ablation can lead, however, to profound estrogen suppression.[14] Using this combination, 2 clinical trials have demonstrated responses equivalent to that observed in the postmenopausal population[15] (**Table 3**).

Masuda and colleagues[16] conducted a randomized, prospective, double-blind NET trial enrolling 197 premenopausal patients. Women were treated with goserelin and were randomized to receive either anastrozole or tamoxifen (STAGE trial). Superior overall tumor response (complete response or partial response) was observed with anastrozole compared with tamoxifen (70.4% vs 50.5%; P = .004), which was confirmed by ultrasound and MRI.

In a small trial reported by Torrisi and colleagues,[17] 32 premenopausal women with T2–T4, N0 breast cancer were treated with letrozole in combination with a gonadotropin-releasing hormone (GnRH) analog. After 4 months of treatment, 1 patient (3%) had a complete clinical response, which was confirmed as a pCR at pathologic examination; 15 patients (47%) obtained a clinical and imaging partial response giving an overall response rate (ORR) of 50%; 16 patients had stable disease stable; and none of the patients progressed during treatment. BCS was performed in 15 patients (47%) whereas 17 patients (53%) underwent mastectomy.

Neoadjuvant Endocrine Treatment in Estrogen Receptor–Positive, HER2-Positive Disease

Both the Immediate Preoperative Anastrozole, Tamoxifen, or Combined With Tamoxifen (IMPACT) and the P024 trials (discussed later) included a small subpopulation of patients whose tumors overexpressed HER2.[18–20] The results indicated that HER2 expression did not impede tumor response to NET; however, the proliferation marker Ki67 was not significantly decreased, as is seen in patients with HER2-negative tumors.

In the P024 study, letrozole was found to be clinically more effective compared with tamoxifen for ER-positive, HER2-positive tumors.[18] In a reanalysis of tumor samples by fluorescence in situ hybridization, approximately 10% of the patients

Table 3
Randomized controlled neoadjuvant endocrine therapy trials (premenopausal women hormone receptor–positive breast cancer)

Source (Trial Name)	No.	Patient Characteristics at Baseline	Study Arms	Duration (wk)	Primary Endpoint	Response (per Primary Endpoint)	Rate of Breast Cancer Surgery
Masuda et al,[16] 2012 (STAGE)	197	ER+/HER2−, operable	A. Tamoxifen + goserelin B. Anastrozole + goserelin	24	OR by caliper measurements	A. 51% B. 70%	A. 68% B. 86%
Torrisi et al,[17] 2007	72	ER+ and/or PR+, operable	A. ECF B. ECF + GnRH analog	9 (≥3 cycles of chemotherapy)	OR by breast ultrasound + mammography and caliper measurements	A. 53% B. 64%	N/A

Abbreviation: ECF, epirubicin, cisplatin, fluorouracil.

were found to have HER2-positive disease, with a 44% to 47% response rate when assessed by mammography or ultrasound. Despite the observed clinical response, NET in the dual positive tumors was not associated with suppression of Ki67.[21]

In the IMPACT trial, 14% of assessed patients had overexpression of HER2.[19] In this subgroup, 7 (58%) of 12 patients treated with anastrozole responded compared with 2 (22%) of 9 patients treated with tamoxifen and 4 (31%) of 13 patients treated with the combination. Additionally, suppression of Ki67 after 2 weeks and 12 weeks was significantly greater with anastrozole than with tamoxifen ($P = .004$ and $P<.001$) but was similar between tamoxifen and the combination ($P = .600$ and $P = .912$).[22] Although the patient population and treatment duration differed between the P024 and the IMPACT studies, the trend in favor of anastrozole reflects that observed with letrozole and reinforces the hypothesis that AIs may be more effective than tamoxifen in the treatment of ER-positive early breast cancer that also overexpresses HER2.

THE MOST EFFICACIOUS ENDOCRINE AGENT

Several trials have been conducted to identify the optimal drug for NET. From these studies the greatest response rates have been observed using AIs (**Table 4**).

Tamoxifen Versus Aromatase Inhibitors

Three randomized clinical trials have compared tamoxifen with AIs for tumor response in postmenopausal women (see **Table 4**). In the P024 study, 4 months of letrozole was compared with tamoxifen in a double-blind, randomized, multicenter study in women with hormone receptor (HR)-positive tumors who were ineligible for BCS. Letrozole was found more effective than tamoxifen in terms of clinical and radiologic (ultrasound and mammography) response rates and in relation to rates of BCS. The IMPACT trial and Preoperative Arimidex Compared to Tamoxifen (PROACT) trial found no significant difference in ORR between treatment with AIs versus tamoxifen.[20,23] A meta-analysis of these studies, including a total of 1160 patients, indicated superior outcomes in terms of clinical objective response rate and breast cancer therapy (BCT) rates with AI compared with tamoxifen.

Comparison of Aromatase Inhibitors

The Z1031 trial was designed to determine which AI (anastrozole, letrozole, or exemestane) should be recommended for future testing against chemotherapy in the neoadjuvant setting.[24] This was a phase II trial that recruited 377 postmenopausal women with clinical stage 2/3 HR-positive disease to receive an AI for 4 months before surgery. No statistical difference in clinical response or surgical outcome was observed between the 3 arms. A major finding was that half of the patients who were considered candidates for mastectomy or were inoperable before neoadjuvant AI had successful BCT.[24]

Selective Estrogen Receptor Down-Regulators Versus Aromatase Inhibitors

Fulvestrant, a selective ER down-regulator, has been evaluated in 2 trials compared with anastrozole. Quenel-Tueux and colleagues[25] studied 108 postmenopausal women with histologically confirmed nonmetastatic breast cancer, ER positive and/or progesterone-receptor positive, not eligible for BCS at baseline, who were HER2 positive or HER2 negative. The objective response rate determined by clinical palpation was 58.9% in the anastrozole arm and 53.8% in the fulvestrant arm. Both drugs were found effective neoadjuvant treatments for

Table 4
Randomized controlled neoadjuvant endocrine therapy trials (postmenopausal women with hormone receptor–positive breast cancer)

Source (Trial Name)	No.	Patient Characteristics at Baseline	Neoadjuvant Endocrine Therapy	Duration (wk)	Primary Endpoint	Response (per Primary Endpoint)	Rate of Breast Cancer Surgery
Eiermann et al,[20] 2001 (P024)	337	ER+ and/or PR+, none eligible for BCS (14% deemed inoperable)	A. Tamoxifen B. Letrozole	16	CR by palpation	A. 36% B. 55%	A. 35% B. 45%
Smith et al,[19] 2005 (IMPACT)	330	ER+, operable (96 eligible for BCS) Locally advanced	A. Tamoxifen B. Anastrozole C. Anastrozole + tamoxifen	12	OR by caliper measurements	A. 36% B. 37% C. 39%	A. 31% B. 44% C. 24%
Cataliotti et al,[24] 2006 (PROACT)	451	ER+ and/or PR+, operable or potentially operable (386 would require mastectomy or were deemed inoperable) Locally advanced	A. Tamoxifen B. Anastrozole	12	OR by ultrasound measurements	A. 35% B. 40%	A. 31 % B. 43%
Ellis et al,[23] 2011 (Z1031)	374	ER+, eligible for mastectomy or inoperable clinical stages II–III	A. Exemestane B. Letrozole C. Anastrozole	16–18	OR by clinical assessment	A. 63% B. 75% C. 69%	A. 48% B. 42% C. 64%
Lerebours et al,[26] 2016 (CARMINA 02)	116	ER+ and/or PR+/HER2−, operable, none eligible for BCS	A. Anastrozole B. Fulvestrant	16	CR by palpation	A. 53% B. 37%	A. 58% B. 50%
Quenel-Tueux et al,[25] 2015	120	ER+ and/or PR+, none eligible for BCS	A. Anastrozole B. Fulvestrant	24	CR by palpation	A. 59% B. 54%	A. 59% B. 50%

postmenopausal patients with large operable or locally advanced ER-positive breast cancers, making BCS a viable option for some women who were not eligible for it initially.

Most recently, showing similar findings, the French trial UNICANCER CARMINA 02[28] evaluated fulvestrant versus anastrozole in 116 postmenopausal women with ER-positive, HER2-negative, operable breast cancers. This was a multicenter, phase 2, randomized trial that evaluated clinical response rate after up to 6 months of endocrine treatment. The clinical response rates at 6 months were 52.6% with anastrozole and 36.8% with fulvestrant. BCS was performed for 57.6% versus 50% of patients treated with anastrozole versus fulvestrant, respectively. The relapse-free survival rates at 3 years were 94.9% with anastrozole and 91.2% with fulvestrant. Both drugs were found effective and well tolerated as NET in postmenopausal women with HR-positive/HER2-negative breast cancer with a trend toward better outcomes with anastrozole (**Table 4**).

DURATION OF TREATMENT

From the available data in studies of postmenopausal women, 4 months to 6 months of an AI seems optimal with modest persistent benefits thereafter (**Table 5**). The relatively slow downstaging with NET relates to the absence of any increase of apoptosis with endocrine therapy and the dependence of response on the antiproliferative effects of estrogen withdrawal.

Dixon and colleagues[27] investigated the potential benefits of prolonged treatment with neoadjuvant letrozole comparing a duration of 3 months versus longer than 3 months. At 3 months, 69.8% of patients had a partial or complete response. The response rate increased to 83.5% with prolonged letrozole treatment. Continuing letrozole beyond 3 months increased the number of women who initially required mastectomy or had locally advanced breast cancer who were subsequently suitable for breast conserving surgery from 60% at 3 months to 72%.

Llombart-Cussac and colleagues[28] evaluated the efficacy of letrozole over a period of 4 months to 1 year in postmenopausal women. The median time to objective response was 3.9 months and the median time to maximum response was 4.2 months, although 37.1% of patients achieved the maximal response within 6 months to 12 months.

Studies from Carpenter and colleagues[29] and Krainick-Strobel and colleagues[30] evaluated the duration of letrozole in patients initially unsuitable for BCS. Carpenter and colleagues[29] found patients suitable for surgery after 7.5 months, whereas Krainick-Strobel and colleagues[30] found that more than half of the patients will be eligible for BCS within 4 months of treatment with letrozole.[29,30]

Similar results were seen with exemestane. Fontein and colleauges[31] found an ORR of 59% at 3 months and 68% ORR at 6 months, although Hojo and colleagues[32] found responses comparable in both the 4-month and 6-month duration treatment groups. The response rates as assessed by clinical examination were 42.3% and 48.0% for 4 months and 6 months of treatment, respectively. Pathologic responses (minimal response or better) were observed in 19.2% and 32.0% of patients, and BCS was performed on 50.0% and 48.0% of patients from the 4-month and 6-month treatment groups, respectively.

The St Gallen International Expert Consensus has endorsed that treatment should be continued until maximal response. However, 4 months to 6 months of NET with an AI seems optimal with modest persistent benefits thereafter.[33]

Table 5
Duration of treatment

Study	No.	Patient Characteristics at Baseline	Neoadjuvant Endocrine Therapy	Duration (Months)	Outcome Measures	Response
Dixon et al,[27] 2009	182	Postmenopausal ER+, operable Large or locally advanced	Letrozole	3 vs >3	OR by caliper and ultrasound measurements	3 mo 70% ORR >3 mo 83% ORR 3 mo 60% BCS >3 mo 72% BCS
Llombart-cussac et al,[28] 2012	70	Postmenopausal ER+ and/or PR+	Letrozole	4–12	Optimal duration of treatment defined as the time required to attain the MR by clinical palpation	Median time to OR was 3.9 mo Median time to MR was 4.2 mo
Carpenter et al,[29] 2014	146	Postmenopausal ER+ and/or PR+, none eligible for BCS	Letrozole	3–12	Optimal duration of treatment that would allow BCS	Median time to achieve tumor response to allow BCS was 7.5 mo
Krainick-Strobel et al,[30] 2008	33	Postmenopausal ER+ and/or PR+, none eligible for BCS (only mastectomy)	Letrozole	4–8	OR (by clinical examination, mammography, and ultrasound) and decisions regarding BCS	4 mo 55% ORR 8 mo 24% ORR 4 mo 71% BCS >4 mo 80% BCS
Fontein et al,[31] 2014	102	Postmenopausal ER+	Exemestane	3 vs 6	CR (by palpation) at 3 and 6 mo	3 mo 59% ORR >3 mo 68% ORR 3 mo 62% BCS >3 mo 71% BCS
Hojo et al,[32] 2013	52	Postmenopausal ER+ and/or PR+	Exemestane	4 vs 6	CR (by palpation) and decisions regarding BCS	4 mo 42% ORR 6 mo 48% ORR 4 mo 50% BCS 6 mo 48% BCS

Abbreviations: CR, clinical response; MR, maximal response; ORR, objective response rate.

PREDICTORS OF RESPONSE AND SURROGATE ENDPOINTS
Pathologic Complete Response

pCR has been the outcome most often assessed in NCT studies, and it is defined as having no residual invasive carcinoma and no in situ carcinoma in the breast and lymph nodes. pCR is rarely achieved, however, in NET trials in patients with ER-positive, HER2-negative disease.[34,35] Although pCR may be observed in 40% to 50% of patients receiving NCT, it is rare after NET (<2%).[36] Thus, it has not been used a predictor of long-term survival in this population. Several studies have attempted to define prognostic markers for NET (**Table 6**).

Ki67

Immunohistochemical assessment of cells staining for the nuclear antigen Ki67, a nuclear marker expressed in all phases of the cell cycle other than the G0 phase,[37] measures the proportion of cells proliferating in a tumor. NET has been shown to cause a significant reduction in Ki67, with the degrees of suppression related to the level of ER expression. Ki67 levels after NET have been shown to be prognostic.[38] The IMPACT trial demonstrated that high Ki67 expression levels after 2 weeks of NET was associated with a poorer recurrence-free survival. DeCensi and colleagues[39] found that after 4 weeks of treatment, Ki67 was a good predictor of recurrence-free survival and overall survival. The risk of death was 5.5-times higher in patients with postdrug Ki67 greater than or equal to 20% than in those with Ki67 less than 20%.[36] At this time, there is an ongoing UK national trial, Perioperative Endocrine Therapy: Individualizing Care (POETIC), which aims to validate whether changes in Ki67 or in gene expression after 2 weeks of treatment with AI may predict long-term outcome and may help select patients who may need further adjuvant chemotherapy.[40]

Preoperative Endocrine Prognostic Index

The preoperative endocrine prognostic index (PEPI) was generated from the P024 study. After 4 months of NET with either letrozole or tamoxifen, it was found that Ki67, pathologic tumor size, nodal status, and ER status were independently associated with recurrence-free survival and overall survival. The Allred scoring system, a clinical instrument based on the percentage of cells that stain by immunohistochemistry for ER (on a scale of 0–5) and the intensity of that staining (on a scale of 0–3, for a possible total score of 8), was used to quantify ER status. Patients with a PEPI score of 0 (pT1/2, pN0, Ki67 ≤2.7%, and Allred >2) have been found to have an extremely low

| Table 6 | |
| **Markers to predict outcome** | |
Markers	**Predicts**
Ki67 on treatment	Endocrine resistance and recurrence risk
PEPI score	Recurrence-free survival
4-gene panel (ER, PR, HER2, and Ki67)	Distinguishes luminal A from luminal B breast cancer subtypes
PAM 50	Relapse-free survival
Oncotype DX 21-gene recurrence score	Recurrence score
	Distant disease recurrence and benefit of adjuvant chemotherapy in ER^+ breast cancer

relapse risk; 3.7% at 5 years versus 14.4% at 5 years for PEPI greater than 0, based on 119 cases[36] (**Table 7**).

Multigene Expression Tests

Prediction analysis of microarray 50
Prediction analysis of microarray 50 (PAM50) is 50-gene quantitative polymerase chain reaction assay developed to identify the intrinsic biological breast cancer subtypes (luminal A/B, HER2 enriched, basal like). A risk of recurrence score is derived from the expression profile of the genes, with special weighting given to a set of proliferation-associated genes, with tumor size also included. The commercial Prosigna test (Nano String Technologies, Inc.) is Food and Drug Administration approved as a prognostic predictor of postmenopausal women with lymph node–negative, HR-positive, and HER2-negative breast cancer treated with adjuvant endocrine therapy.[41]

Four-gene panel
Recently it has been demonstrated that a 4-marker immunohistochemistry panel (ER, PR, HER2, and Ki67), distinguishes luminal A from luminal B breast cancer subtypes and may be useful in selecting adjuvant therapy and predicting long-term outcomes.[42] Although it is an inexpensive test with prognostic utility, the lack of reproducibility of the 4-marker immunohistochemistry panel is problematic. Differences can occur because of variability in several factors, including fixation, antigen retrieval, reagents, and interpretation.[43]

Oncotype DX 21-gene recurrence score
Oncotype DX is an reverse transcription–polymerase chain reaction–based multi-gene analysis that predicts recurrence in ER-positive, lymph node–negative breast

Table 7
The preoperative endocrine prognostic index score

Pathology, Biomarker Status	Recurrence-free Survival		Breast Cancer–specific Survival	
	Hazard Ratio	Points	Hazard Ratio	Points
Tumor size				
T 1/2	—	0	—	0
T 3/4	2.8	3	4.4	3
Node status				
Negative	—	0	—	0
Positive	3.2	3	3.9	3
Ki67 level				
0%–2.7%	—	0	—	0
>2.7%–7.3%	1.3	1	1.4	1
>7.3%–19.7%	1.7	1	2.0	2
>19.7%–53.1%	2.2	2	2.7	3
>53.1%	2.9	3	3.8	3
ER status, Allred score				
0–2	2.8	3	7.0	3
3–8	—	0	—	0

cancer patients. It is composed of 21 genes, 16 cancer-related genes and 5 housekeeping genes (proliferation: Ki67, STK15, survivin, cyclin B1, and MYBL2; invasion: stromolysin 3 and cathepsin L2; HER2: GRB7 and HER2; estrogen: ER, PR, Bcl-2, and SCUBE2; and other: GSTM1, CD68, and BAG1) and 5 reference genes ([beta]-actin, GAPDH, RPLPO, GUS, and TFRC). The cumulative result of this test is the recurrence score (0–100), which can be categorized into low-risk (score <18), intermediate-risk (score 18–30), and high-risk (score ≥31) groups.[44]

WHO BENEFITS MOST?

The advantage of the NET approach is the ability to assess clinical and molecular responses of an individual patient's tumor to an endocrine agent. It has been shown that evaluating biomarkers after a short course of NET can guide treatment. In the IMPACT trial,[38,45] pretreatment values of Ki67 have not been shown to be prognostic, whereas a decrease in Ki67 after 2 weeks of hormonal therapy seems to predict recurrence-free survival. The preoperative Window of Endocrine Therapy Provides Information to Increase Compliance (POWERPINC) study tested the impact of 1 week of tamoxifen on Ki67.[46] The decrease in proliferation was similar to that seen in other studies using 2 weeks of NET.[22] This strategy allows an early identification of high-risk patients with endocrine resistant tumors.[36]

The 21-gene recurrence score has also been shown to have predict value. Ueno and colleagues[47] evaluated pretreatment and post-treatment tumor tissue from patients with estrogen-positive tumors treated with neoadjuvant exemestane. The clinical response rate was 59% in patients with a low recurrence score compared with 20% in patients with a high recurrence score. Recurrence scores were highly correlated in the pretreatment and post-treatment samples.

In the Z1031 trial, PAM50 analysis identified AI-unresponsive nonluminal subtypes in 3% of patients with ER-rich cancers.[24] This will likely prove helpful in the future to exclude uncommon nonluminal intrinsically endocrine therapy–resistant tumors.

RESIDUAL DISEASE CONSEQUENCES

As discussed previously, achievement of pCR with preoperative endocrine therapy is rare. Although pCR is associated with improved outcomes in patients with ER-negative disease, it may not have an appreciable impact on outcomes in those with ER-positive disease.[48–50] Some investigators have shown that gene alterations after NET include decrease in proliferation genes and up-regulation of immune function and extracellular matrix remodeling genes.[51] These molecular changes may be more relevant endpoints in patients treated with NET.

There are currently several trials addressing the optimal treatment of patients with residual disease after NET. The New Primary Endocrine-therapy Origination Study (NEOS), a multicenter phase III randomized trial, will assess the need for adjuvant chemotherapy in postmenopausal women with stage T1c-T2N0M0, HR-positive tumors who responded to neoadjuvant letrozole.[52]

The Alliance for Clinical Trials in Oncology has an ongoing phase III neoadjuvant clinical trial (Alternate Approaches for Clinical Stage II or III Estrogen Receptor Positive Breast Cancer Neoadjuvant Treatment [ALTERNATE]), which will assess a biomarker treatment strategy to identify women at low risk of disease recurrence based on Ki67 after 2 and 12 weeks of NET and PEPI score at surgery after 6 months of NET.

FUTURE DIRECTIONS
Neoadjuvant Endocrine Therapy in Combination with Other Drugs

Endocrine therapy has been tested in combination with a variety of other drugs as neoadjuvant therapy in patients with breast cancer. The Celecoxib Anti-Aromatase Neoadjuvant (CAAN) trial evaluated the efficacy of combing an AI and cyclooxygenase-2 inhibitor as neoadjuvant therapy in postmenopausal patients with invasive hormone-sensitive breast cancer.[53] Patients were randomly assigned to receive exemestane plus celecoxib, exemestane, or letrozole. All groups showed clinical responses; however there was no significant difference in clinical response seen with the addition of celecoxib.

Baselga and colleagues[54] explored whether sensitivity to letrozole was enhanced with the mechanism target of rapamycin (mTOR) inhibitor, everolimus. Postmenopausal women with operable ER-positive breast cancer received neoadjuvant treatment with letrozole and either everolimus or placebo. The response rate by clinical palpation in the everolimus arm was higher than that with letrozole alone (68.1% v 59.1%). Furthermore, an antiproliferative response (reduction in Ki67 expression to natural logarithm of percentage positive Ki67 of <1 at day 15), occurred in 57% of patients in the everolimus arm and in 30% in the placebo arm ($P<.01$). Thus, everolimus increased letrozole efficacy in the neoadjuvant setting.

Lapatinib, a dual inhibitor of the tyrosine kinase activity of EGFR and HER2, in combination with letrozole was evaluated by Guarneri and colleagues[55] as neoadjuvant therapy in postmenopausal women with HR-positive/HER2-negative tumors. Patients received either letrozole plus lapatinib or letrozole plus placebo. The clinical response rates of both groups were similar, with the letrozole plus lapatinib combination group having slightly better response results (70% for letrozole + lapatinib and 63% for letrozole + placebo).

The NeoPalAna trial reported by Ma and colleagues[56] assessed the antiproliferative activity of the CDK4/6 inhibitor palbociclib in patients with clinical stage II/III, ER-positive, HER2-negative breast cancer. They received anastrozole daily for 4 weeks, followed by the addition of palbociclib daily for four 28-day cycles. Anastrozole was continued until surgery. The primary endpoint was complete cell-cycle arrest: central Ki67 $\leq 2.7\%$ (CCCA). The CCCA rate was significantly higher after adding palbociclib to anastrozole, demonstrating additional proliferation suppression with combination therapy (**Table 8**).

Current Ongoing Clinical Trials

NET has been used to downstage tumors prior to surgery, assess response for prognostic information, investigate mechanisms of endocrine resistance, and facilitate novel trial design. NET in postmenopausal women with locally advanced ER-positive breast cancer may result in a reduction in tumor size either improving the chances of BCT or rendering an inoperable tumor operable. Patients in neoadjuvant endocrine studies who switch to NCT after a poor response to endocrine therapy have low pCR rates, suggesting that AI resistance in ER-rich tumors is not associated with an enhanced chemotherapy response.[36]

The ability to identify good and poor responses to NET early in treatment provides a strategy to triage poor responders into clinical trials of targeted agents to address endocrine resistance. Multiple trials are ongoing that combine molecularly targeted agents with endocrine therapy in the neoadjuvant setting. NeoPalAna is enrolling the endocrine-resistant population based on high Ki67 on endocrine therapy to receive the combination of the CDK4/6 inhibitor palbociclib and anastrozole to

Table 8
Neoadjuvant endocrine therapy in combination with other drugs

Source (Trial Name)	No.	Patient Characteristics	Study Arms	Duration (Wk)	Primary Endpoint	Response (per Primary Endpoint)
Chow et al,[53] 2008 (CAAN)	82	Postmenopausal ER+ and/or PR+	A. Exemestane B. Exemestane + celecoxib C. Letrozole	12	OR by caliper measurements	A. 55% B. 59% C. 62%
Baselga et al,[54] 2009	270	Postmenopausal ER+, operable	A. Letrozole + everolimus B. Letrozole + placebo	16	CR by palpation	A. 68.1% B. 59.1%
Guarneri et al,[55] 2014	92	Post-menopausal HR+/HER2− operable	A. Letrozole + lapatinib B. Letrozole + placebo	24	OR by ultrasound measurements	A. 70% B. 63%
Ma et al,[56] 2017 (NeoPalAna)	50	ER+/HER2−	Anastrozole (+ goserelin if premenopausal) followed by palbociclib (C1D1) for four 28-d cycles	25	CCCA after adding palbociclib to anastrozole	C1D1 26% vs C1D15 87%

Abbreviations: C1D1, cycle 1 day 1; C1D15, cycle 1 day 15.

Table 9
Current ongoing clinical trials

Clinical Trial	Study Arms	Phase	Sponsor
Neoadjuvant Endocrine Therapy vs Chemotherapy in Premenopausal Patients With ER+ & HER2− Breast Cancer	A. Goserelin + tamoxifen + AI B. EC + fluorouracil	3	Peking University
Neoadjuvant Aromatase Inhibitor With Ovarian Suppression vs Chemotherapy in Premenopausal Breast Cancer Patients (COMPETE)	A. Goserelin + exemestane or anastrozole B. Docetaxel + EC	3	Ruijin Hospital
Letrozole Plus Ribociclib or Placebo as Neo-adjuvant Therapy in ER-positive, HER2-negative Early Breast Cancer (FELINE)	A. Letrozole + placebo B. Letrozole + ribociclib	2	University of Kansas Medical Center
Endocrine Treatment Alone for Elderly Patients With Estrogen Receptor Positive Operable Breast Cancer and Low Recurrence Score	A. Goserelin B. Anastrozole C. Exemestane D. Fulvestrant E. Tamoxifen	2	Washington University School of Medicine
Durvalumab and Endocrine Therapy in ER+/Her2− Breast Cancer After CD8+ Infiltration Effective Immune-Attractant Exposure (ULTIMATE)	A. Tremelimumab + exemestane B. Durvalumab + exemestane	2	UNICANCER
Fulvestrant and/or Anastrozole in Treating Postmenopausal Patients With Stage II-III Breast Cancer Undergoing Surgery	A. Fulvestrant + anastrozole B. Anastrozole C. Fulvestrant	3	Alliance for Clinical Trials in Oncology
Neoadjuvant Letrozole Plus Metformin vs Letrozole Plus Placebo for ER-positive Postmenopausal Breast Cancer	A. Letrozole + metformin B. Letrozole + placebo	2	Seoul National University Hospital
Neoadjuvant Lenvatinib Combined With Letrozole in Hormone Receptor Positive Breast Cancer	A. Lenvatinib + letrozole	1, 2	National University Hospital, Singapore
A Trial of Neoadjuvant Everolimus Plus Letrozole vs FEC in Women With ER-positive, HER2-negative Breast Cancer	A. Everolimus + letrozole B. Fluorouracil + EC	2	Sun Yat-Sen Memorial Hospital of Sun Yat-Sen University
Neoadjuvant Trastuzumab and Letrozole for Postmenopausal Women (HERAKLES)	A. Trastuzumab + letrozole	2	Gangnam Severance Hospital
A Phase II Randomized Study Evaluating the Biological and Clinical Effects of the Combination of Palbociclib With Letrozole as Neoadjuvant Therapy in Post-Menopausal Women With Estrogen-Receptor Positive Primary Breast Cancer (PALLET)	A. Letrozole + palbociclib	2	NSABP Foundation Inc

Data from https://clinicaltrials.gov/. Accessed May 1, 2017.

overcome endocrine resistance (NCT01723774). An in-depth understanding of endocrine resistance mechanisms is needed for successful development of targeted agents. The neoadjuvant setting provides a unique research platform to expedite the evaluation of novel therapeutics to improve the outcome of patients with ER-positive breast cancer (**Table 9**).

SUMMARY

NET can be effective at downstaging patients with ER-positive tumors and identifying those tumors that are endocrine sensitive and endocrine resistant. The optimal prognostic markers for stratification are under investigation. Use of NET allows the identification of patients with ER-positive tumors with a good response to endocrine therapy who might avoid chemotherapy and those who may benefit from additional treatment based on endocrine resistance.

REFERENCES

1. Chia YH, Ellis MJ, Ma CX. Neoadjuvant endocrine therapy in primary breast cancer: indications and use as a research tool. Br J Cancer 2010;103(6):759–64.
2. Chiba A, Hoskin TL, Heins CN, et al. Trends in neoadjuvant endocrine therapy use and impact on rates of breast conservation in hormone receptor-positive breast cancer: a national cancer data base study. Ann Surg Oncol 2017;24(2): 418–24.
3. Hind D, Wyld L, Reed MW. Surgery, with or without tamoxifen, vs tamoxifen alone for older women with operable breast cancer: cochrane review. Br J Cancer 2007;96(7):1025–9.
4. Preece PE, Wood RA, Mackie CR, et al. Tamoxifen as initial sole treatment of localised breast cancer in elderly women: a pilot study. Br Med J (Clin Res Ed) 1982;284(6319):869–70.
5. Horobin JM, Preece PE, Dewar JA, et al. Long-term follow-up of elderly patients with locoregional breast cancer treated with tamoxifen only. Br J Surg 1991;78(2): 213–7.
6. Bergman L, van Dongen JA, van Ooijen B, et al. Should tamoxifen be a primary treatment choice for elderly breast cancer patients with locoregional disease? Breast Cancer Res Treat 1995;34(1):77–83.
7. Gradishar WJ, Anderson BO, Balassanian R, et al. NCCN guidelines insights: breast cancer, version 1.2017. J Natl Compr Canc Netw 2017;15(4):433–51.
8. Cheang MC, Martin M, Nielsen TO, et al. Defining breast cancer intrinsic subtypes by quantitative receptor expression. Oncologist 2015;20(5):474–82.
9. Early Breast Cancer Trialists' Collaborative Group (EBCTCG), Davies C, Godwin J, Gray R, et al. Relevance of breast cancer hormone receptors and other factors to the efficacy of adjuvant tamoxifen: patient-level meta-analysis of randomised trials. Lancet 2011;378(9793):771–84.
10. Charehbili A, Fontein DBY, Kroep JR, et al. Neoadjuvant hormonal therapy for endocrine sensitive breast cancer: a systematic review. Cancer Treat Rev 2014;40(1):86–92.
11. Semiglazov VF, Semiglazov VV, Dashyan GA, et al. Phase 2 randomized trial of primary endocrine therapy versus chemotherapy in postmenopausal patients with estrogen receptor-positive breast cancer. Cancer 2007;110(2):244–54.
12. Alba E, Calvo L, Albanell J, et al. Chemotherapy (CT) and hormonotherapy (HT) as neoadjuvant treatment in luminal breast cancer patients: results from the

GEICAM/2006-03, a multicenter, randomized, phase-II study. Ann Oncol 2012; 23(12):3069–74.

13. Palmieri C, Cleator S, Kilburn LS, et al. NEOCENT: a randomised feasibility and translational study comparing neoadjuvant endocrine therapy with chemotherapy in ER-rich postmenopausal primary breast cancer. Breast Cancer Res Treat 2014; 148(3):581–90.

14. Stein RC, Dowsett M, Hedley A, et al. The clinical and endocrine effects of 4-hydroxyandrostenedione alone and in combination with goserelin in premenopausal women with advanced breast cancer. Br J Cancer 1990;62(4):679–83.

15. Gazet JC, Coombes RC, Ford HT, et al. Assesssment of the effect of pretreatment with neoadjuvant therapy on primary breast cancer. Br J Cancer 1996;73(6): 758–62.

16. Masuda N, Sagara Y, Kinoshita T, et al. Neoadjuvant anastrozole versus tamoxifen in patients receiving goserelin for premenopausal breast cancer (STAGE): a double-blind, randomised phase 3 trial. Lancet Oncol 2012;13(4):345–52.

17. Torrisi R, Bagnardi V, Pruneri G, et al. Antitumour and biological effects of letrozole and GnRH analogue as primary therapy in premenopausal women with ER and PgR positive locally advanced operable breast cancer. Br J Cancer 2007;97(6):802–8.

18. Ellis MJ, Coop A, Singh B, et al. Letrozole is more effective neoadjuvant endocrine therapy than tamoxifen for ErbB-1- and/or ErbB-2-positive, estrogen receptor-positive primary breast cancer: evidence from a phase III randomized trial. J Clin Oncol 2001;19(18):3808–16.

19. Smith IE, Dowsett M, Ebbs SR, et al. Neoadjuvant treatment of postmenopausal breast cancer with anastrozole, tamoxifen, or both in combination: the Immediate Preoperative Anastrozole, Tamoxifen, or Combined with Tamoxifen (IMPACT) multicenter double-blind randomized trial. J Clin Oncol 2005;23(22):5108–16.

20. Eiermann W, Paepke S, Appfelstaedt J, et al. Preoperative treatment of postmenopausal breast cancer patients with letrozole: a randomized double-blind multicenter study. Ann Oncol 2001;12:1527–32.

21. Ellis MJ, Tao Y, Young O, et al. Estrogen-independent proliferation is present in estrogen-receptor HER2-positive primary breast cancer after neoadjuvant letrozole. J Clin Oncol 2006;24(19):3019–25.

22. Dowsett M, Ebbs SR, Dixon JM, et al. Biomarker changes during neoadjuvant anastrozole, tamoxifen, or the combination: influence of hormonal status and HER-2 in breast cancer–a study from the IMPACT trialists. J Clin Oncol 2005; 23(11):2477–92.

23. Ellis MJ, Suman VJ, Hoog J, et al. Randomized phase II neoadjuvant comparison between letrozole, anastrozole, and exemestane for postmenopausal women with estrogen receptor-rich stage 2 to 3 breast cancer: clinical and biomarker outcomes and predictive value of the baseline PAM50-based intrinsic subtype–ACOSOG Z1031. J Clin Oncol 2011;29(17):2342–9.

24. Cataliotti L, Buzdar A, Noguchi S, et al. Comparison of anastrazole versus tamoxifen as preoperative therapy in postmenopausal women with hormone receptor-positive breast cancer: the pre-operative "Arimidex" compared to tamoxifen (PROACT) trial. Cancer 2006;106(10):2095–103.

25. Quenel-Tueux N, Debled M, Rudewicz J, et al. Clinical and genomic analysis of a randomised phase II study evaluating anastrozole and fulvestrant in postmenopausal patients treated for large operable or locally advanced hormone-receptor-positive breast cancer. Br J Cancer 2015;113(4):585–94.

26. Lerebours F, Rivera S, Mouret-Reynier M, et al. Randomized phase 2 neoadjuvant trial evaluating anastrozole and fulvestrant efficacy for postmenopausal, estrogen receptor–positive, human epidermal growth factor receptor 2–negative breast cancer patients: Results of the UNICANCER CARMINA 02 French trial (UCBG 0609). Cancer 2016;122:3032–40.

27. Dixon J, Renshaw L, Macaskill E, et al. Increase in response rate by prolonged treatment with neoadjuvant letrozole. Breast Cancer Res Treat 2009;113(1): 145–51.

28. Llombart-Cussac A, Guerrero Á, Galán A, et al. Phase II trial with letrozole to maximum response as primary systemic therapy in postmenopausal patients with ER/PgR [+] operable breast cancer. Clin Transl Oncol 2012;14(2):125–31.

29. Carpenter R, Doughty J, Cordiner C, et al. Optimum duration of neoadjuvant letrozole to permit breast conserving surgery. Breast Cancer Res Treat 2014; 144(3):569–76.

30. Krainick-Strobel UE, Lichtenegger W, Wallwiener D, et al. Neoadjuvant letrozole in postmenopausal estrogen and/or progesterone receptor positive breast cancer: a phase IIb/III trial to investigate optimal duration of preoperative endocrine therapy. BMC Cancer 2008;8(1):62.

31. Fontein DB, Charehbili A, Nortier JW, et al. Efficacy of six month neoadjuvant endocrine therapy in postmenopausal, hormone receptor-positive breast cancer patients–a phase II trial. Eur J Cancer 2014;50(13):2190–200.

32. Hojo T, Kinoshita T, Imoto S, et al. Use of the neo-adjuvant exemestane in postmenopausal estrogen receptor-positive breast cancer: a randomized phase II trial (PTEX46) to investigate the optimal duration of preoperative endocrine therapy. Breast 2013;22(3):263–7.

33. Goldhirsch A, Winer EP, Coates AS, et al. Personalizing the treatment of women with early breast cancer: highlights of the St Gallen International Expert Consensus on the Primary Therapy of Early Breast Cancer 2013. Ann Oncol 2013;24(9):2206–23.

34. Von Minckwitz G, Untch M, Blohmer J, et al. Definition and impact of pathologic complete response on prognosis after neoadjuvant chemotherapy in various intrinsic breast cancer subtypes. J Clin Oncol 2012;30(15):1796–804.

35. Tan MC, Al Mushawah F, Gao F, et al. Predictors of complete pathological response after neoadjuvant systemic therapy for breast cancer. Am J Surg 2009;198(4):520–5.

36. Ellis MJ, Suman VJ, Hoog J, et al. Ki67 proliferation index as a tool for chemotherapy decisions during and after neoadjuvant aromatase inhibitor treatment of breast cancer: results from the American College of Surgeons Oncology Group Z1031 Trial (Alliance). Clin Oncol 2017;35(10):1061–9.

37. Gerdes J, Lemke H, Baisch H, et al. Cell cycle analysis of a cell proliferation-associated human nuclear antigen defined by the monoclonal antibody Ki-67. J Immunol 1984;133(4):1710–5.

38. Dowsett M, Smith IE, Ebbs SR, et al, IMPACT Trialists Group. Prognostic value of Ki67 expression after short-term presurgical endocrine therapy for primary breast cancer. J Natl Cancer Inst 2007;99:167–70.

39. DeCensi A, Guerrieri-Gonzaga A, Gandini S, et al. Prognostic significance of Ki-67 labeling index after short-term presurgical tamoxifen in women with ER-positive breast cancer. Ann Oncol 2011;22(3):582–7.

40. Dowsett M, Smith I, Robertson J, et al. Endocrine therapy, new biologicals, and new study designs for presurgical Studies in breast cancer. J Natl Cancer Inst Monogr 2011;43:120–3.

41. Parker J, Mullins M, Cheang M, et al. Supervised risk predictor of breast cancer based on intrinsic subtypes. J Clin Oncol 2009;27(8):1160–7.

42. Cheang MC, Chia SK, Voduc D, et al. Ki67 index, HER2 status, and prognosis of patients with luminal B breast cancer. J Natl Cancer Inst 2009x;101(10):736–50.

43. Cuzick J, Dowsett M, Pineda S, et al. Prognostic value of a combined estrogen receptor, progesterone receptor, Ki-67, and human epidermal growth factor receptor 2 immunohistochemical score and comparison with the genomic health recurrence score in early breast cancer. J Clin Oncol 2011;29(32):4273–8.

44. Paik S, Shak S, Tang G, et al. A multigene assay to predict recurrence of tamoxifen-treated, node-negative breast cancer. N Engl J Med 2004;351: 2817–26.

45. Dowsett M, Nielsen TO, A'Hern R, et al, International Ki-67 in Breast Cancer Working Group. Assessment of Ki67 in breast cancer: recommendations from the International Ki67 in Breast Cancer working group. J Natl Cancer Inst 2011;103(22): 1656–64.

46. Cohen AL, Factor RE, Mooney K, et al. POWERPIINC (PreOperative Window of Endocrine TheRapy Provides Information to IncreaseCompliance) trial: Changes in tumor proliferation index and quality of life with 7 days of preoperative tamoxifen. Breast 2017;31:219–23.

47. Ueno T, Masuda N, Yamanaka T, et al. Evaluating the 21-gene assay Recurrence Score® as a predictor of clinical response to 24 weeks of neoadjuvant exemestane in estrogen receptor-positive breast cancer. Int J Clin Oncol 2014;19(4): 607–13.

48. Ring A, Smith I, Ashley S, et al. Oestrogen receptor status, pathological complete response and prognosis in patients receiving neoadjuvant chemotherapy for early breast cancer. Br J Cancer 2004;91:2012–7.

49. Liedtke C, Mazouni C, Hess K, et al. Response to neoadjuvant therapy and long-term survival in patients with triple-negative breast cancer. J Clin Oncol 2008;26: 1275–81.

50. Colleoni M, Gelber S, Coates AS, et al. Influence of endocrine-related factors on response to perioperative chemotherapy for patients with node-negative breast cancer. J Clin Oncol 2001;19:4141–9.

51. Arthur LM, Turnbull AK, Webber VL, et al. Molecular changes in lobular breast cancers in response to endocrine therapy. Cancer Res 2014;74(19):5371–6.

52. Iwata H. Neoadjuvant endocrine therapy for postmenopausal patients with hormone receptor-positive early breast cancer: a new concept. Breast Cancer 2011;18(2):92–7.

53. Chow LW, Yip AY, Loo WT, et al. Celecoxib anti-aromatase neoadjuvant (CAAN) trial for locally advanced breast cancer. J Steroid Biochem Mol Biol 2008; 111(1–2):13–7.

54. Baselga J, Semiglazov V, van Dam P, et al. Phase II randomized study of neoadjuvant everolimus plus letrozole compared with placebo plus letrozole in patients with estrogen receptor-positive breast cancer. J Clin Oncol 2009;27(16):2630–7.

55. Guarneri V, Generali DG, Frassoldati A, et al. Double-blind, placebo-controlled, multicenter, randomized, phase IIb neoadjuvant study of letrozole-lapatinib in postmenopausal hormone receptor-positive, human epidermal growth factor receptor 2-negative, operable breast cancer. J Clin Oncol 2014;32(10):1050–7.

56. Ma CX, Gao F, Luo J, et al. NeoPalAna: neoadjuvant palbociclib, a cyclin-dependent kinase 4/6 inhibitor, and anastrozole for clinical stage 2 or 3 estrogen receptor-positive breast cancer. Clin Cancer Res 2017;23(15):4055–65.

Triple-Negative Breast Cancer

Who Should Receive Neoadjuvant Chemotherapy?

Lubna N. Chaudhary, MD, MS, K. Hope Wilkinson, MD, MS,
Amanda Kong, MD, MS*

KEYWORDS

- Triple-negative breast cancer • Neoadjuvant chemotherapy
- Breast-conserving surgery

KEY POINTS

- Progress in the treatment of triple-negative breast cancer (TNBC) remains an important challenge.
- Given the aggressive biology and high risk of distant recurrence, systemic chemotherapy is warranted in most patients.
- Neoadjuvant chemotherapy benefits patients with locally advanced disease by downsizing the tumor and increasing the probability of breast-conserving surgery.
- Clinical and pathologic responses provide important prognostic information, which makes neoadjuvant therapy an attractive approach for all patients with TNBC.
- Clinical research in the neoadjuvant setting is focused on improvement in pathologic complete response rates and outcomes of patients with residual disease.

INTRODUCTION

With advances in genetic studies, breast cancer has been identified as a heterogeneous disease with distinct subtypes that respond variably to different therapies. The concept of classifying breast tumors into subtypes was first described by Perou and colleagues,[1] who used gene expression profiling and identified 4 subtypes, including estrogen receptor (ER)–positive luminal-like, basal-like (BL), human epidermal growth factor receptor 2 (HER2)-positive, and normal breast. Triple-negative breast cancer (TNBC) is commonly defined as the absence of estrogen, progesterone, and HER2 receptors (ER-negative, progesterone receptor [PR]-negative, and HER2-negative), with estrogen and progesterone negativity defined as less than 1% of tumor cells staining using the current American Society of Clinical Oncology (ASCO) and College of American Pathologists guidelines.[2] When TNBCs are evaluated

The author has nothing to disclose.
Department of Surgery, Medical College of Wisconsin, Milwaukee, WI, USA
* Corresponding author.
E-mail address: akong@mcw.edu

histopathologically, they are often, but not always, BL (approximately 85%).[3] Therefore, TNBCs are often erroneously thought of as interchangeable with the BL subtype although they are not the same entity. TNBC is a heterogeneous disease in itself and Lehmann and colleagues[4] identified 6 specific subtypes of TNBC using gene expression profiles from 21 breast cancer data sets, including 2 BLs (BL1 and BL2), an immunomodulatory, a mesenchymal, a mesenchymal stem–like, and a luminal androgen receptor (LAR). The investigators concluded that these subtypes of TNBC demonstrate distinct phenotypes with diverse gene expression patterns with variable sensitivity to different targeted therapies.

INCIDENCE AND CLINICAL PRESENTATION

Approximately 10% to 17% of breast cancers are classified as TNBCs based on standard immunohistochemical staining for ER, PR, and HER2.[5,6] In contrast to hormone receptor (HR)-positive tumors, they are more often high-grade invasive ductal carcinomas of no special type that have higher mitotic indices with central necrotic zones and lymphocytic infiltration.[7] They are more likely to present as a palpable mass[5,7,8] and tend to develop as interval breast cancers, which are invasive tumors that become clinically apparent between annual screening mammograms.[9,10] They are more responsive to chemotherapy compared with luminal tumors.

Despite their overall aggressive behavior, several studies have found that TNBCs are less likely to metastasize to the axillary lymph nodes.[5,11,12] In terms of metastatic disease, TNBCs more often spread to the brain and lungs.[5,13,14] Distant recurrences also tend to appear earlier than other subtypes. Dent and colleagues[15] studied a cohort of 1601 women with breast cancer of whom 180 had TNBC. They found that these women had an increased likelihood of death (hazard ratio 3.2; 95% CI, 2.3–4.5; $P<.001$) within 5 years of diagnosis compared with all other subtypes. They also demonstrated that the risk of distant recurrence peaked at approximately 3 years with a rapid decline thereafter compared with the other subtypes, where the risk of recurrence was constant. In a follow-up study, the same group also found that women with TNBC were 4 times more likely to experience a visceral metastasis within 5 years of diagnosis compared with all other subtypes.[14] Using the National Comprehensive Cancer Network (NCCN) Breast Cancer Outcomes Database, Lin and colleagues[5] found that TNBC was associated with worse breast cancer–specific survival (BCSS) and overall survival (OS) (hazard ratio for BCSS 2.99; 95% CI, 2.59–3.45; $P<.0001$; and hazard ratio for OS 2.72; 95% CI, 2.39–3.10; $P<.0001$) compared with HR-positive, HER2-negative tumors. TNBC was also associated with a dramatic increase in the risk of death within 2 years of diagnosis in this study, which likely reflects the tendency for these tumors to develop distant recurrence within this time period.

EPIDEMIOLOGY

TNBC disproportionately affects younger, premenopausal women.[5–8,16] In particular, those with a high body mass index are at higher risk.[5,17] The data regarding standard risk factors for the development of breast cancer, such as parity, oral contraceptive use, age at menarche, and their relationship to TNBC, are still not clear.[18]

TNBC is more frequently diagnosed in African American women as well as women of African descent compared with other breast cancer subtypes.[5,6,8,16,19] The Carolina Breast Cancer Study found that the BL breast cancer subtype was more prevalent among premenopausal African American women compared with postmenopausal African American women as well as women of other ethnicities of any age with a shorter survival compared with other subtypes.[16] Using California Cancer Registry data,

Bauer and colleagues[6] identified that TNBCs were more likely to be found in women under age 40 and non-Hispanic black or Hispanic women. These women had poorer survival compared with women with other breast cancer subtypes regardless of stage, although these women also belonged to a lower socioeconomic status.

Several studies have also confirmed that patients with BRCA1 mutations more often develop TNBC.[20,21] Approximately 60% to 90% of BRCA1-associated tumors and 16% to 23% of BRCA2-associated tumors are TNBC.[20–22] Only approximately 15% of TNBCs, however, are associated with a BRCA1 or BRCA2 mutation.[23]

ADJUVANT VERSUS NEOADJUVANT CHEMOTHERAPY

Despite the poor prognosis of TNBC, studies have demonstrated that TNBC is more responsive to chemotherapy than other molecular subtypes.[24–26] Because common treatments used for patients with HR-positive and/or HER2-positive breast cancers are ineffective in TNBC, both NCCN and the European Society for Medical Oncology (ESMO) guidelines recommend the use of third-generation chemotherapy.[27,28]

A series of large randomized clinical trials have established that adjuvant (after surgery) and neoadjuvant (before surgery) administration of the same chemotherapy regimen yields similar results in disease-free survival (DFS) and OS.[29] In the National Surgical Adjuvant Breast and Bowel Project (NSABP) B-18 trial, there was no survival benefit for receiving doxorubicin and cyclophosphamide in the neoadjuvant setting compared with the adjuvant setting.[30] NSABP B-27 compared AC with preoperative or postoperative docetaxel and showed a significant increase in pathologic complete responses (pCRs) with the addition of preoperative docetaxel (26% vs 13%; $P<.0001$), but there was no significant difference in DFS or OS.[31,32] A meta-analysis of 9 randomized clinical trials also demonstrated no difference in OS, disease progression, or distant recurrence for women with breast cancer receiving adjuvant versus neoadjuvant chemotherapy.[33]

There is a lack of robust prospective data in TNBC restricted trial populations. Most clinical data have been derived from retrospective exploratory subgroup analyses, which suggested high sensitivity to chemotherapy in TNBC. These studies established the efficacy of anthracycline and taxane–based regimens and formed the basis of more recent clinical trials, particularly in the neoadjuvant setting for TNBC patients.

Although subgroup analyses of some individual trials have indicated mixed results for anthracycline-based therapy in TNBC subpopulations, most studies indicate a favorable effect in TNBC, including a meta-analysis of 5 randomized clinical trials.[34,35] Findings from multiple subgroup analyses of large phase III adjuvant trials support a role for taxanes in the adjuvant treatment of TNBC.[36–40] At this time, an anthracycline and taxane–based regimen remains standard of care for TNBC patients. Nonanthracycline regimens, such as taxane with cyclophosphamide, may be an appropriate choice for some patients, such as older patients and those with considerable comorbidities and cardiac risks.

Benefits of Neoadjuvant Chemotherapy

Neoadjuvant chemotherapy, initially used only for locally advanced or inflammatory breast cancer, has become more common for patients with operable disease, especially in patients with TNBC.[30,31,41–45] This treatment approach allows more individuals to undergo breast-conserving surgery (BCS) and provides an assessment of response to treatment. In an era where individualization of therapy is highly valued, neoadjuvant chemotherapy allows the activity of novel agents or therapeutic combinations to be studied in vivo in a much shorter timeframe than with adjuvant trials.[46,47]

Surgical Outcomes

Neoadjuvant chemotherapy allows reduction of tumor volume in the primary tumor and the regional nodes, which can facilitate more options for surgical treatment. Several trials have demonstrated that tumors can be downsized with neoadjuvant chemotherapy, allowing for increased rates of BCS. In the NSABP B-18 trial, where patients were randomized to preoperative versus postoperative chemotherapy, lumpectomy was performed more frequently in the preoperative chemotherapy group compared with the postoperative group (67% vs 60%; $P = .002$).[48] In a retrospective study of 1242 patients treated at the Memorial Sloan Kettering Cancer Center with pathologic T1-2N0 TNBC, those who underwent BCS were compared with those who underwent total mastectomy without radiation. There was no significant difference in local recurrence, distant metastasis, overall recurrence, DFS, or OS between the 2 groups.[49] Although none of these patients received neoadjuvant chemotherapy, it can be extrapolated that similar results would be found in the neoadjuvant population because the NSABP trials established that there is no difference in survival based on the timing of chemotherapy delivery.

Pathologic Response to Chemotherapy

pCR is defined as the absence of residual invasive cancer on pathologic evaluation of the resected breast primary and regional lymph nodes after neoadjuvant therapy. Several neoadjuvant trials have shown that pCR predicts for long-term outcomes and is, therefore, a potential surrogate marker for DFS and OS. Achieving a pCR is more common in highly proliferating carcinomas like TNBC or HER2-positive tumors compared with luminal tumors.[50] A large pooled analysis comprised of 12 randomized clinical trials of neoadjuvant chemotherapy in breast cancer conducted by the Collaborative Trials in Neoadjuvant Breast Cancer international working group showed longer event-free survival (EFS) and OS in patients who achieved a pCR.[51] The association between pCR and long-term outcomes was strongest in patients with TNBC and in those with HER2-positive, HR-negative tumors who received trastuzumab.

Liedtke and colleagues[26] reported results from the MD Anderson Cancer Center for stages I to III breast cancer patients who received neoadjuvant chemotherapy. Patients with TNBC had significantly higher pCR rates compared with non-TNBC (22% vs 11%; $P = .034$), and those with a pCR had excellent survival, which was similar to non-TNBC patients. In contrast, patients with residual disease after chemotherapy had worse OS if they had TNBC compared with non-TNBC ($P<.0001$). A recently published cohort study with prospective follow-up of patients treated with an anthracycline and taxane–based neoadjuvant chemotherapy regimen demonstrated an estimated 10-year relapse-free survival of 86% for TNBC patients who achieved pCR versus only 23% for those with significant residual disease after chemotherapy.[52]

A summary of pCR rates from selected randomized clinical trials of neoadjuvant chemotherapy is shown in **Table 1**. In the GeparTrio trial, Huober and colleagues[53] reported a pCR rate of 38.9% in TNBC patients compared with 23.6% in HER2-positive disease and 11.2% in HR-positive patients. The attainment of a pCR predicted for improved DFS in TNBC patients (hazard ratio 6.67, $P<0.001$).[54] Similarly, in the Preoperative Epirubicin, Paclitaxel, Darbepoetin (PREPARE) trial, patients with a pCR had a significantly improved DFS rate (hazard ratio 2.27; $P = .001$).[55] The NeoAdjuvant Treatment (NATT) Trial study also showed significantly improved EFS and OS in patients with a pCR ($P = .03$ and $P = 0.04$, respectively).[56]

Overall, the available data suggest that pCR is associated with improved long-term outcomes and is an acceptable endpoint for neoadjuvant clinical trials. The pCR rates

Table 1
Selected randomized controlled trials of neoadjuvant chemotherapy in breast cancer

Study/Y	Tumor Size	Chemotherapy Regimen	Number of Patients Treated	Pathologic Complete Response (%)[b]	Pathologic Complete Response in Triple-Negative Breast Cancer (%)[b]
GeparDuo/2005[80]	T2–T3	AC-Doc vs ADoc	913	14.3% vs 7% (P<.001)	22.8% (P = .0001)
GeparTrio/2010[53]	T2–T4	TAC	2072	20.5%	38.9% (P = .0015)
GeparQuattro/2010[81]	T1–T4	EC-T	1421	22.3%	17.6%
Preoperative Epirubicin, Paclitaxel, Darbepoetin (PREPARE)/2011[82]	T2–T4	ddE-ddT-CMF vs EC-T	733	18.7% vs 13.2% (P = .04)	44.6% vs 30.4% (P = .12)
Investigation of Serial Studies to Predict Your Therapeutic Response With Imaging and Molecular Analysis (I-SPY) 1/2012[83]	≥3 cm	AC-T[a]	221	27%	35%
European Organisation for Research and Treatment of Cancer (EORTC) 10994/2014[84]	T2–T4	FEC-T vs Doc-EDoc	1289	18%	31%
NeoAdjuvant Treatment Trial (NATT)/2016[56,85]	T2–T4	TAC vs TC	96	17.6 vs 6.8% (P = .11)	15.4% vs 4.3% (P = .35)

Abbreviations: AC, doxorubicin/cyclophosphamide; CMF, C-cyclophosphamide, M-Methotrexate, F-5-flourouracil; dd, dose-dense; Doc, docetaxel; E, epirubicin; TAC, docetaxel/doxorubicin/cyclophosphamide; TC, taxane with cyclophosphamide.
[a] 95% patients received a taxane after AC.
[b] pCR comparisons between the 2 chemotherapy regimens used in that trial.

in TNBC range from approximately 30% to 40% with anthracycline and taxane–based regimens. Efforts to further maximize pCR rates are under way by assessing the addition of different chemotherapeutic agents to standard regimens, including drugs, such as capecitabine, 5-Fluorouracil, vinorelbine, bevacizumab, everolimus, gemcitabine, and platinum agents.

Role of Platinum Agents in Triple-Negative Breast Cancer

Preclinical data suggest that TNBC tumors are more sensitive to DNA-damaging agents, such as platinum analogs, because of deficiencies in the BRCA-associated DNA repair mechanism.[57]

The Cancer and Leukemia Group B (CALGB) 40603 trial[58] showed that the addition of carboplatin to the standard neoadjuvant regimen of dose dense AC and T significantly increased pCR rates in the breast (60% vs 44%; P = .0018) as well as the axilla (54% v 41%; P = .0029). This study was not powered to assess EFS or OS and did not demonstrate any significant differences in these measures, although EFS did trend in the direction expected for the increase in the pCR rate seen with the addition of carboplatin.

The GeparSixto 66 study used a novel chemotherapy regimen consisting of weekly paclitaxel, nonpegylated liposomal doxorubicin and bevacizumab for 18 weeks and administered carboplatin weekly.[59] In addition to the improvement in pCR rates (37% to 53% with carboplatin; $P = .005$), similar to what was observed in the CALGB 40603 trial, GeparSixto also showed an improvement in DFS, specifically in TNBC patients randomized to the carboplatin arm (85.8% with carboplatin and 76.1% without; hazard ratio for consistency in the paper (HR) = 0.56; $P = .035$).

At this time, the role of carboplatin in the neoadjuvant setting for TNBC remains controversial and it is unclear whether its potential benefits outweigh the increase in hematologic toxicities. Given the improvement in responses, however, it is reasonable to consider its addition in high risk patients. Clinical trials are ongoing to further evaluate the role of platinum agents in patients with both BRCA and non-BRCA mutated TNBCs (NCT02413320 and NCT02547987).

Response-Guided Therapy

Neoadjuvant trials allow rapid assessment of drug efficacy and could theoretically expedite development and approval of treatments for breast cancer.[60] Neoadjuvant chemotherapy provides the opportunity to discontinue or change treatment in cases of nonresponsiveness. It also provides the opportunity for additional adjuvant therapy in patients with significant residual disease after neoadjuvant chemotherapy. There are few data, however, with these approaches. Response-guided therapy is a promising strategy to optimize and individualize treatment of breast cancer.

The CREATE-X study, a phase III trial, randomized patients with HER2-negative breast cancer and residual invasive disease after neoadjuvant chemotherapy with an anthracycline and/or taxane to adjuvant treatment with capecitabine at 1250 mg/m^2 twice daily, 2 weeks on/1 week off, for up to 8 cycles.[61] The estimated 5-year DFS was 74.1% with capecitabine compared with 67.7% in the control arm ($P = .005$). OS rates were 89.2% and 83.9%, respectively ($P < .01$). The TNBC subgroup experienced a 42% reduction in risk of death with capecitabine. Although there were more adverse events with capecitabine use, it is reasonable to consider this approach in high risk patients with significant residual disease especially in TNBC patients where there are no other standard adjuvant therapy options after completion of neoadjuvant chemotherapy.

An ongoing phase III trial is evaluating the role of adjuvant platinum-based chemotherapy, capecitabine, or observation in TNBC patients with residual disease after neoadjuvant chemotherapy (NCT02445391). Other approaches, such as genomically directed therapy (NCT02101385), immunomodulatory agents (NCT02954874), and vaccine strategies (NCT02427581), are being assessed in clinical trials in patients with residual TNBC after neoadjuvant chemotherapy.

SMALL TUMORS

Patients with breast cancer who have T1a,b ($\leq$1-cm) node-negative tumors generally have an excellent prognosis, with BCSS at 10 years exceeding 95%.[62,63] Outcomes for these patients vary, however, by biologic subtype.[64–69] The potential benefit of chemotherapy in small TNBCs remains unclear.

In a series of 194 TNBC patients from Memorial Sloan Kettering Cancer Center, both local-regional and distant recurrence-free survival were similar in T1mic/T1a and T1b tumors (94.5% vs 95.5%, respectively; $P = .81$). There were no differences in outcomes based on receipt of chemotherapy (95.9 vs 94.5%).[70] A recently published prospective cohort study within the NCCN reported on clinical outcomes of 4113 women with T1a,b node-negative breast cancer of all subtypes with overall favorable prognosis.[71] For TNBCs, the 5-year distant relapse-free survival for T1a tumors was 93% without chemotherapy versus 100% with chemotherapy and for T1b tumors; it was 90% without chemotherapy compared with 96% with chemotherapy.

Patel et al.[72] recently reported survival outcomes in 13,065 patients with small TNBCs using the National Cancer Database. Tumor size was a strong predictor of survival. Compared with T1a tumors, hazard ratio for death was 1.43 (95% CI, 0.86–2.37) for T1b tumors and 3.00 (95% CI, 1.86–4.83) for T1c tumors. This study demonstrated a statistically significant 4-year OS benefit in patients with T1b and T1c tumors who received adjuvant chemotherapy compared with those who did not (97.1% vs 91.9% for T1b and 94.4% vs 80.6% for T1c, respectively; $P<.0001$ for both) whereas for T1a tumors, there was no significant difference seen (98.3% vs 93.7%; $P = .14$).

The NCCN guidelines do not recommend adjuvant chemotherapy for T1a TNBCs.[27] For T1b tumors, chemotherapy can be considered and there is a strong recommendation for chemotherapy in T1c tumors. In contrast, the St. Gallen 2015[73,74] and ESMO[28] guidelines recommend chemotherapy for all TNBCs regardless of the tumor size.

Patients with small TNBCs can undergo surgery first to fully assess the extent of disease and decide if chemotherapy is indicated. If a decision is to treat with chemotherapy before surgery based on other factors, such as young age, high grade, high Ki-67, and so forth, however, then the neoadjuvant approach can be considered for even small tumors given the prognostic information it provides with response assessment.

FUTURE DIRECTIONS

Currently, chemotherapy is used as systemic treatment in patients with TNBC; however, research is ongoing to identify actionable targets. TNBC is an aggressive subtype of breast cancer with a heterogeneous response to therapy. Lehmann and colleagues[75] reported that BL1 TNBC cell lines were the most sensitive to cisplatin and that the mesenchymal and mesenchymal stem–like lines were most sensitive to the Abl/Src inhibitor dasatinib. The clinical validity of the genomic subclassification of TNBC was confirmed by Masuda and colleagues[76] with a retrospective analysis of the response to neoadjuvant chemotherapy. The overall pCR in this study was 28%. In the BL1 subtype, the pCR was the highest (51%), in comparison with 0 in the BL2 subtype and 10% in the LAR subtype, clearly demonstrating the need to develop alternative treatments for some subgroups.

Potential targets and approaches, including DNA damage and repair, immunomodulation, HR modulation, and signaling pathway inhibition, are being evaluated to improve treatment and outcomes in TNBC. Although no biologic therapies are currently part of standard neoadjuvant therapy for TNBC, the poly ADP ribose polymerase (PARP) inhibitor veliparib is being studied in this setting. In a pilot study, the addition of carboplatin and veliparib doubled the pCR rate achieved with weekly paclitaxel and dose-dense AC in TNBC (51% vs 26% in control),[77] which led to an ongoing international randomized study comparing this combination to the control chemotherapy regimen with or without carboplatin (NCT02032277). The PD-1 inhibitor pembrolizumab is also being assessed in a phase III trial with neoadjuvant chemotherapy in TNBC patients to assess response rates (NCT03036488). The benefit of androgen blockage in the LAR subtype of TNBC has been shown in metastatic setting.[78,79] This approach is now being studied in the neoadjuvant setting with a phase II trial of enzalutamide, an antiandrogen drug, in combination with weekly paclitaxel for androgen receptor positive TNBC (NCT02689427).

SUMMARY

Progress in the treatment of TNBC remains an important challenge. Given the aggressive biology and high risk of distant recurrence, systemic chemotherapy is warranted in most patients. Neoadjuvant chemotherapy benefits patients with locally advanced disease by downsizing the tumor and increasing the probability of BCS. Clinical and pathologic responses provide important prognostic information, which makes neoadjuvant therapy an attractive approach for all patients with TNBC. Clinical research in the neoadjuvant setting is focused on improvement in pCR rates and outcomes of patients with residual disease. New targeted treatments and immunotherapeutic drugs are under development. The challenge is to conduct more focused studies due to the importance of heterogeneity in TNBC subtypes. Given the advantages neoadjuvant treatment offers, all patients with TNBC who are believed to be candidates for systemic chemotherapy should be considered for treatment in the neoadjuvant setting.

REFERENCES

1. Perou CM, Sorlie T, Eisen MB, et al. Molecular portraits of human breast tumours. Nature 2000;406(6797):747–52.
2. Hammond ME, Hayes DF, Dowsett M, et al. American Society of Clinical Oncology/College Of American Pathologists guideline recommendations for immunohistochemical testing of estrogen and progesterone receptors in breast cancer. J Clin Oncol 2010;28(16):2784–95.
3. Reis-Filho JS, Tutt AN. Triple negative tumours: a critical review. Histopathology 2008;52(1):108–18.
4. Lehmann BD, Bauer JA, Chen X, et al. Identification of human triple-negative breast cancer subtypes and preclinical models for selection of targeted therapies. J Clin Invest 2011;121(7):2750–67.
5. Lin NU, Vanderplas A, Hughes ME, et al. Clinicopathologic features, patterns of recurrence, and survival among women with triple-negative breast cancer in the National Comprehensive Cancer Network. Cancer 2012;118(22):5463–72.
6. Bauer KR, Brown M, Cress RD, et al. Descriptive analysis of estrogen receptor (ER)-negative, progesterone receptor (PR)-negative, and HER2-negative invasive breast cancer, the so-called triple-negative phenotype: a population-based study from the California cancer Registry. Cancer 2007;109(9):1721–8.
7. Newman LA, Reis-Filho JS, Morrow M, et al. The 2014 Society of Surgical Oncology Susan G. Komen for the Cure Symposium: triple-negative breast cancer. Ann Surg Oncol 2015;22(3):874–82.
8. Jones T, Neboori H, Wu H, et al. Are breast cancer subtypes prognostic for nodal involvement and associated with clinicopathologic features at presentation in early-stage breast cancer? Ann Surg Oncol 2013;20(9):2866–72.
9. Dogan BE, Gonzalez-Angulo AM, Gilcrease M, et al. Multimodality imaging of triple receptor-negative tumors with mammography, ultrasound, and MRI. AJR Am J Roentgenol 2010;194(4):1160–6.
10. Kojima Y, Tsunoda H. Mammography and ultrasound features of triple-negative breast cancer. Breast Cancer 2011;18(3):146–51.
11. Crabb SJ, Cheang MC, Leung S, et al. Basal breast cancer molecular subtype predicts for lower incidence of axillary lymph node metastases in primary breast cancer. Clin Breast Cancer 2008;8(3):249–56.

12. Ugras S, Stempel M, Patil S, et al. Estrogen receptor, progesterone receptor, and HER2 status predict lymphovascular invasion and lymph node involvement. Ann Surg Oncol 2014;21(12):3780–6.
13. Smid M, Wang Y, Zhang Y, et al. Subtypes of breast cancer show preferential site of relapse. Cancer Res 2008;68(9):3108–14.
14. Dent R, Hanna WM, Trudeau M, et al. Pattern of metastatic spread in triple-negative breast cancer. Breast Cancer Res Treat 2009;115(2):423–8.
15. Dent R, Trudeau M, Pritchard KI, et al. Triple-negative breast cancer: clinical features and patterns of recurrence. Clin Cancer Res 2007;13(15 Pt 1):4429–34.
16. Carey LA, Perou CM, Livasy CA, et al. Race, breast cancer subtypes, and survival in the Carolina Breast Cancer Study. JAMA 2006;295(21):2492–502.
17. Pierobon M, Frankenfeld CL. Obesity as a risk factor for triple-negative breast cancers: a systematic review and meta-analysis. Breast Cancer Res Treat 2013;137(1):307–14.
18. Boyle P. Triple-negative breast cancer: epidemiological considerations and recommendations. Ann Oncol 2012;23(Suppl 6):vi7–12.
19. Stark A, Kleer CG, Martin I, et al. African ancestry and higher prevalence of triple-negative breast cancer: findings from an international study. Cancer 2010; 116(21):4926–32.
20. Foulkes WD, Metcalfe K, Sun P, et al. Estrogen receptor status in BRCA1- and BRCA2-related breast cancer: the influence of age, grade, and histological type. Clin Cancer Res 2004;10(6):2029–34.
21. Atchley DP, Albarracin CT, Lopez A, et al. Clinical and pathologic characteristics of patients with BRCA-positive and BRCA-negative breast cancer. J Clin Oncol 2008;26(26):4282–8.
22. Stevens KN, Vachon CM, Couch FJ. Genetic susceptibility to triple-negative breast cancer. Cancer Res 2013;73(7):2025–30.
23. Couch FJ, Hart SN, Sharma P, et al. Inherited mutations in 17 breast cancer susceptibility genes among a large triple-negative breast cancer cohort unselected for family history of breast cancer. J Clin Oncol 2015;33(4):304–11.
24. Rouzier R, Perou CM, Symmans WF, et al. Breast cancer molecular subtypes respond differently to preoperative chemotherapy. Clin Cancer Res 2005; 11(16):5678–85.
25. Carey LA, Dees EC, Sawyer L, et al. The triple negative paradox: primary tumor chemosensitivity of breast cancer subtypes. Clin Cancer Res 2007;13(8): 2329–34.
26. Liedtke C, Mazouni C, Hess KR, et al. Response to neoadjuvant therapy and long-term survival in patients with triple-negative breast cancer. J Clin Oncol 2008;26(8):1275–81.
27. Gradishar W, Salerno KE. NCCN guidelines update: breast cancer. J Natl Compr Canc Netw 2016;14(5 Suppl):641–4.
28. Senkus E, Kyriakides S, Ohno S, et al. Primary breast cancer: ESMO clinical practice guidelines for diagnosis, treatment and follow-up. Ann Oncol 2015; 26(Suppl 5):v8–30.
29. Mieog JS, van der Hage JA, van de Velde CJ. Preoperative chemotherapy for women with operable breast cancer. Cochrane Database Syst Rev 2007;(2):CD005002.
30. Wolmark N, Wang J, Mamounas E, et al. Preoperative chemotherapy in patients with operable breast cancer: nine-year results from National Surgical Adjuvant Breast and Bowel Project B-18. J Natl Cancer Inst Monogr 2001;(30):96–102.
31. Bear HD, Anderson S, Smith RE, et al. Sequential preoperative or postoperative docetaxel added to preoperative doxorubicin plus cyclophosphamide for

operable breast cancer:National Surgical Adjuvant Breast and Bowel Project Protocol B-27. J Clin Oncol 2006;24(13):2019–27.

32. Rastogi P, Anderson SJ, Bear HD, et al. Preoperative chemotherapy: updates of National Surgical Adjuvant Breast and Bowel Project Protocols B-18 and B-27. J Clin Oncol 2008;26(5):778–85.

33. Mauri D, Pavlidis N, Ioannidis JP. Neoadjuvant versus adjuvant systemic treatment in breast cancer: a meta-analysis. J Natl Cancer Inst 2005;97(3):188–94.

34. Gluz O, Nitz UA, Harbeck N, et al. Triple-negative high-risk breast cancer derives particular benefit from dose intensification of adjuvant chemotherapy: results of WSG AM-01 trial. Ann Oncol 2008;19(5):861–70.

35. Di Leo A, Desmedt C, Bartlett JM, et al. HER2 and TOP2A as predictive markers for anthracycline-containing chemotherapy regimens as adjuvant treatment of breast cancer: a meta-analysis of individual patient data. Lancet Oncol 2011; 12(12):1134–42.

36. Hugh J, Hanson J, Cheang MC, et al. Breast cancer subtypes and response to docetaxel in node-positive breast cancer: use of an immunohistochemical definition in the BCIRG 001 trial. J Clin Oncol 2009;27(8):1168–76.

37. Sparano JA, Wang M, Martino S, et al. Weekly paclitaxel in the adjuvant treatment of breast cancer. N Engl J Med 2008;358(16):1663–71.

38. Ellis P, Barrett-Lee P, Johnson L, et al. Sequential docetaxel as adjuvant chemotherapy for early breast cancer (TACT): an open-label, phase III, randomised controlled trial. Lancet 2009;373(9676):1681–92.

39. Martin M, Rodriguez-Lescure A, Ruiz A, et al. Molecular predictors of efficacy of adjuvant weekly paclitaxel in early breast cancer. Breast Cancer Res Treat 2010; 123(1):149–57.

40. Hayes DF, Thor AD, Dressler LG, et al. HER2 and response to paclitaxel in node-positive breast cancer. N Engl J Med 2007;357(15):1496–506.

41. Schick P, Goodstein J, Moor J, et al. Preoperative chemotherapy followed by mastectomy for locally advanced breast cancer. J Surg Oncol 1983;22(4): 278–82.

42. Sorace RA, Bagley CS, Lichter AS, et al. The management of nonmetastatic locally advanced breast cancer using primary induction chemotherapy with hormonal synchronization followed by radiation therapy with or without debulking surgery. World J Surg 1985;9(5):775–85.

43. Bonadonna G, Veronesi U, Brambilla C, et al. Primary chemotherapy to avoid mastectomy in tumors with diameters of three centimeters or more. J Natl Cancer Inst 1990;82(19):1539–45.

44. Hortobagyi GN, Ames FC, Buzdar AU, et al. Management of stage III primary breast cancer with primary chemotherapy, surgery, and radiation therapy. Cancer 1988;62(12):2507–16.

45. Schwartz GF, Birchansky CA, Komarnicky LT, et al. Induction chemotherapy followed by breast conservation for locally advanced carcinoma of the breast. Cancer 1994;73(2):362–9.

46. Colleoni M, Goldhirsch A. Neoadjuvant chemotherapy for breast cancer: any progress? Lancet Oncol 2014;15(2):131–2.

47. Thompson AM, Moulder-Thompson SL. Neoadjuvant treatment of breast cancer. Ann Oncol 2012;23(Suppl 10):x231–6.

48. Fisher B, Brown A, Mamounas E, et al. Effect of preoperative chemotherapy on local-regional disease in women with operable breast cancer: findings from National Surgical Adjuvant Breast and Bowel Project B-18. J Clin Oncol 1997; 15(7):2483–93.

49. Zumsteg ZS, Morrow M, Arnold B, et al. Breast-conserving therapy achieves locoregional outcomes comparable to mastectomy in women with T1-2N0 triple-negative breast cancer. Ann Surg Oncol 2013;20(11):3469–76.

50. von Minckwitz G, Untch M, Blohmer JU, et al. Definition and impact of pathologic complete response on prognosis after neoadjuvant chemotherapy in various intrinsic breast cancer subtypes. J Clin Oncol 2012;30(15):1796–804.

51. Cortazar P, Zhang L, Untch M, et al. Pathological complete response and long-term clinical benefit in breast cancer: the CTNeoBC pooled analysis. Lancet 2014;384(9938):164–72.

52. Symmans WF, Wei C, Gould R, et al. Long-term prognostic risk after neoadjuvant chemotherapy associated with residual cancer burden and breast cancer subtype. J Clin Oncol 2017;35(10):1049–60.

53. Huober J, von Minckwitz G, Denkert C, et al. Effect of neoadjuvant anthracycline-taxane-based chemotherapy in different biological breast cancer phenotypes: overall results from the GeparTrio study. Breast Cancer Res Treat 2010;124(1): 133–40.

54. von Minckwitz G, Blohmer JU, Costa SD, et al. Response-guided neoadjuvant chemotherapy for breast cancer. J Clin Oncol 2013;31(29):3623–30.

55. Untch M, von Minckwitz G, Konecny GE, et al. PREPARE trial: a randomized phase III trial comparing preoperative, dose-dense, dose-intensified chemotherapy with epirubicin, paclitaxel, and CMF versus a standard-dosed epirubicin-cyclophosphamide followed by paclitaxel with or without darbepoetin alfa in primary breast cancer–outcome on prognosis. Ann Oncol 2011;22(9):1999–2006.

56. Chen X, Ye G, Zhang C, et al. Non-anthracycline-containing docetaxel and cyclophosphamide regimen is associated with sustained worse outcome compared with docetaxel, anthracycline and cyclophosphamide in neoadjuvant treatment of triple negative and HER2-positive breast cancer patients: updated follow-up data from NATT study. Chin J Cancer Res 2016;28(6):561–9.

57. Hurley J, Reis IM, Rodgers SE, et al. The use of neoadjuvant platinum-based chemotherapy in locally advanced breast cancer that is triple negative: retrospective analysis of 144 patients. Breast Cancer Res Treat 2013;138(3):783–94.

58. Sikov WM, Berry DA, Perou CM, et al. Impact of the addition of carboplatin and/or bevacizumab to neoadjuvant once-per-week paclitaxel followed by dose-dense doxorubicin and cyclophosphamide on pathologic complete response rates in stage II to III triple-negative breast cancer: CALGB 40603 (Alliance). J Clin Oncol 2015;33(1):13–21.

59. von Minckwitz G, Schneeweiss A, Loibl S, et al. Neoadjuvant carboplatin in patients with triple-negative and HER2-positive early breast cancer (GeparSixto; GBG 66): a randomised phase 2 trial. Lancet Oncol 2014;15(7):747–56.

60. Prowell TM, Pazdur R. Pathological complete response and accelerated drug approval in early breast cancer. N Engl J Med 2012;366(26):2438–41.

61. San Antonio Breast Cancer Symposium; 2015; San Antonio T. San Antonio, TX, December 8–15, 2015.

62. Hanrahan EO, Gonzalez-Angulo AM, Giordano SH, et al. Overall survival and cause-specific mortality of patients with stage T1a,bN0M0 breast carcinoma. J Clin Oncol 2007;25(31):4952–60.

63. Tabar L, Fagerberg G, Day NE, et al. Breast cancer treatment and natural history: new insights from results of screening. Lancet 1992;339(8790):412–4.

64. Fisher B, Dignam J, Tan-Chiu E, et al. Prognosis and treatment of patients with breast tumors of one centimeter or less and negative axillary lymph nodes. J Natl Cancer Inst 2001;93(2):112–20.

65. Fehrenbacher L, Capra AM, Quesenberry CP Jr, et al. Distant invasive breast cancer recurrence risk in human epidermal growth factor receptor 2-positive T1a and T1b node-negative localized breast cancer diagnosed from 2000 to 2006: a cohort from an integrated health care delivery system. J Clin Oncol 2014;32(20):2151–8.

66. Curigliano G, Viale G, Bagnardi V, et al. Clinical relevance of HER2 overexpression/amplification in patients with small tumor size and node-negative breast cancer. J Clin Oncol 2009;27(34):5693–9.

67. Gonzalez-Angulo AM, Litton JK, Broglio KR, et al. High risk of recurrence for patients with breast cancer who have human epidermal growth factor receptor 2-positive, node-negative tumors 1 cm or smaller. J Clin Oncol 2009;27(34): 5700–6.

68. Park YH, Kim ST, Cho EY, et al. A risk stratification by hormonal receptors (ER, PgR) and HER-2 status in small (< or = 1 cm) invasive breast cancer: who might be possible candidates for adjuvant treatment? Breast Cancer Res Treat 2010;119(3):653–61.

69. Amar S, McCullough AE, Tan W, et al. Prognosis and outcome of small (<=1 cm), node-negative breast cancer on the basis of hormonal and HER-2 status. Oncologist 2010;15(10):1043–9.

70. Ho AY, Gupta G, King TA, et al. Favorable prognosis in patients with T1a/T1bN0 triple-negative breast cancers treated with multimodality therapy. Cancer 2012; 118(20):4944–52.

71. Vaz-Luis I, Ottesen RA, Hughes ME, et al. Outcomes by tumor subtype and treatment pattern in women with small, node-negative breast cancer: a multi-institutional study. J Clin Oncol 2014;32(20):2142–50.

72. Patel. Abstract p5-14-02 San Antonio Breast Cancer Symposium; San Antonio, TX, December 6–10, 2016.

73. Esposito A, Criscitiello C, Curigliano G. Highlights from the 14(th) St Gallen International Breast Cancer Conference 2015 in Vienna: dealing with classification, prognostication, and prediction refinement to personalize the treatment of patients with early breast cancer. Ecancermedicalscience 2015;9:518.

74. Untch M, Harbeck N, Huober J, et al. Primary therapy of patients with early breast cancer: evidence, controversies, consensus: opinions of german specialists to the 14th St. Gallen International Breast Cancer Conference 2015 (Vienna 2015). Geburtshilfe Frauenheilkd 2015;75(6):556–65.

75. Lehmann BD, Pietenpol JA. Identification and use of biomarkers in treatment strategies for triple-negative breast cancer subtypes. J Pathol 2014;232(2):142–50.

76. Masuda H, Baggerly KA, Wang Y, et al. Differential response to neoadjuvant chemotherapy among 7 triple-negative breast cancer molecular subtypes. Clin Cancer Res 2013;19(19):5533–40.

77. Rugo HS, Olopade OI, DeMichele A, et al. Adaptive randomization of veliparib-carboplatin treatment in breast cancer. N Engl J Med 2016;375(1):23–34.

78. Gucalp A, Tolaney S, Isakoff SJ, et al. Phase II trial of bicalutamide in patients with androgen receptor-positive, estrogen receptor-negative metastatic breast cancer. Clin Cancer Res 2013;19(19):5505–12.

79. Arce-Salinas C, Riesco-Martinez MC, Hanna W, et al. Complete response of metastatic androgen receptor-positive breast cancer to bicalutamide: case report and review of the literature. J Clin Oncol 2016;34(4):e21–4.

80. von Minckwitz G, Raab G, Caputo A, et al. Doxorubicin with cyclophosphamide followed by docetaxel every 21 days compared with doxorubicin and docetaxel

every 14 days as preoperative treatment in operable breast cancer: the GEPAR-DUO study of the German Breast Group. J Clin Oncol 2005;23(12):2676–85.

81. von Minckwitz G, Rezai M, Loibl S, et al. Capecitabine in addition to anthracy-cline- and taxane-based neoadjuvant treatment in patients with primary breast cancer: phase III GeparQuattro study. J Clin Oncol 2010;28(12):2015–23.

82. Untch M, Fasching PA, Konecny GE, et al. PREPARE trial: a randomized phase III trial comparing preoperative, dose-dense, dose-intensified chemo-therapy with epirubicin, paclitaxel and CMF versus a standard-dosed epirubi-cin/cyclophosphamide followed by paclitaxel +/- darbepoetin alfa in primary breast cancer–results at the time of surgery. Ann Oncol 2011;22(9):1988–98.

83. Esserman LJ, Berry DA, DeMichele A, et al. Pathologic complete response pre-dicts recurrence-free survival more effectively by cancer subset: results from the I-SPY 1 TRIAL–CALGB 150007/150012, ACRIN 6657. J Clin Oncol 2012;30(26): 3242–9.

84. Bonnefoi H, Litiere S, Piccart M, et al. Pathological complete response after neo-adjuvant chemotherapy is an independent predictive factor irrespective of simpli-fied breast cancer intrinsic subtypes: a landmark and two-step approach analyses from the EORTC 10994/BIG 1-00 phase III trial. Ann Oncol 2014; 25(6):1128–36.

85. Chen X, Ye G, Zhang C, et al. Superior outcome after neoadjuvant chemotherapy with docetaxel, anthracycline, and cyclophosphamide versus docetaxel plus cyclophosphamide: results from the NATT trial in triple negative or HER2 positive breast cancer. Breast Cancer Res Treat 2013;142(3):549–58.

Intraoperative Margin Assessment in Breast Cancer Management

Chantal Reyna, MD[a], Sarah M. DeSnyder, MD[b],*

KEYWORDS

- Breast cancer • Breast-conserving surgery • Breast-conserving therapy
- Lumpectomy • Re-excision • Margin • Intraoperative assessment

KEY POINTS

- Rates of margin re-excision vary widely in the literature.
- Efforts to reduce re-excision rates must begin at the time of diagnosis with high-quality imaging, minimally invasive breast biopsy, and multidisciplinary planning.
- A variety of techniques to reduce rates of re-excision have been described; however, careful tracking of re-excision rates and cosmetic outcomes must be undertaken when using these techniques.

INTRODUCTION: NATURE OF THE PROBLEM

Numerous trials have demonstrated equivalent survival outcomes for mastectomy and breast-conserving therapy (BCT) in early-stage breast cancer.[1–6] For patients with unifocal, early-stage breast cancer, BCT is often the preferred treatment. The goal of breast-conserving surgery (BCS) is to excise the tumor with negative margins while providing satisfactory cosmesis. Positive margins after BCS represent a significant risk factor for recurrence and patients with positive margins have rates of ipsilateral breast tumor recurrence twice those of patients with negative margins.[7] Patients who choose to undergo BCT are counseled about the possibility of having to return to surgery for re-excision of positive or close margins. The rates of re-excision reported in the literature range from less than 10% to greater than 50%.[8–15] Importantly, this variability is not explained by characteristics of either the patients or their disease.

Disclosure Statement: Dr S.M. DeSnyder works in a consulting role at MD Anderson Physician's Network. Dr C. Reyna has nothing to disclose.

[a] Breast Surgical Oncology, The University of Texas MD Anderson Cancer Center, 1515 Holcombe Boulevard, Unit 1639, Houston, TX 77030, USA; [b] Breast Surgical Oncology, The University of Texas MD Anderson Cancer Center, 1400 Pressler Street, Unit 1434, Houston, Texas 77030, USA
* Corresponding author.
E-mail address: sgainer@mdanderson.org

Achieving a negative margin at initial surgical intervention spares patients from undergoing additional operative intervention, thus sparing patients additional cost and risk. A return to the operating room for margin re-excision results in additional exposure to the risks of anesthesia, increased surgical complications including increased surgical site infections, increased health care costs, and even increased conversion to bilateral mastectomies.[16–19]

The definition of a negative margin has varied widely over time and across practices. The National Surgical Adjuvant Breast and Bowel Project B-06 trial defined a negative margin as "no ink on tumor," whereas the Milan trials required quadrantectomy with a 2-cm to 3-cm gross margin.[1,2] For patients undergoing BCS, the margin width required for a negative margin has varied widely in clinical practice.[20,21] These different definitions of margin negativity influence re-excision rates. The Society of Surgical Oncology–American Society for Radiation Oncology (SSO-ASTRO) consensus guideline on margins for BCS with whole-breast irradiation in patients with stages I and II invasive breast cancer suggest that "no ink on tumor" be considered the standard for a negative margin.[22] This guideline is based on 33 studies that included more than 28,000 patients with analysis failing to indicate an association between increased margin width and decreased risk of local recurrence. Some investigators have suggested, however, that physicians should consider each case individually, taking into account clinical, pathologic, and treatment variables to determine the need for re-excision rather than using solely margin width.[23] Soon after publication of the guideline, a survey of members of the American Society of Breast Surgeons revealed that a majority of surgeons did not perform re-excision of margins when tumor was not touching the inked margins, but for more complex margin scenarios individual surgeon judgment was used to determine if re-excision was needed.[24] The recently published SSO–ASTRO–American Society of Clinical Oncology consensus guideline on margins for BCS with whole-breast irradiation in patients with ductal carcinoma in situ (DCIS) suggested that a 2-mm margin be considered the standard for a negative margin in these patients.[25] This guideline is based on 20 studies that included 7883 patients with analysis indicating that a 2-mm margin decreased the risk of local recurrence in comparison to smaller margins.

Although eliminating re-excisions for patients undergoing BCS is not feasible, several intraoperative margin assessment strategies are available to reduce the need for re-excision. It is important to recognize, however, that this effort must start at the time of diagnosis. High-quality diagnostic mammography must be performed with supplemental imaging when necessary, the diagnostic biopsy should be obtained in a minimally invasive manner, and multidisciplinary discussions should be undertaken especially for those patients receiving neoadjuvant therapy.[26]

PREOPERATIVE LOCALIZATION

Since the introduction of the SSO-ASTRO guideline of "no ink on tumor," attention to margin status has increased, particularly in regards to intraoperative techniques.[22] Breast cancers removed by segmental mastectomy most commonly require preoperative localization to identify the lesion to be removed. After resection, regardless of which preoperative localization modality is used, meticulous attention to proper specimen orientation is critical. It is recommended that 3 or more margins are labeled to ensure accuracy and improve results.[26] Positive margins increase the risk of local recurrence and proper preoperative localization is critical to ensuring complete excision.[22,27] A variety of techniques to localize breast lesions have been implemented, ranging from needle localization to radioguidance to electromagnetics.

NEEDLE LOCALIZATION
Stereotactic-Guided Needle Localization

On the day of surgery, the patient is taken to the radiology department. If using mammography (stereotactic approach), the breast is placed in compression paddles with an alpha-numeric grid targeting the area of concern with the shortest skin to lesion distance. A needle introducer with wire is placed into the breast parallel to the chest wall. Once placement is confirmed by medial-lateral and cranial-caudal views, the wire is deployed into the tissue. Post-placement images, typically with markers on the skin, are performed to help the surgeon determine the distance to the lesion and the best incision site (**Fig. 1**). After excision of the specimen, a radiograph is taken to confirm excision of the lesion (**Fig. 2**).[28]

Ultrasound-Guided Needle Localization

With ultrasound-guided needle localization, the patient is taken to the radiology department and placed in either a supine or lateral decubitus position. The lesion is visualized with the ultrasound probe and under direct visualization the needle and wire combination is placed into or surrounding the lesion. A post-procedure mammogram is performed. Some surgeons perform wire localization under ultrasound guidance in the operating room.

Important Considerations for Needle Localization

Needle localization is the most common and oldest method of localization. Regardless of which method is used, needle localization requires same-day placement of a wire into the lesion followed by the surgical removal of the wire and lesion. Excellent coordination between radiology and surgery is necessary. Several drawbacks occur, however, with this method. First, wire placement may affect incision location, resulting in undermining, excess removal of tissue, and poor cosmetic results compared

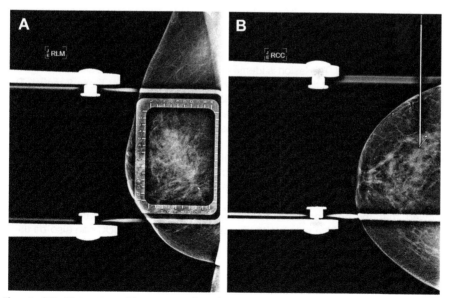

Fig. 1. (*A*) Mammographic compression for needle localization. (*B*) Mammographic compression for needle localization after wire placement.

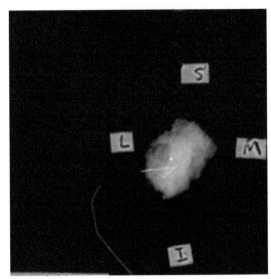

Fig. 2. Specimen radiograph after surgical excision by needle localization. A, anterior; I, inferior; L, lateral; M, medial; P, posterior; S, superior.

with other methods.[29] More importantly, needle localization has been associated with higher re-excision rates.[30] For larger lesions, needle bracketing techniques can be used, but these are associated with more residual disease and incomplete resection.[31]

INTRAOPERATIVE ULTRASOUND

Intraoperative ultrasound (IOUS) may be performed by breast imaging specialists or by surgeons. The patient is taken to the operating room and placed under anesthesia. IOUS can be performed either before the patient is prepped and draped or after the sterile field has been created. If IOUS is done in the sterile field, then an ultrasound probe cover and sterile gel are required. The lesion is identified with the ultrasound and skin markings are created on either end of the probe and a line is drawn to connect these 2 marks. The probe is then turned 90° and the lesion is identified again. The ends of the probe are marked and a second line is created transecting the previous line, which identifies the lesion. For large lesions, the edges of the lesion can be marked.[32] This technique eliminates the need for radiology involvement; however, IOUS does require the lesion to be seen under ultrasound and can be operator dependent. For lesions not visible by ultrasound, a dissolvable marker or iatrogenic hematoma may allow for use of IOUS.[33]

For DCIS patients, margin status and re-excision rates between IOUS and needle localization have been demonstrated to be equivalent.[34] A recent meta-analysis showed that for both palpable and nonpalpable lesions, localization with IOUS resulted in fewer positive margins than needle localization.[35] IOUS can also be used as an adjunct to needle localization.[36]

RADIOGUIDED SURGERY

Radioguided surgery has also become an alternative to needle localization. It consists of either radioactive seed localization (RSL) or radiocolloid injection into the lesion and a gamma probe utilized to guide excision. RSL is used more in the United States and is focused on in this article. This technique is similar to needle localization. Under either stereotactic or ultrasound guidance, a needle is placed into the lesion. Once in place, a titanium clip containing an iodine-125 I seed is placed into the lesion. For larger lesions, several seeds may be placed for bracketing localization. A gamma probe is used to obtain a numeric response, which correlates with distance to the seed. The numbers are higher close to the radioactive seed and decrease sharply when away from the target. The excised specimen must be accurately labeled with a radioactive label and the receiving pathology team must handle and dispose of the radioactive seed properly. A specimen radiograph is obtained to ensure excision of the seed and lesion (**Fig. 3**).

Importantly, RSL uncouples the need for radiology and surgery to be coordinated on the same day because the seed can be placed up to 5 days prior to surgery.[37] Early studies showed RSL to have fewer positive margins compared with needle localization.[29,37] Although a meta-analysis showed fewer positive margins, smaller resection volumes, and shorter operative times, only 1 of the included study addressed RSL.[38] Recent studies show that there is no difference between RSL and needle localization regarding rates of positive margins, length of operation, or excision volumes.[39] In addition, RSL is reported by patients to be more convenient and less painful.[40] RSL requires, however, onsite nuclear medicine support, a strict chain of custody, and regulations for disposal of the seeds. This may make set-up of an RSL program cumbersome for many facilities.[41]

INTRAOPERATIVE ASSESSMENT TECHNIQUES

Several intraoperative assessment techniques have been described in the literature, each of which has been used to reduce re-excision rates.

Gross Assessment

Gross examination of the whole specimen is performed by both the pathologist and the surgeon. India ink is used to define each of the 6 margins and the specimen is then serially sectioned. Margins are interpreted grossly by the pathologist as well as the surgeon. Intraoperative re-excision of any suspicious margin is performed.

Mixed results with this technique have been reported. Balch and colleagues[8] reported a 25% re-excision rate despite utilization of gross margin assessment. Another study demonstrated no reduction in the need for a second operation for re-excision.[42] Less residual disease was noted, however, within re-excision specimens collected at the time of second operation in those who had undergone gross assessment with subsequent appropriate intraoperative margin re-excision. In contrast, Fleming and colleagues[43] demonstrated that gross margin evaluation with appropriate

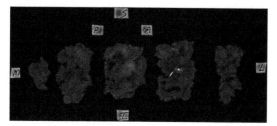

Fig. 3. Specimen radiograph confirming excision of the radioactive seed and targeted lesion.

intraoperative re-excision decreased the need for a second operation to 9.1% from 21.4%. Both lobular subtype and larger tumor size were demonstrated to be predictors of the need for a second operation for re-excision.

Specimen Radiograph

Although specimen imaging should be used for all BCS cases to document excision of the targeted lesion, some investigators have suggested use of specimen radiograph to guide intraoperative re-excision.[44] The excised specimen is oriented by the surgeon in the operating room and then delivered to the pathology suite where orientation is discussed by the pathologist and the surgeon. Specimen radiography of the whole specimen is performed to identify the targeted lesion and biopsy clip. India ink is used to define each of the 6 margins. Some investigators have reported using the whole specimen imaged from various angles to guide intraoperative margin re-excision.[45–49] Many of these studies have demonstrated poor sensitivity for this technique with 1 even reporting higher rates of positive margins with use of intraoperative specimen radiograph.[45–47] Other investigators have reported, however, decreased rates of second surgeries for re-excision of margins.[48,49]

Some investigators have advocated for additional intraoperative specimen processing with specimen radiograph.[50,51] This technique requires serial sectioning of the specimen, followed by placement of the sections on a radiograph plate based on anatomic orientation (**Fig. 4**). In addition to gross examination of the margins, the sections are submitted for specimen radiography. The specimen radiograph of the serially sectioned specimen is examined by the radiologist, pathologist, and surgeon. If tumor or suspicious calcifications are noted at or in close proximity to the margin, the pathologist, radiologist, and surgeon discuss immediate re-excision versus frozen section analysis. One series of patients with DCIS reported that use of this technique eliminated the need for a second surgery for re-excision in 28.4% of patients,[50] although another series, which included those with both invasive and in situ disease, reported that 24.2% of patients avoided a second surgery for re-excision.[51]

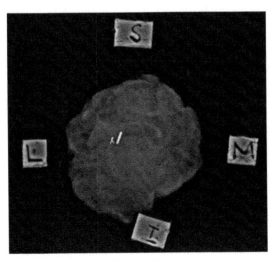

Fig. 4. Radiograph of serially sectioned BCS specimen.

Frozen Section

Intraoperative assessment with frozen section analysis has been described as a method to reduce rates of re-excision. This technique has been described as either excising tissue circumferentially from the lumpectomy specimen or excising tissue from each of the 6 margins of the lumpectomy cavity and submitting these specimens for intraoperative frozen section analysis. A recent systematic review of the literature, which included 37 studies that examined more than 3600 tumors analyzed by intraoperative frozen section, reported a decrease in re-excision rates from 26% to 4% with this technique.[52] Several studies have also demonstrated intraoperative frozen section evaluation to be cost effective.[53,54]

Cavity Shave Margins

Another intraoperative technique used to reduce the number of positive margins is cavity shaving. This technique uses removal of additional circumferential or selected tissue margins after excision of the original specimen. The number of cavity shave margins can vary from 1 (specific margin) to 6 (circumferential). Reported margin widths range from no ink on tumor to 5 mm.[55] Recently, a randomized controlled study showed that cavity shaving reduces the rates of positive margins and the rates of re-excision by up to 50%.[56] This supports previous studies that demonstrated that cavity shaved margins reduced reoperation rates.[57–60] Debate remains, however, on the overall benefit of cavity shaving. Cavity shaving makes it difficult to assess the final width of the lesion and difficult to accurately measure the final margin width. In addition, cavity shaving results in excess tissue removal, which may affect cosmesis.[61]

INVESTIGATIONAL DEVICES

As an alternative to cytology and routine cavity shaving, new intraoperative methods are being investigated, including SAVI SCOUT (Cianna Medical, Aliso Viejo, CA), Magseed (Endomag, Austin, TX), and MarginProbe (DUNE Medical Devices, Alpharetta, GA). For SAVI SCOUT and Magseed, the process is similar to RSL. The device is placed under radiologic guidance and a handheld probe is used to localize the marker intraoperatively. The SAVI SCOUT uses an infrared electromagnetic wave reflector to localize the breast lesion. A recent study shows that SAVI SCOUT is feasible for the localization and removal of breast lesions.[62] Similarly, Magseed sends a reply to the alternating magnetic fields sent from the probe creating an audible and numeric response to guide excision. Magseed can be placed into the breast up to 30 days before surgery still allowing for the uncoupling of radiology and surgery. It is undergoing clinical investigation but has been cleared by the Food and Drug Administraion for segmental mastectomies. Lastly, MarginProbe is a new technology being assessed to help intraoperative evaluation of margins. Based on radiofrequency spectroscopy, it allows intraoperative assessment with a handheld device to identify positive margins. It has been shown to identify positive margins as well as decrease positive margins rates, reducing the need for re-excision.[63,64] It has a specificity up to 70% and a false-negative rate of approximately 25%, however, based on certain studies.[64,65] It has also been found to have a high false-positive rate, which may lead to excess tissue removal.[64]

SUMMARY

Although re-excision rates have varied widely in reports of the literature, national databases have reported a range of 20% to 24%.[8–15] When institutional re-excision rates are noted to be at or above these reported national database averages, consideration should be given to using 1 or more of these techniques and to tracking the resulting re-excision rates. It is also important to ensure that cosmetic outcomes remain appropriate when steps are taken to reduce re-excision rates for those undergoing BCS.[26]

REFERENCES

1. Fisher B, Redmond C, Poisson R, et al. Eight-year results of a randomized clinical trial comparing total mastectomy and lumpectomy with or without irradiation in the treatment of breast cancer. N Engl J Med 1989;320(13):822–8.
2. Veronesi U, Cascinelli N, Mariani L, et al. Twenty-year follow-up of a randomized study comparing breast-conserving surgery with radical mastectomy for early breast cancer. N Engl J Med 2002;347(16):1227–32.
3. Blichert-Toft M, Nielsen M, During M, et al. Long-term results of breast conserving surgery vs. mastectomy for early stage invasive breast cancer: 20-year follow-up of the Danish randomized DBCG-82TM protocol. Acta Oncol 2008;47(4):672–81.
4. Jacobson JA, Danforth DN, Cowan KH, et al. Ten-year results of a comparison of conservation with mastectomy in the treatment of stage I and II breast cancer. N Engl J Med 1995;332(14):907–11.
5. Sarrazin D, Le MG, Arriagada R, et al. Ten-year results of a randomized trial comparing a conservative treatment to mastectomy in early breast cancer. Radiother Oncol 1989;14(3):177–84.
6. van Dongen JA, Bartelink H, Fentiman IS, et al. Randomized clinical trial to assess the value of breast-conserving therapy in stage I and II breast cancer, EORTC 10801 trial. J Natl Cancer Inst Monogr 1992;(11):15–8.
7. Houssami N, Macaskill P, Marinovich ML, et al. The association of surgical margins and local recurrence in women with early-stage invasive breast cancer treated with breast-conserving therapy: a meta-analysis. Ann Surg Oncol 2014; 21(3):717–30.
8. Balch GC, Mithani SK, Simpson JF, et al. Accuracy of intraoperative gross examination of surgical margin status in women undergoing partial mastectomy for breast malignancy. Am Surg 2005;71(1):22–7 [discussion: 27–8].
9. Thompson M, Henry-Tillman R, Margulies A, et al. Hematoma-directed ultrasound-guided (HUG) breast lumpectomy. Ann Surg Oncol 2007;14(1):148–56.
10. Margenthaler JA, Gao F, Klimberg VS. Margin index: a new method for prediction of residual disease after breast-conserving surgery. Ann Surg Oncol 2010;17(10): 2696–701.
11. Singh M, Singh G, Hogan KT, et al. The effect of intraoperative specimen inking on lumpectomy re-excision rates. World J Surg Oncol 2010;8:4.
12. Jeevan R, Cromwell DA, Trivella M, et al. Reoperation rates after breast conserving surgery for breast cancer among women in England: retrospective study of hospital episode statistics. BMJ 2012;345:e4505.
13. McCahill LE, Single RM, Aiello Bowles EJ, et al. Variability in reexcision following breast conservation surgery. JAMA 2012;307(5):467–75.
14. Landercasper J, Whitacre E, Degnim AC, et al. Reasons for re-excision after lumpectomy for breast cancer: insight from the American Society of Breast Surgeons Mastery(SM) database. Ann Surg Oncol 2014;21(10):3185–91.
15. Wilke LG, Czechura T, Wang C, et al. Repeat surgery after breast conservation for the treatment of stage 0 to II breast carcinoma: a report from the National Cancer Data Base, 2004-2010. JAMA Surg 2014;149(12):1296–305.
16. Boughey JC, Hieken TJ, Jakub JW, et al. Impact of analysis of frozen-section margin on reoperation rates in women undergoing lumpectomy for breast cancer:

evaluation of the National Surgical Quality Improvement Program data. Surgery 2014;156(1):190–7.

17. Greenup RA, Peppercorn J, Worni M, et al. Cost implications of the SSO-ASTRO consensus guideline on margins for breast-conserving surgery with whole breast irradiation in stage I and II invasive breast cancer. Ann Surg Oncol 2014;21(5): 1512–4.

18. King TA, Sakr R, Patil S, et al. Clinical management factors contribute to the decision for contralateral prophylactic mastectomy. J Clin Oncol 2011;29(16): 2158–64.

19. Olsen MA, Nickel KB, Margenthaler JA, et al. Increased risk of surgical site infection among breast-conserving surgery re-excisions. Ann Surg Oncol 2015;22(6): 2003–9.

20. Taghian A, Mohiuddin M, Jagsi R, et al. Current perceptions regarding surgical margin status after breast-conserving therapy: results of a survey. Ann Surg 2005;241(4):629–39.

21. Azu M, Abrahamse P, Katz SJ, et al. What is an adequate margin for breast-conserving surgery? Surgeon attitudes and correlates. Ann Surg Oncol 2010; 17(2):558–63.

22. Moran MS, Schnitt SJ, Giuliano AE, et al. Society of Surgical Oncology-American Society for Radiation Oncology consensus guideline on margins for breast-conserving surgery with whole-breast irradiation in stages I and II invasive breast cancer. Ann Surg Oncol 2014;21(3):704–16.

23. Hunt KK, Smith BD, Mittendorf EA. The controversy regarding margin width in breast cancer: enough is enough. Ann Surg Oncol 2014;21(3):701–3.

24. DeSnyder SM, Hunt KK, Smith BD, et al. Assessment of practice patterns following publication of the SSO-ASTRO consensus guideline on margins for breast-conserving therapy in stage I and II invasive breast cancer. Ann Surg Oncol 2015;22(10):3250–6.

25. Morrow M, Van Zee KJ, Solin LJ, et al. Society of Surgical Oncology-American Society for Radiation Oncology-American Society of Clinical Oncology Consensus Guideline on margins for breast-conserving surgery with whole-breast irradiation in ductal carcinoma in situ. J Clin Oncol 2016;34(33):4040–6.

26. Landercasper J, Attai D, Atisha D, et al. Toolbox to reduce lumpectomy reoperations and improve cosmetic outcome in breast cancer patients: the American Society of Breast Surgeons Consensus Conference. Ann Surg Oncol 2015;22(10): 3174–83.

27. Harness JK, Giuliano AE, Pockaj BA, et al. Margins: a status report from the Annual Meeting of the American Society of Breast Surgeons. Ann Surg Oncol 2014;21(10):3192–7.

28. Kopans DB, Lindfors K, McCarthy KA, et al. Spring hookwire breast lesion localizer: use with rigid-compression mammographic systems. Radiology 1985; 157(2):537–8.

29. Lovrics PJ, Goldsmith CH, Hodgson N, et al. A multicentered, randomized, controlled trial comparing radioguided seed localization to standard wire localization for nonpalpable, invasive and in situ breast carcinomas. Ann Surg Oncol 2011;18(12):3407–14.

30. Dua SM, Gray RJ, Keshtgar M. Strategies for localisation of impalpable breast lesions. Breast 2011;20(3):246–53.

31. Edwards SB, Leitman IM, Wengrofsky AJ, et al. Identifying factors and techniques to decrease the positive margin rate in partial mastectomies: have we missed the mark? Breast J 2016;22(3):303–9.

32. Harlow SP, Krag DN, Ames SE, et al. Intraoperative ultrasound localization to guide surgical excision of nonpalpable breast carcinoma. J Am Coll Surg 1999;189(3):241–6.

33. Klein RL, Mook JA, Euhus DM, et al. Evaluation of a hydrogel based breast biopsy marker (HydroMARK(R)) as an alternative to wire and radioactive seed localization for non-palpable breast lesions. J Surg Oncol 2012;105(6):591–4.

34. James TA, Harlow S, Sheehey-Jones J, et al. Intraoperative ultrasound versus mammographic needle localization for ductal carcinoma in situ. Ann Surg Oncol 2009;16(5):1164–9.

35. Ahmed M, Douek M. Intra-operative ultrasound versus wire-guided localization in the surgical management of non-palpable breast cancers: systematic review and meta-analysis. Breast Cancer Res Treat 2013;140(3):435–46.

36. Rahusen FD, Bremers AJ, Fabry HF, et al. Ultrasound-guided lumpectomy of nonpalpable breast cancer versus wire-guided resection: a randomized clinical trial. Ann Surg Oncol 2002;9(10):994–8.

37. Gray RJ, Pockaj BA, Karstaedt PJ, et al. Radioactive seed localization of nonpalpable breast lesions is better than wire localization. Am J Surg 2004;188(4): 377–80.

38. Ahmed M, van Hemelrijck M, Douek M. Systematic review of radioguided versus wire-guided localization in the treatment of non-palpable breast cancers. Breast Cancer Res Treat 2013;140(2):241–52.

39. Langhans L, Tvedskov TF, Klausen TL, et al. Radioactive seed localization or wire-guided localization of nonpalpable invasive and in situ breast cancer: a randomized, multicenter, open-label trial. Ann Surg 2017;266(1):29–35.

40. Bloomquist EV, Ajkay N, Patil S, et al. A randomized prospective comparison of patient-assessed satisfaction and clinical outcomes with radioactive seed localization versus wire localization. Breast J 2016;22(2):151–7.

41. Rao R, Moldrem A, Sarode V, et al. Experience with seed localization for nonpalpable breast lesions in a public health care system. Ann Surg Oncol 2010;17(12): 3241–6.

42. Bolger JC, Solon JG, Khan SA, et al. A comparison of intra-operative margin management techniques in breast-conserving surgery: a standardised approach reduces the likelihood of residual disease without increasing operative time. Breast Cancer 2015;22(3):262–8.

43. Fleming FJ, Hill AD, Mc Dermott EW, et al. Intraoperative margin assessment and re-excision rate in breast conserving surgery. Eur J Surg Oncol 2004;30(3):233–7.

44. Silverstein MJ, Recht A, Lagios MD, et al. Special report: consensus conference III. Image-detected breast cancer: state-of-the-art diagnosis and treatment. J Am Coll Surg 2009;209(4):504–20.

45. Kaufman CS, Jacobson L, Bachman BA, et al. Intraoperative digital specimen mammography: rapid, accurate results expedite surgery. Ann Surg Oncol 2007;14(4):1478–85.

46. Britton PD, Sonoda LI, Yamamoto AK, et al. Breast surgical specimen radiographs: how reliable are they? Eur J Radiol 2011;79(2):245–9.

47. Layfield DM, May DJ, Cutress RI, et al. The effect of introducing an in-theatre intra-operative specimen radiography (IOSR) system on the management of palpable breast cancer within a single unit. Breast 2012;21(4):459–63.

48. Bathla L, Harris A, Davey M, et al. High resolution intra-operative two-dimensional specimen mammography and its impact on second operation for re-excision of positive margins at final pathology after breast conservation surgery. Am J Surg 2011;202(4):387–94.

49. Ciccarelli G, Di Virgilio MR, Menna S, et al. Radiography of the surgical specimen in early stage breast lesions: diagnostic reliability in the analysis of the resection margins. Radiol Med 2007;112(3):366–76.
50. Chagpar A, Yen T, Sahin A, et al. Intraoperative margin assessment reduces re-excision rates in patients with ductal carcinoma in situ treated with breast-conserving surgery. Am J Surg 2003;186(4):371–7.
51. Cabioglu N, Hunt KK, Sahin AA, et al. Role for intraoperative margin assessment in patients undergoing breast-conserving surgery. Ann Surg Oncol 2007;14(4): 1458–71.
52. Esbona K, Li Z, Wilke LG. Intraoperative imprint cytology and frozen section pathology for margin assessment in breast conservation surgery: a systematic review. Ann Surg Oncol 2012;19(10):3236–45.
53. Osborn JB, Keeney GL, Jakub JW, et al. Cost-effectiveness analysis of routine frozen-section analysis of breast margins compared with reoperation for positive margins. Ann Surg Oncol 2011;18(11):3204–9.
54. Boughey JC, Keeney GL, Radensky P, et al. Economic implications of widespread expansion of frozen section margin analysis to guide surgical resection in women with breast cancer undergoing breast-conserving surgery. J Oncol Pract 2016;12(4):e413–22.
55. Gray RJ, Pockaj BA, Garvey E, et al. Intraoperative margin management in breast-conserving surgery: a systematic review of the literature. Ann Surg Oncol 2017. [Epub ahead of print].
56. Chagpar AB, Killelea BK, Tsangaris TN, et al. A randomized, controlled trial of cavity shave margins in breast cancer. N Engl J Med 2015;373(6):503–10.
57. Kobbermann A, Unzeitig A, Xie XJ, et al. Impact of routine cavity shave margins on breast cancer re-excision rates. Ann Surg Oncol 2011;18(5):1349–55.
58. Hequet D, Bricou A, Koual M, et al. Systematic cavity shaving: modifications of breast cancer management and long-term local recurrence, a multicentre study. Eur J Surg Oncol 2013;39(8):899–905.
59. Rizzo M, Iyengar R, Gabram SG, et al. The effects of additional tumor cavity sampling at the time of breast-conserving surgery on final margin status, volume of resection, and pathologist workload. Ann Surg Oncol 2010;17(1):228–34.
60. Marudanayagam R, Singhal R, Tanchel B, et al. Effect of cavity shaving on reoperation rate following breast-conserving surgery. Breast J 2008;14(6):570–3.
61. Moo TA, Choi L, Culpepper C, et al. Impact of margin assessment method on positive margin rate and total volume excised. Ann Surg Oncol 2014;21(1):86–92.
62. Mango V, Ha R, Gomberawalla A, et al. Evaluation of the SAVI SCOUT surgical guidance system for localization and excision of nonpalpable breast lesions: a feasibility study. AJR Am J Roentgenol 2016;(207):W1–4.
63. Allweis TM, Kaufman Z, Lelcuk S, et al. A prospective, randomized, controlled, multicenter study of a real-time, intraoperative probe for positive margin detection in breast-conserving surgery. Am J Surg 2008;196(4):483–9.
64. Schnabel F, Boolbol SK, Gittleman M, et al. A randomized prospective study of lumpectomy margin assessment with use of MarginProbe in patients with nonpalpable breast malignancies. Ann Surg Oncol 2014;21(5):1589–95.
65. Karni T, Pappo I, Sandbank J, et al. A device for real-time, intraoperative margin assessment in breast-conservation surgery. Am J Surg 2007;194(4):467–73.

Oncoplastic Breast Reconstruction
Should All Patients be Considered?

Mehran Habibi, MD, MBA[a], Kristen P. Broderick, MD[b],
Mohamad E. Sebai, MBBS, MD[c], Lisa K. Jacobs, MD, MSPH[d],*

KEYWORDS

- Breast cancer • Breast preservation • Oncoplastic surgery • Reconstructive surgery
- Cosmesis

KEY POINTS

- Partial mastectomy with radiation therapy results in a poor cosmetic outcome requiring additional surgery in up to 30% of patients.
- Poor cosmetic outcome after partial mastectomy can be due to either volume loss, scar contracture, or malalignment of the nipple areolar complex.
- Oncoplastic techniques can be used in all sizes of tissue defects after partial mastectomy to reduce the poor cosmetic outcome.
- Collaborating with a plastic surgeon can increase the number of patients that are candidates for breast preservation and allow larger volumes of resection and contralateral symmetry procedures.
- Oncoplastic surgery focuses on maintaining the normal breast contour and the blood supply and position of the nipple and areola.

INTRODUCTION: NATURE OF THE PROBLEM

Surgical techniques involving breast cancer have recently evolved in 3 important areas: patient recovery, oncological safety, and optimal cosmetic outcome.[1] The first recorded surgical management of breast cancer dates back to 3000 to 2500 BC as described in *The Edwin Smith Surgical Papyrus*, the oldest known surgical treatise.[2]

Disclosure Statement: The authors have nothing to disclose.
[a] Department of Surgery, Johns Hopkins University, 4940 Eastern Avenue, Room A-562, Baltimore, MD 21224, USA; [b] Department of Plastic and Reconstructive Surgery, Johns Hopkins University, 4940 Eastern Avenue, Suite A 520, Baltimore, MD 21224, USA; [c] Department of Surgery, Johns Hopkins University School of Medicine, 4940 Eastern Avenue, Building A 5th Floor-Room 562, Baltimore, MD 21224, USA; [d] Department of Surgery, Johns Hopkins University, Blalock 607, Baltimore, MD 21287, USA
* Corresponding author.
E-mail address: Ljacob14@jhmi.edu

Surg Oncol Clin N Am 27 (2018) 167–180
http://dx.doi.org/10.1016/j.soc.2017.07.007
1055-3207/18/© 2017 Elsevier Inc. All rights reserved.

No significant advancements took place until the first century AD when a Greek physician named Leonidas developed a surgical approach through incision and cautery.[1] For the next few centuries, progress was minimal and few individuals contributed to the improvement of mastectomy. Some of those who contributed were Galen, Jean Louis Petit, Joseph Pancoast, and Samuel Gross.[1,3] Due to high mortality rates from infection and the intolerable postoperative pain, mastectomy was not popular until the introduction of anesthesia in the nineteenth century. Dr William Halsted[4] is credited with developing the technique to safely perform a radical mastectomy. Dr Halsted used anesthesia and the concept of sterilization and disinfection to dramatically improve the outcome of the procedure. From that time on, procedures for breast cancer gained momentum and breast cancer surgical therapy started to evolve toward less invasive approaches while maintaining optimal oncologic outcomes; for example, Patey[5] and Handley[6] described the modified radical mastectomy, sparing the pectoralis major muscle.

In the twentieth century, surgical management of the breast further evolved to breast conservation therapy, taking advantage of increased understanding and use of hormonal therapy, chemotherapy, and radiotherapy.[7–9] This change in surgical management was made possible by the completion of large randomized clinical trials in the 1970s and 1980s, which demonstrated that in specific patient populations the less extensive surgical approach of partial mastectomy has equivalent oncological outcomes to mastectomy when performed with appropriate adjuvant therapy.[7,10]

The improvements in surgical techniques have not only addressed survival but also cosmesis. Breast reconstruction after mastectomy is available to most women. One of the earliest records of breast reconstruction after mastectomy is from the French surgeon Verneuil in 1887, who performed autologous tissue transfer from the healthy breast to the diseased breast.[11] Since then, other approaches have been developed, including both autologous and prosthetic reconstruction. The initial efforts focused on reconstruction of mastectomy defects. Only recently has reconstruction of the breast after partial mastectomy been considered important. Surgeons are now expanding the indications for breast preservation, resulting in more extensive partial mastectomies that increase the risk for cosmetic deformity.[12]

A critical aspect that should be considered when performing breast cancer surgery, either partial mastectomy or mastectomy with reconstruction, is to maintain the natural look and shape of the breast, anticipating the effects of radiation on the partial mastectomy cavity and the mastectomy flaps. It has been reported that up to 30% of women undergoing partial mastectomy with radiation therapy will develop breast disfigurement requiring further surgical correction.[13] To address the cosmetic defects that result from partial mastectomy, breast reconstruction procedures have been developed or adapted from breast cosmetic procedures. In the early 1990s, Audretsch[14] suggested integrating plastic surgery principles with breast conservative surgeries.[14–16] Currently, integrating oncological surgical techniques and plastic surgery techniques is referred to as oncoplastic breast surgery, which aims to provide the optimal oncological safety outcomes in addition to achieving a favorable breast cosmesis for patients undergoing breast preservation. The term oncoplastic is Greek in origin for molding of tumor.[17] John Bostwick III introduced the term tumor-specific immediate reconstruction in 1996 and proposed his classification for oncoplastic breast surgery.[18,19]

Four main factors influence the extent of breast deformity after breast conservation: (1) tumor location, (2) tumor to breast size ratio, (3) use of radiotherapy, and (4) surgical resection approach.[16] Oncoplastic breast surgical approaches have evolved over the years. To achieve optimal outcomes, patient selection criteria and several surgical approaches were studied and proposed. It is vital for all surgical oncologists approaching breast cancer to consider these factors. Each will be considered in describing the available oncoplastic procedures. The indications for oncoplastic procedures and when to pursue preoperative plastic surgery consultation is discussed based on those factors.

SURGICAL TECHNIQUE
Preoperative Planning

The decision of which surgical approach to be used for the oncoplastic procedure is heavily based on patient and tumor characteristics (**Fig. 1**). Mansfield and colleagues[17] reported the following factors for consideration before surgery: volume of tissue to be excised, tumor location, breast size and glandular density, adjuvant therapies, and patient-related risk factors, particularly smoking, obesity, diabetes, and previous surgery. The patient's clinical disease presentation, imaging, pathologic test review, anticipated adjuvant therapy needs, anticipated skin resection, and appropriateness for breast conservation therapy are thoroughly evaluated. Other considerations include prior breast surgery and surgical scars, prior radiation history (partial breast radiation therapy for prior breast cancers and mantle radiation for prior lymphomas), and bra cup size (both current and desired), as well as back or neck pain due to large breasts, intertriginous rashes, breast ptosis, body mass index, smoking history, and lactation history. These factors guide surgeons in selecting those patients who will benefit from oncoplastic surgery and what extent of tissue rearrangement will be optimal. The most obvious example is a large-breasted woman with back and neck pain, intertriginous rashes, and a small tumor in the lower pole of the breast, who would obviously benefit from a breast reduction at the time of the partial mastectomy, with the tumor being removed as part of the reduction specimen. More complex decision-making is required for a woman with prior breast augmentation who has parenchymal atrophy and may require a mastopexy technique to redistribute the parenchyma evenly with respect to the nipple areolar position. In this case, it may be preferable to perform mastectomy and implant removal with immediate total breast reconstruction, allowing avoidance of radiation-associated capsular contracture.[20] Women with tumors in the upper quadrants and lactational breast deflation may benefit from oncoplastic techniques to prevent deformity due to ptosis or

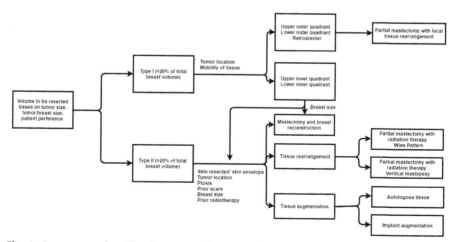

Fig. 1. A summary algorithm for approaches to performing oncoplastic procedures.

pseudoptosis. Each of the previous examples describes patients with significant benefit from plastic surgery consultation and oncoplastic surgery. However, most women will have smaller defects that can be closed primarily without breast distortion and do not need plastic surgery assistance. In patients with smaller defects, there are still advantages to locally rearranging the remaining breast tissue. This tissue rearrangement is done to reduce the scar contraction, tethering of the skin, and distortion of the location of the nipple and areola.

Preoperative considerations for surgical planning include the previously discussed 4 main factors that affect the extent of deformity and several others. The location of the tumor will dictate the available local tissue that can be used to close the defect. Tumors in the upper outer quadrant generally have ample surrounding tissue that can be used to close the defect and tissue loss in this location is less cosmetically noticeable. Tumors in the upper inner quadrant have little surrounding tissue to close the defect; scarring in this location is more noticeable because it is a more visible location in the breast.

The use of radiation therapy after partial mastectomy significantly reduces the risk of tumor recurrence in the breast and is recommended in all but rare exceptions. The cosmetic effect of the radiation therapy results in less pliable skin, firmness of the breast parenchyma, and scar contraction. The location of the defect combined with the radiation therapy can result in asymmetry of the breast volume and asymmetry in the position of the nipple and areola. Tumor to breast size ratio will influence the volume loss, resulting in breast size discrepancies. The larger the tumor and the smaller the breast, the more significant the volume deficit. Patient's with more than a 20% volume loss should have a preoperative plastic surgery consultation. Similar to the breast size to tumor ratio, the planned skin resection to skin envelope ratio is a key measure for cosmetic outcome. The location of the skin resection will affect the location of the nipple areolar complex and symmetry with the contralateral breast. Surgical scars may limit the oncoplastic techniques available if the blood supply to portions of the parenchyma or nipple areolar complex have previously been disrupted and may require a more sophisticated analysis of a volume replacement strategy to prevent postoperative ischemic necrosis. Patients with prior history of smoking, previous radiation, obesity, or a high body mass index will be at higher risk of postoperative complications. Previous mantle irradiation is a contraindication for breast preservation in some cases, depending on the location of the tumor and the prior radiation fields. Patients with previous partial breast radiation therapy may still be candidates for breast preservation depending on the site of the recurrent tumor. In cases in which breast preservation after prior radiation is considered an option, tissue rearrangement using oncoplastic techniques may be necessary to maintain the contour of the breast and the position of the nipple areolar complex. Each of these factors should be considered preoperatively in determining the need for plastic surgery consultation and in planning the location of incisions and tissue rearrangement needed to close the partial mastectomy defect.

Anticipated Breast Deformities After Partial Mastectomy

Anticipating the deformity created is the first step to understanding when to use oncoplastic techniques. Excised breast tissue volume has been reported to be the most predictive factor for breast deformity, especially when the resected volume is greater than 20% of the total breast tissue volume.[21] Risk of deformity is also associated with location of the tumor within the breast. Tumors in the upper outer quadrants have more favorable results, whereas tumors in the upper inner quadrants or in the lower pole have higher risks of deformity.[22] In the upper inner quadrant, the volume loss creates an unfavorable concavity of the medial cleavage of the breast. In the lower quadrants, the nipple can settle into a downward position overhanging a concavity in the lower pole, creating a bird-beak deformity.

Nipple Areolar Location

One key element involved in planning oncoplastic reconstruction involves maintenance of the relationship of the nipple-areolar complex (NAC) to the breast mound. Partial mastectomy defects, once irradiated, can create movement of the NAC toward the defect. Both the surgical scar and the partial mastectomy cavity will contract, creating contour deformities and possible nipple malposition. By preserving or relocating the NAC strategically within the skin envelope in a central position, and rearranging the breast parenchyma to fill the partial mastectomy defect, the effects of radiation and scarring on the breast mound can be mitigated.[20,22] This problem can occur with all lumpectomies and, therefore, some consideration for tissue rearrangement to reduce the partial mastectomy defect should be considered.

With planned incisions and parenchymal reconstructions, the pertinent blood supply to the nipple areolar complex must be considered. Skin incisions should be personalized with respect to skin quality, amount of breast ptosis, and prior surgical incisions. For larger volume resections or for patients with factors that predict a poor cosmetic outcome, coordination with a plastic surgeon can facilitate joint planning of incisions to best access the tumor while maximizing perfusion to the critical components of the breast. In addition, many patients will benefit from a symmetry procedure on the contralateral breast. Kronowitz and colleagues[20] described a management algorithm for reconstructing partial mastectomy defects, based on the location of the tumor within the breast, and did recommend a multidisciplinary breast team to guide the patient to determine the best approach.

PREPPING AND PATIENT POSITIONING

All patients should be marked in a standing position before surgery by the plastic surgeon and the oncologic surgeon. Midline, lateral and inframammary breast folds, and breast meridians should be marked. Tumor location, nipple location (both current and anticipated location), and planned incisions, including skin resections and dermoglandular pedicles, should also be marked. One advantage to using the vertical mastopexy or Wise-pattern skin incisions is the access gained to the axilla for sentinel node and axillary node dissections.[23] However, there is a valid argument that, in some cases, undermining the lateral Wise skin flap can compromise blood supply to the skin closure and should be discussed by the surgeons.[20]

The patient is positioned supine under general anesthesia. Care should be made to ensure symmetric shoulder and arm height. Arms are abducted to 90°, secured on armboards in supination to avoid ulnar nerve compression, padded, and wrapped appropriately. This allows access to the axilla for lymph node evaluation and protects the patient during the seated position of the procedure, which is performed to check symmetry and nipple height. The patient should be situated at the proper location over the break in the bed to allow the back of the bed to raise the patient to an upright position. This should be tested by sitting the patient up while asleep but before prepping and draping.

SURGICAL APPROACH

Clough and colleagues[22] described a commonly used approach for oncoplastic procedures. They classified the surgical approach into 2 levels based on the resected volume from the breast with a level I procedure requiring less the 20% volume resection from the breast. Following skin incision, the skin and/or nipple areolar complex are undermined and the full glandular thickness is resected. After completing the resection, the glandular tissue is closed by reapproximation. This is an appropriate technique for smaller volumes of resection in which the location of the nipple and areola will remain symmetric to the contralateral breast (**Figs. 2** and **3**). Level II procedures are cases requiring more than 20% volume resection from the breast or patients with ptosis or glandular atrophy. Level II procedures are more complex and are described as 2 groups of procedures: volume displacement and volume replacement (**Figs. 4** and **5**). For volume replacement techniques, the glandular gap is filled with either autologous tissue from another site (latissimus dorsi flaps) or with a breast implant.[24–26] Volume displacement procedures use mammoplasty techniques to fill the resulting glandular defect. This is done by mobilizing the locoregional glandular and fatty tissue, which results in a redistribution of breast tissue and equal reduction of the breast volume as a whole and not just at the tumor area.

SURGICAL PROCEDURE
Level II Volume Displacement Procedures

The key to these procedures involves planning the pedicle of the NAC as a separate entity from the skin envelope and planning incisions considering the location of the tumor.[20,23] The tumor is removed using the oncoplastic incisions. Sufficient tissue

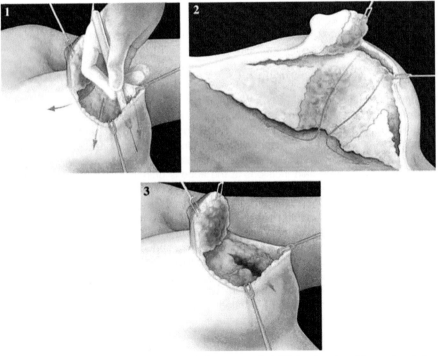

Fig. 2. Level I oncoplastic surgery: surgical concept. 1. Initial extensive skin undermining. 2. Excision of the lesion from subcutaneous tissue to pectoralis fascia. 3. Reapproximation and suturing of the gland. (*From* Clough KB, Kaufman GJ, Nos C, et al. Improving breast cancer surgery: a classification and quadrant per quadrant atlas for oncoplastic surgery. Ann Surg Oncol 2010;17(5):1378; with permission.)

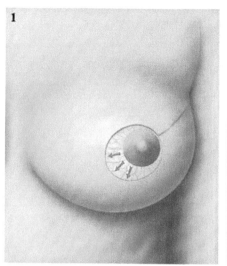
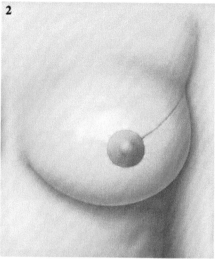

Fig. 3. Level I oncoplastic surgery: nipple recentralization. 1. A skin crescent is de-epithelialized opposite to the lumpectomy bed in the upper-outer quadrant. 2. NAC is recentralized to avoid NAC deviation postlumpectomy. (*From* Clough KB, Kaufman GJ, Nos C, et al. Improving breast cancer surgery: a classification and quadrant per quadrant atlas for oncoplastic surgery. Ann Surg Oncol 2010;17(5):1378; with permission.)

should be removed to increase the likelihood of achieving negative margins. The primary tumor is processed in the same manner as a standard partial mastectomy. After removal of the primary tumor, the skin envelope is elevated with a thick layer of subcutaneous tissue, the breast parenchyma is reapproximated to recreate the breast mound, and limited undermining is performed to maximize perfusion to the parenchyma and minimize postoperative fat necrosis.[20] The skin is then redraped over the breast mound and closed. There are several skin incision patterns that have been described to do this, depending on the amount of skin resection needed, the desired movement of the nipple areolar complex, and the location of the primary tumor. These include the Wise-pattern type for larger skin resections, and the vertical scar or Lejour type. The NAC pedicle can be from virtually any direction, based on tumor location. Other techniques described are round block or Benelli technique (for upper pole tumors) and Grisotti flaps (for central tumors).[17]

Level II Volume Displacement Techniques by Tumor Locations

Lower pole tumors
In women with grade II breast ptosis or higher, either a Wise-pattern or vertical scar should be used. The location of the tumor (medial, central, or lateral) in the lower pole will help determine the proper NAC pedicle. For central lower tumors, a superior or superomedial pedicle is used (see **Fig. 4**). The lower pole skin and some additional parenchyma may be resected and closed to fill the defect. Modifications to the inferior pedicle may be made to accommodate the desired volume of tissue resection for tumors located in the medial and lateral lower poles. This will help avoid the flattened medial cleavage that sometimes occurs with an inferior pedicle.[20]

Upper pole tumors
In cases of upper pole tumors, an inferiorly based pedicle is used (see **Fig. 5**). The Wise pattern or vertical scar is created, maintaining the dermal plexus on the inferior

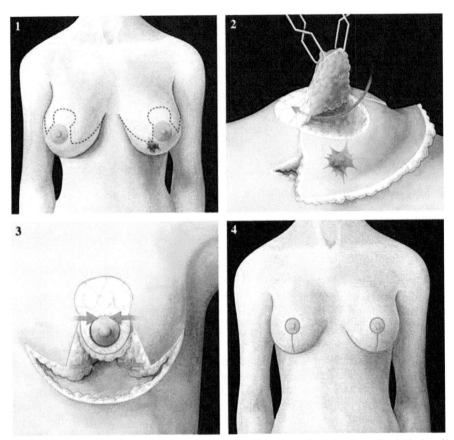

Fig. 4. Level II oncoplastic surgery: superior pedicle mammoplasty for lower pole lesion (6 o'clock). 1. Preoperative drawings. 2. Superior pedicle de-epithelialized and elevated. 3. Re-approximation of medial and lateral glandular flaps after wide excision. 4. Final result after reshaping and contralateral symmetrization. (*From* Clough KB, Kaufman GJ, Nos C, et al. Improving breast cancer surgery: a classification and quadrant per quadrant atlas for oncoplastic surgery. Ann Surg Oncol 2010;17(5):1380; with permission.)

pedicle. The upper pole tumor defect is filled with the upper aspect of the pedicle and the nipple repositioned. For minimal ptosis, a vertical skin excision can be used. Another option is a crescent mastopexy or Benelli mastopexy incision in which a wider periareolar incision is made and de-epithelialized. The skin envelope is undermined in the mastectomy plane to complete the excision of the tumor. For upper medial defects, the medial portion of the inferior breast pedicle can be extended to fill the defect or a laterally based pedicle can be used. Lateral upper quadrant tumors are in an area where breast parenchyma is usually resected during breast reductions. Often, the tissue needs only to be resected and the superomedial or inferior pedicle used to relocate the nipple areolar complex.

Central tumors
Centrally located tumors that are not amenable to NAC preservation due to oncologic factors also benefit from oncoplastic techniques.[27] Previously, these central or retro-areolar tumors were not thought to be amenable to partial mastectomy; however,

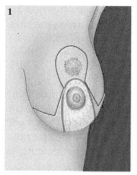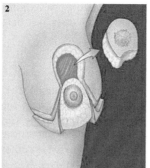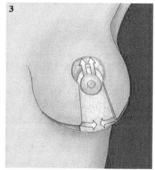

Fig. 5. Level II oncoplastic surgery: Inferior pedicle mammoplasty for 12 o'clock tumors. 1. Preoperative drawings. Inferior pedicle de-epithelialized. 2. Tumor resection. Complementary resection of medial and lateral pillars. 3. Advancement of inferior pedicle into the defect and skin closure. (*From* Clough KB, Kaufman GJ, Nos C, et al. Improving breast cancer surgery: a classification and quadrant per quadrant atlas for oncoplastic surgery. Ann Surg Oncol 2010;17(5):1384; with permission.)

oncologic safety is comparable to mastectomy.[28–30] Depending on the size of the breast and degree of ptosis, several techniques can be used. For smaller breasted women with minimal ptosis, a periareolar incision, with limited undermining of the surrounding tissue can be performed to allow closure of the defect in a straight horizontal line. Alternatively, a circular periareolar incision can be used and then closed in a pursestring.[27] For women with larger degrees of ptosis, the Wise-pattern skin excision is used, the tumor removed centrally, and the lateral wings of the upper breast parenchyma undermined along the chest wall to close the parenchyma inferiorly, resulting in an inverted-T scar.[20,27] An additional modification preserves a circular island of skin on an inferomedial pedicle to replace the skin where the nipple areolar complex was resected. The vertical or Wise-pattern skin incisions are closed around the skin. This paddle of skin placed centrally will maintain the natural pout of the breast and a nipple can be created from this skin at a later date.[27]

OBESE PATIENTS

The Wise-pattern skin excision combined with a pedicled nipple areolar complex is found to have fewer complications in obese women when compared with total breast reconstruction.[31]

Level II Volume Replacement Techniques

Volume replacement techniques fill the glandular defect with either autologous tissue from another site (latissimus dorsi flaps) or with an implant.[24–26] These are best performed at the time of initial partial mastectomy but are also used after a deformity has developed after radiation. Unfortunately, these often result in donor site scars and less than satisfactory cosmetic results when compared with immediate reconstruction because the fibrosis from radiation is often difficult to counteract.[20,26]

POSTOPERATIVE CARE

The patients with larger resections are often observed overnight due to the risk of postoperative hematoma. Smaller resections are discharged the same day. Surgical bras are used at the preference of the surgeons. Drains are not typically required. Surgical healing time depends on the extent of the reconstruction but typically is complete by 4 to 6 weeks and does not delay postoperative radiation therapy.

RECOVERY AND REHABILITATION

Most patients do well and require minimal assistance with rehabilitation. Occupational or physical therapists familiar with postoperative breast cancer therapy can be helpful with range of motion exercises and chest wall massage. Scar tissue may contract with time and chest wall massage can minimize deformities. Massage techniques for cutaneous nerve desensitization are helpful for the hyperesthesia related to parenchymal dissections in the breast and lymph node resections. After the effects of radiation therapy mature, some patients develop tightened parenchyma and chest wall and shoulder tightness, which will improve with proper therapy.

POSTOPERATIVE SURGICAL COMPLICATIONS

Postoperative complications after oncoplastic procedures have been reported to be between 15% and 30%.[32–35] These include surgical site morbidity of skin, flap, or fat necrosis; nipple areolar complex necrosis; and infection, seroma, hematoma, and wound dehiscence, which might require interventional procedures or reoperation.[36] Necrosis is the most prominent complication with the volume displacement approach.[17,22] However, donor site morbidity is prominent when autologous tissue is used for the volume replacement approach.[17,22] Complications arising after the surgery might affect patient recovery and ultimately cause delays in receiving adjuvant therapy; however, this is unlikely. As such, it is important to screen patients based on the criteria previously discussed to insure optimal outcomes. Evaluating the glandular density and fatty composition of the breast is critical to minimize complications related to surgical manipulation of the tissue. Higher glandular density is associated with lower risk for fat necrosis and, conversely, higher fat density has a higher risk for fat necrosis after surgical reshaping.[22] Nonetheless, good outcomes have been reported using oncoplastic principles in both large tumor to breast volume ratios, obese patients, and for patient with tumors in difficult locations.[23,27,31,37]

DELAYED RECONSTRUCTION FOR PARTIAL MASTECTOMY DEFECTS

Unfortunately, acquired deformities after partial mastectomy and whole breast radiation are often difficult to correct, requiring extensive surgery[20] with high complication rates.[20] If a woman develops a delayed deformity after breast conservation therapy, the 2 main options to correct the deformity include autologous tissue flaps and completion mastectomy with total breast reconstruction. There is often a contracted partial mastectomy cavity, with focal parenchymal volume loss; tethering of the overlying skin to the cavity; and tight, contracted skin that is at very high risk for mastectomy skin necrosis after undermining. Depending on the location of the defect, the nipple areolar complex can also be malpositioned toward the defect because the tethered skin and parenchyma pulls the nipple toward the defect as it contracts. Conversely, extensive volume and skin loss also occur.[26] The irradiated tissue is not easily amenable to local tissue rearrangement, with a complication rate as high as 50%.[20] Implant placement in these defects is not usually effective unless the woman has a central partial mastectomy defect with a simple size discrepancy with the contralateral breast and no true skin, parenchyma, or nipple distortion. Lateral thoracic or abdominally based flaps bring nonirradiated tissue into the breast to facilitate healing and fill the contracted cavities.[20,26] They also replace skin in cases in which the skin is distorted, contracted, or causing nipple areolar distortion. In some cases, the distortion is so severe that a completion mastectomy and total breast reconstruction is required.

ONCOLOGICAL OUTCOMES

Several studies have reported the oncological safety of oncoplastic breast procedures. Several randomized controlled clinical trials, prospective studies, and systematic reviews have reported high 5-year overall and disease-free survival, low recurrence rates, and that complications did not affect delivery of adjuvant therapy.[36,38–41] As such, current evidence suggests that oncoplastic procedures do provide the oncological safety that they were designed to do.

PARTIAL MASTECTOMY MARGIN STATUS

Some patients present with tumors whose margins may be involved after partial mastectomy. The risk of positive margins is increased in women with extensive ductal carcinoma in situ, large tumor to breast size ratio, and those with multifocal tumors. When volume replacement techniques are used and in type I defects closed by reapproximation of local tissue, new parenchyma is simply interposed into the defect and the margins of the cavity remain in the same location relative to the rest of the breast. For the type II defects treated with oncoplastic techniques, positive margins create a significant problem. Most reconstructive techniques involve some manipulation of the partial mastectomy cavity, making it difficult to identify by the surgeon during reexcision of the margins and by the radiation oncologist when planning a radiation therapy boost dose. However, in larger reconstructions, such as a breast reduction using a superomedial pedicle and wise pattern skin resection for a lower pole tumor, these volume replacement techniques may result in more extensive manipulation of the parenchyma and movement of the walls of the cavity. This will make re-excisions for positive margins a challenge surgically because the borders of the cavity may have been shifted. In cases in which there is a high risk for positive margins, immediate reconstruction may not be indicated but can safely be achieved once any re-excisions are performed and margin status is clear. For this reason, the authors recommend preoperative consultation with plastic surgery, preferably before partial mastectomy, in women who meet the criteria for an oncoplastic procedure and have a high risk of positive margins. In some patients, the decision to pursue an oncoplastic procedure is determined after the original partial mastectomy is done showing positive margins. If consultation was not done preoperatively, it is needed before radiation is begun.

COSMETIC AND QUALITY OF LIFE OUTCOMES

There are limited studies looking into cosmetic and quality of life outcomes after oncoplastic breast procedures. Cosmetic outcomes have been assessed subjectively without standardized validated methodology. With those limitations, several studies reported good cosmetic outcomes after oncoplastic procedures in 84% to 89% of subjects.[38,42–44] Quality of life outcomes have been studied using standardized questionnaires, such as BREAST-Q, Short Form-36, and the Rosenberg Self-Esteem Scale, and have reported that the quality of life outcomes for oncoplastic procedures are higher and superior to breast conservative surgery alone.[10,45,46]

SUMMARY

The goal of oncoplastic surgery is to improve the cosmesis for women undergoing partial mastectomy with radiation therapy. All patients treated with breast preservation should have attempts made to reduce the parenchymal defect within the breast. Scarring in the breast due to both the parenchymal defect and radiation therapy can result in volume loss, tethering of the skin, and distortion of the location of the nipple areolar complex. Reapproximating the breast tissue and reshaping the breast with awareness of the position of the nipple and areola on the breast mound results in good cosmetic outcomes and improved quality of life with equivalent survival and local control. Therefore, oncoplastic surgery should be attempted in all patients who undergo breast preservation for breast cancer.

REFERENCES

1. Laronga C, Lewis JD, Smith PD. The changing face of mastectomy: an oncologic and cosmetic perspective. Cancer Control 2012;19(4):286–94.
2. Feldman RP, Goodrich JT. The Edwin Smith Surgical Papyrus. Childs Nerv Syst 1999;15(6):281–4.
3. Lewison EF. The surgical treatment of breast cancer: an historical and collective review. Surgery 1953;34(5):904–53.
4. Halsted WS. The results of operations for the cure of cancer of the breast performed at the Johns Hopkins Hospital from June, 1889, to January, 1894. Ann Surg 2016;20(5):497.
5. Patey DH, Dyson WH. The prognosis of carcinoma of the breast in relation to the type of operation performed. Br J Cancer 1948;2(3):7–13.
6. Handley RS, Thackray AC. Conservative radical mastectomy (Patey's operation). Ann Surg 1963;157:162.
7. Fisher B, Redmond C, Poisson R, et al. Eight-year results of a randomized clinical trial comparing total mastectomy and lumpectomy with or without irradiation in the treatment of breast cancer. N Engl J Med 1989;320(13):822–8.
8. Lakhtakia R. A brief history of breast cancer: part I: surgical domination reinvented. Sultan Qaboos Univ Med J 2014;14(2):9.
9. Veronesi U, Volterrani F, Luini A, et al. Quadrantectomy versus lumpectomy for small size breast cancer. Eur J Cancer Clin Oncol 1990;26(6):671–3.
10. Veiga DF, Veiga-Filho J, Ribeiro LM, et al. Quality-of-life and self-esteem outcomes after oncoplastic breast-conserving surgery. Plast Reconstr Surg 2010; 125(3):811–7.
11. Rozen WM, Rajkomar AK, Anavekar NS, et al. Post-mastectomy breast reconstruction: a history in evolution. Clin Breast Cancer 2009;9(3):145–54.
12. Gabka CJ, Maiwald G, Baumeister RG. Expanding the indications spectrum for breast saving therapy of breast carcinoma by oncoplastic operations. Langenbecks Arch Chir Suppl Kongressbd 1997;114:1224–7 [in German].
13. Clough KB, Cuminet J, Fitoussi A, et al. Cosmetic sequelae after conservative treatment for breast cancer: classification and results of surgical correction. Ann Plast Surg 1998;41(5):471.
14. Audretsch W. Space-holding technic and immediate reconstruction of the female breast following subcutaneous and modified radical mastectomy. Arch Gynecol Obstet 1987;241(Suppl):9 [in German].
15. Elliot FL. Surgery of the breast: principles and art. Plast Reconstr Surg 2000; 105(5):1891.

16. Losken A, Hamdi M. Partial breast reconstruction techniques in oncoplastic surgery. Boca Raton (FL): CRC Press; 2009.
17. Mansfield L, Agrawal A, Cutress RI. Oncoplastic breast conserving surgery. Gland Surg 2013;2(3):158–62.
18. Audretsch WP, Rezai M, Kolotas C, et al. Tumor-specific immediate reconstruction in breast cancer patients. Perspect Plast Surg 1998;11(01):71–100.
19. Losken A, Elwood ET, Styblo TM, et al. The role of reduction mammaplasty in reconstructing partial mastectomy defects. Plast Reconstr Surg 2002;109(3): 968–75 [discussion: 976–7].
20. Kronowitz SJ, Kuerer HM, Buchholz TA, et al. A management algorithm and practical oncoplastic surgical techniques for repairing partial mastectomy defects. Plast Reconstr Surg 2008;122(6):1631–47.
21. Bulstrode NW, Shrotria S. Prediction of cosmetic outcome following conservative breast surgery using breast volume measurements. Breast 2001;10(2):124–6.
22. Clough KB, Kaufman GJ, Nos C, et al. Improving breast cancer surgery: a classification and quadrant per quadrant atlas for oncoplastic surgery. Ann Surg Oncol 2010;17(5):1375–91.
23. Fitoussi AD, Berry MG, Famà F, et al. Oncoplastic breast surgery for cancer: analysis of 540 consecutive cases [outcomes article]. Plast Reconstr Surg 2010; 125(2):454–62.
24. Rainsbury RM. Breast-sparing reconstruction with latissimus dorsi miniflaps. Eur J Surg Oncol 2002;28(8):891–5.
25. Yang JD, Kim MC, Lee JW, et al. Usefulness of oncoplastic volume replacement techniques after breast conserving surgery in small to moderate-sized breasts. Arch Plast Surg 2012;39(5):489–96.
26. Levine JL, Soueid NE, Allen RJ. Algorithm for autologous breast reconstruction for partial mastectomy defects. Plast Reconstr Surg 2005;116(3):762–7.
27. Huemer GM, Schrenk P, Moser F, et al. Oncoplastic techniques allow breast-conserving treatment in centrally located breast cancers. Plast Reconstr Surg 2007;120(2):390–8.
28. Horiguchi J, Koibuchi Y, Iijima K, et al. Local control by breast-conserving surgery with nipple resection. Anticancer Res 2005;25(4):2957–9.
29. Pezzi CM, Kukora JS, Audet IM, et al. Breast conservation surgery using nipple-areolar resection for central breast cancers. Arch Surg 2004;139(1):32–7 [discussion: 38].
30. Simmons RM, Brennan MB, Christos P, et al. Recurrence rates in patients with central or retroareolar breast cancers treated with mastectomy or lumpectomy. Am J Surg 2001;182(4):325–9.
31. Tong WM, Baumann DP, Villa MT, et al. Obese women experience fewer complications after oncoplastic breast repair following partial mastectomy than after immediate total breast reconstruction. Plast Reconstr Surg 2016;137(3):777–91.
32. Bajaj AK, Kon PS, Oberg KC, et al. Aesthetic outcomes in patients undergoing breast conservation therapy for the treatment of localized breast cancer. Plast Reconstr Surg 2004;114(6):1442–9.
33. Kronowitz SJ, Feledy JA, Hunt KK, et al. Determining the optimal approach to breast reconstruction after partial mastectomy. Plast Reconstr Surg 2006; 117(1):1.
34. Munhoz AM, Montag E, Arruda EG, et al. Critical analysis of reduction mammaplasty techniques in combination with conservative breast surgery for early breast cancer treatment. Plast Reconstr Surg 2006;117(4):1091.

35. Peled AW, Sbitany H, Foster RD, et al. Oncoplastic mammoplasty as a strategy for reducing reconstructive complications associated with postmastectomy radiation therapy. Breast J 2014;20(3):302–7.

36. Piper ML, Esserman LJ, Sbitany H, et al. Outcomes following oncoplastic reduction mammoplasty: a systematic review. Ann Plast Surg 2016;76(Suppl 3):6.

37. Barnea Y, Friedman O, Arad E, et al. An oncoplastic breast augmentation technique for immediate partial breast reconstruction following breast conservation. Plast Reconstr Surg 2017;139(2):348e–57e.

38. Clough KB, Lewis JS, Couturaud B, et al. Oncoplastic techniques allow extensive resections for breast-conserving therapy of breast carcinomas. Ann Surg 2003; 237(1):26–34.

39. Clough KB, Soussaline M, Campana F, et al. Mammoplasty combined with irradiation: conservative treatment of breast cancer localized in the lower quadrant. Ann Chir Plast Esthet 1990;35(2):117–22 [in French].

40. McIntosh J, O'Donoghue JM. Therapeutic mammaplasty–a systematic review of the evidence. Eur J Surg Oncol 2012;38(3):196–202.

41. Piper M, Peled AW, Sbitany H. Oncoplastic breast surgery: current strategies. Gland Surg 2015;4(2):154–63.

42. Chan SWW, Cheung PS, Lam SH. Cosmetic outcome and percentage of breast volume excision in oncoplastic breast conserving surgery. World J Surg 2010; 34(7):1447–52.

43. Meretoja TJ, Svarvar C, Jahkola TA. Outcome of oncoplastic breast surgery in 90 prospective patients. Am J Surg 2010;200(2):224–8.

44. Yang JD, Bae SG, Chung HY, et al. The usefulness of oncoplastic volume displacement techniques in the superiorly located breast cancers for Korean patients with small to moderate-sized breasts. Ann Plast Surg 2011;67(5):474–80.

45. Haloua MH, Krekel NM, Winters HA, et al. A systematic review of oncoplastic breast-conserving surgery: current weaknesses and future prospects. Ann Surg 2013;257(4):609–20.

46. Kim KDD, Kim Z, Kuk JC, et al. Long-term results of oncoplastic breast surgery with latissimus dorsi flap reconstruction: a pilot study of the objective cosmetic results and patient reported outcome. Ann Surg Treat Res 2016;90(3):117–23.

Alternatives to Standard Fractionation Radiation Therapy After Lumpectomy

Hypofractionated Whole-Breast Irradiation and Accelerated Partial-Breast Irradiation

Nisha Ohri, MD, Bruce G. Haffty, MD*

KEYWORDS

- Breast cancer • Breast-conserving therapy • Lumpectomy • Standard fractionation
- Hypofractionation • Accelerated partial-breast irradiation

KEY POINTS

- Adjuvant whole-breast irradiation after lumpectomy has been an established standard of care to optimize local tumor control for decades.
- Standard-fractionation whole-breast irradiation delivered over 5 to 7 weeks can achieve durable tumor control with low toxicity and favorable cosmesis but can be inconvenient and cost ineffective.
- Hypofractionated whole-breast irradiation can be completed in 3 to 4 weeks and is the preferred standard of care in appropriately selected patients.
- Accelerated partial breast irradiation can be delivered using even shorter treatment regimens, and early results suggest it is an effective alternative to WBI in select patients.
- Results from ongoing hypofractionated whole-breast irradiation and accelerated partial breast irradiation trials will help establish their roles in the adjuvant management of early stage breast cancer.

INTRODUCTION

Breast-conservation therapy, or breast-conserving surgery (BCS) followed by adjuvant radiation therapy (RT), was established as an acceptable alternative to mastectomy after multiple randomized trials conducted in the 1970s and 1980s demonstrated equivalent high survival rates with both approaches.[1,2] In 2005, the

Disclosure Statement: The authors have nothing to disclose.
Department of Radiation Oncology, Rutgers Cancer Institute of New Jersey, 195 Little Albany Street, New Brunswick, NJ 08901, USA
* Corresponding author.
E-mail address: hafftybg@cinj.rutgers.edu

Early Breast Cancer Trialists' Collaborative Group meta-analysis further established breast-conservation therapy as the standard of care for early-stage breast cancer. The most commonly used radiation regimen in these randomized trials was 50 Gy in 25 fractions to the whole breast with or without a boost, now referred to as a *standard fractionation whole-breast irradiation* (SF-WBI).[3]

The radiobiological rationale in support of SF-WBI is that smaller doses of radiation per fraction can spare normal tissues, such as the breast, muscle, ribs, and lung, without compromising tumor control. Some of the challenges of SF-WBI, however, include the cost and inconvenience of 5 to 7 weeks of daily radiation treatment. As a result, there has been growing interest in establishing alternate methods of delivering adjuvant RT using shorter and more convenient regimens. This article reviews hypofractionated WBI (HF-WBI) and accelerated partial breast irradiation (APBI) as accepted alternate approaches to SF-WBI in appropriately selected patients with early-stage breast cancer.

HYPOFRACTIONATED WHOLE-BREAST IRRADIATION

HF-WBI refers to the delivery of adjuvant whole-breast RT in a shortened 3- to 4-week course of treatment. The evidence in support of HF-WBI comes from a series of large randomized trials showing equivalence in efficacy, toxicity, and long-term cosmesis compared with SF-WBI. Key features and results of each trial are summarized in **Tables 1** and **2**.

EFFICACY OF HYPOFRACTIONATED WHOLE-BREAST IRRADIATION

One of the earlier HF-WBI trials was initiated in 1986 at the Royal Marsden Hospital and Gloucester Oncology Center (RMH/GOC) in the United Kingdom. This was a pilot trial that included 1410 patients younger than 75 years of age with T1-3, N0-1, M0 breast cancer who underwent BCS with complete macroscopic resection of invasive

Table 1
Key features of randomized breast hypofractionation trials

Variable	RMH/GOC	START A	START B	Canadian
Patients enrolled	1410	2236	2215	1234
Study years	1986–1998	1998–2002	1999–2001	1993–1996
Median follow-up (y)	9.7	9.3	9.9	12.0
Stage	T1-3, N0-1, M0	T1-3a, N0-1, M0	T1-3a, N0-1, M0	T1-2, N0, M0
Surgery				
Lumpectomy, N (%)	1410 (100)	1900 (85)	2038 (92)	1234 (100)
Mastectomy, N (%)	0	336 (15)	117 (8)	0
Treatment arms (Gy/fractions)	50/25 (5 wk) 42.9/13 (5 wk) 39/13 (5 wk)	50/25 (5 wk) 41.6/13 (5 wk) 39/13 (5 wk)	50/25 (5 wk) 40/15 (3 wk)	50/25 (5 wk) 42.5/16 (3.2 wk)
Boost				
N (%)	1051 (75)	1159 (61)	875 (43)	0
Dose (Gy/fractions)	14/7	10/5	10/5	
Regional nodal irradiation, N (%)	290 (21)	318 (14)	161 (7)	0
Chemotherapy, N (%)	196 (14)	793 (35)	491 (22)	135 (11)

Table 2
Key results of randomized breast hypofractionation trials

	RMH/GOC			START A			START B			Canadian		
10-y Endpoints	50 Gy (%)	42.9 Gy (%)	39 Gy (%)	P Value	50 Gy (%)	41.6 Gy (%)	39 Gy (%)	P Value	50 Gy (%)	40 Gy (%)	P Value	50 Gy (%)	42.5 Gy (%)	P Value
Local recurrence	12.1	9.6	14.8	NS[a]	6.7	5.6	8.1	NS	5.2	3.8	NS	6.7	6.2	NS
Distant metastasis	—	—	—	—	14.7	16.8	18.0	NS	16.0	12.3	.014	—	—	—
All-cause mortality	—	—	—	—	19.8	18.4	20.3	NS	19.2	15.9	.042	15.6	15.4	NS

Abbreviation: NS, not significant.
[a] Not significant when each experimental arm was compared with the control arm.

carcinoma. Patients were randomly assigned to 3 radiation dose schedules all delivered over 5 weeks. The control arm consisted of 50 Gy in 25 daily fractions. The 2 experimental HF-WBI arms delivered 42.9 Gy in 13 fractions (3.3 Gy per fraction) and 39 Gy in 13 fractions (3 Gy per fraction), with 2 to 3 fractions delivered per week. A subrandomization to a 14-Gy electron boost in 7 fractions was also performed. The risk of ipsilateral tumor recurrence at 10 years was 12.1% in the 50-Gy arm, 9.6% in the 42.9-Gy arm, and 14.8% in the 39-Gy arm. There was no significant difference in local recurrence when comparing each HF-WBI arm with the SF-WBI arm.[4]

The UK Standardization of Breast Radiotherapy Trial A (START A) included 2236 women with operable T1-3a, N0-1, M0 invasive breast cancer who underwent surgical resection with clear ≥1-mm margins. Although both BCS and mastectomy were allowed, only 15% of enrolled patients underwent mastectomy. Patients were randomly assigned to receive 50 Gy in 25 fractions (control arm), or 41.6 Gy in 13 fractions, or 39 Gy in 13 fractions (experimental arms). All treatments were delivered over 5 weeks, similar to the RMH/GOC study. Boost (10 Gy/5 fractions) was delivered at the discretion of the treating physician in about 61% of patients. About 14% of patients received regional nodal irradiation (supraclavicular nodes ± axillary nodes), and about 35% received adjuvant chemotherapy before radiation. Rates of local relapse at 10 years were 6.7% in the 50-Gy arm, 5.6% in the 41.6-Gy arm, and 8.1% in the 39-Gy arm (P value, not significant). Both disease-free survival (DFS) and overall survival (OS) were similar among all arms.[5,6]

The START B trial had similar inclusion criteria and randomized 2215 patients to 50 Gy in 25 fractions or 40 Gy in 15 fractions. Unlike in the RMH/GOC and START A trials, patients on the HF-WBI arm completed radiation treatment in only 3 weeks. A total of 8% of patients underwent mastectomy, 43% received a boost, 7% received regional nodal irradiation, and 22% received adjuvant chemotherapy. The 10-year local relapse rate was 5.2% in the 50-Gy arm and 3.8% in the 40-Gy arm (P value, not significant). Surprisingly, distant relapse, DFS, and OS were all significantly improved in the 40-Gy arm. It is unclear what drove the improvement in DFS and OS, as the difference in local tumor control was likely too small to translate into a survival benefit.[6,7]

The Canadian trial randomly assigned 1234 patients with T1-2, N0, M0 invasive breast cancer to SF-WBI with 50 Gy in 25 fractions delivered over 5 weeks or HF-WBI with 42.5 Gy in 16 fractions delivered in just more than 3 weeks. Unlike previous trials, patients who underwent mastectomy and those with node-positive disease were not eligible, and lumpectomy boost and nodal irradiation were not allowed. Most patients (75%) were older than 50 years of age, and only 11% received adjuvant chemotherapy. At 10 years, local recurrence rates were 6.7% in the SF-WBI arm and 6.2% in the HF-WBI arm (P value, not significant). Ten-year OS rates were also nearly identical (84.4% and 84.6%, respectively). In an unplanned subgroup analysis, both treatment regimens were equally effective regardless of patient age, tumor size, estrogen receptor status, or receipt of systemic therapy. In patients with high-grade disease, however, 10-year local recurrence was higher in the HF-WBI arm (15.6% vs 4.7%; P = .01).[8]

Long-term Toxicity and Cosmesis of Hypofractionated Whole-Breast Irradiation

In the RMH/GOC trial, long-term rates of fair or poor cosmesis, breast shrinkage, breast distortion, breast edema, and induration were lowest in the 39-Gy arm, although a direct comparison with the 50-Gy arm was not made.[9]

Long-term physician-assessed tissue effects in the START A trial showed similar rates of breast shrinkage, shoulder stiffness, and arm edema among all treatment arms at 10 years. The 39-Gy arm had significantly lower rates of breast edema and telangiectasias compared with the 50-Gy arm. There were no significant differences between the 41.6-Gy and 50-Gy arms. Similar results were seen in START B, with lower rates of breast edema, telangiectasia, and breast shrinkage in the 40-Gy arm. Rates of other late adverse effects including symptomatic rib fracture, symptomatic lung fibrosis, ischemic heart disease, and brachial plexopathy were low (<3%) among all treatment arms in the START A and START B trials.[6]

In the Canadian trial, rates of skin and subcutaneous tissue toxicity at 10 years were similar in the 50-Gy and 42.5-Gy arms. An excellent or good cosmetic outcome was achieved in 69.8% of patients in the HF-WBI arm compared with 71.3% of patients in the SF-WBI arm.

Consensus statement on hypofractionated whole-breast irradiation
In 2011, the American Society for Radiation Oncology (ASTRO) consensus guidelines endorsed HF-WBI as an equally effective regimen compared with SF-WBI for select patients with early-stage breast cancer. Patients were candidates for HF-WBI if they were age 50 years or older at the time of diagnosis, had pathologic T1-2, N0 disease treated with BCS, and did not receive chemotherapy. During treatment planning, it was recommended that the dose within the breast along the central axis should not be lower than 93% or higher than 107% of the prescription dose. For patients who did not meet all criteria, there was no consensus recommendation for or against HF-WBI.[10] ASTRO is currently developing an updated consensus statement on WBI fractionation that is anticipated to be released later this year.

Clinical considerations for hypofractionated whole-breast irradiation
Hypofractionated whole-breast irradiation and boost Although a considerable number of patients enrolled on the RMH/GOC and START A and B trials received a boost, as summarized in **Table 1**, the ASTRO guidelines did not provide a consensus opinion regarding the integration of a breast boost into a HF-WBI regimen. Approximately half of the patients enrolled on the RMH/GOC trial underwent a second randomization for a boost versus no boost, and the remaining half received an elective boost of 14 Gy in 7 fractions. A 10 Gy/5 fraction boost was planned in 61% of patients in the START A trial and 43% of patients in the START B trial. In 2013, post-hoc subgroup analyses compared the combined hypofractionated regimens with the control arms in the RMH/GOC, START A, and START B trials. Tumor control and normal tissue outcomes were similar irrespective of tumor bed boost, suggesting that a breast boost can safely be incorporated into a HF-WBI regimen. These data were published after the 2011 ASTRO guidelines.[6,10]

Hypofractionated whole-breast irradiation and regional nodal irradiation Current guidelines do not endorse HF-WBI in node-positive patients who require regional nodal irradiation.[10] A small proportion of patients enrolled on the RMH/GOC (21%), START A (14%), and START B (7%) trials did receive hypofractionated regional nodal irradiation (see **Table 1**). There was no evidence of increased late adverse effects with regard to shoulder stiffness, arm edema, brachial plexopathy, and lung fibrosis in these trials. However, the most clinically relevant HF-WBI schedule was used in the START B trial in which treatment was completed in 3 weeks, and only 7% of patients received regional nodal irradiation in this analysis.[6]

A recent prospective single arm phase II postmastectomy hypofractionation trial treating the chest wall and regional lymphatics using a novel 3-week fractionation scheme showed acceptable toxicity and outcomes.[11] To further evaluate the safety and efficacy of hypofractionation to the regional nodes, the Alliance Cooperative Group has launched a phase III trial randomly assigning node-positive patients who have undergone modified radical mastectomy with reconstruction to standard fractionation versus hypofractionation (42.5 Gy in 16 daily fractions) to the chest wall/breast and regional lymphatics.[12]

Hypofractionated whole-breast irradiation and chemotherapy The proportion of patients who received chemotherapy in the RMH/GOC, START A, START B, and Canadian trials ranged from 11% to 35% (see **Table 1**), with an even smaller number of patients in the START A and START B trials receiving anthracycline-containing and taxane-containing regimens. Long-term combined results from the RMH/GOC, START A, and START B trials again showed no change in tumor control and normal tissue outcomes with chemotherapy receipt. Although the 2011 ASTRO guidelines did not reach consensus on the use of HF-WBI after chemotherapy, most task force members reported they commonly used HF-WBI after systemic chemotherapy. Additional long-term data on chemotherapy were not available at the time of the 2011 ASTRO consensus.[6,10] The use of HF-WBI after chemotherapy will likely be revisited in the updated consensus guidelines currently under development.

Hypofractionated whole-breast irradiation and ductal carcinoma in-situ Multiple large randomized trials have found the benefits of adjuvant SF-WBI after BCS in reducing the risk of local recurrence for ductal carcinoma in-situ (DCIS).[13-16] The available data in support of HF-WBI for adjuvant management of DCIS comes largely from single and multi-institutional retrospective series.[17-20] A meta-analysis of 2534 patients from 4 studies comparing HF-WBI with SF-WBI for DCIS showed no difference in local recurrence rates with HF-WBI.[21] Although the randomized Canadian trial did include patients with a DCIS component, patients with only DCIS were not studied. In clinical practice, the use of HF-WBI for DCIS is extrapolated from randomized data on invasive carcinoma.

Utilization of hypofractionated whole-breast irradiation
HF-WBI has the potential to reduce treatment cost and increase patient convenience while maintaining tumor control and long-term normal tissue toxicity. In 2013, the American Society of Radiation Oncology encouraged the Choosing Wisely initiative, which is a national campaign in the United States aimed at reducing low-value health care, to discuss the use of HF-WBI in appropriately selected patients with early-stage breast cancer.[22,23]

National cancer registry data show an overall increase in the utilization of HF-WBI. A National Cancer Data Base analysis showed an increase in HF-WBI utilization from 5.4% in 2004 to 22.8% in 2011.[24] Similarly, a Surveillance, Epidemiology, and End Results (SEER) analysis found that the use of HF-WBI increased from 3.8% in 2006 to 13.6% in 2010.[25] Another analysis using administrative claims data showed an increase in HF-WBI from 10.6% in 2008 to 34.5% in 2013 among patients for whom HF-WBI was endorsed by the 2011 ASTRO guidelines. Adjusted mean total health care expenditures 1 year after diagnosis were nearly $3000 lower for patients who received HF-WBI compared with SF-WBI ($28,747 vs $31,641), translating into a mean total health care expenditure savings of 9.1%.[26]

Although national utilization rates of HF-WBI have increased substantially over recent years, a significant proportion of patients with early-stage breast cancer continue to receive SF-WBI. The reluctance of clinicians to adopt HF-WBI as a standard of care may stem, in part, from several remaining questions regarding the safety and efficacy of HF-WBI in certain clinical scenarios, as previously discussed. However, a utilization rate of only 34.5% in patients for whom HF-WBI was endorsed suggests additional factors, such as reimbursement rates, may also play a role.

Accelerated Partial Breast Irradiation

Accelerated partial breast irradiation (APBI) targets RT to the breast tissue surrounding the postlumpectomy surgical cavity, which is considered to be the region at highest risk for recurrence. In addition to treating a smaller target volume, APBI can be delivered using shorter treatment regimens compared with SF-WBI and HF-WBI. A variety of techniques can be used for the delivery of APBI, including multicatheter interstitial brachytherapy, balloon catheter brachytherapy, 3-dimensional conformal RT (3D-CRT), and intraoperative RT (IORT).

Multicatheter interstitial brachytherapy

Multicatheter interstitial brachytherapy was the earliest technique developed for treatment of the partial breast with the longest available follow-up data. The Radiation Therapy Oncology Group (RTOG) 95-17 trial was a multi-institutional prospective phase II study that enrolled patients with stage I or II unifocal breast cancer less than 3 cm in size after lumpectomy with negative margins. Axillary dissection was required with a minimum of 6 lymph nodes recovered. Patients with up to 3 positive lymph nodes without extracapsular extension were allowed. Patients with DCIS, invasive lobular carcinoma, or extensive intraductal component were excluded. Patients who received low-dose-rate (LDR) brachytherapy were treated to a dose of 45 Gy in 3.5 to 5 days, and those who received high-dose-rate (HDR) brachytherapy were treated to a dose of 34 Gy in 10 fractions delivered twice daily. Long-term results from 98 evaluable patients showed a 10-year ipsilateral breast recurrence (IBR) rate of 5.2%. Ten-year DFS and OS rates were 69.8% and 78.0%, respectively.[27]

A smaller phase I/II protocol included 48 patients with T1, N0, M0 breast cancer who received LDR after lumpectomy to doses of 50 Gy, 55 Gy, and 60 Gy. The treatment volume included the lumpectomy cavity with a 3-cm margin. The 12-year IBR rate from this study was 14.6%. Two-thirds of patients reported good or excellent cosmesis.[28] A third series included 45 patients with T1, N0-N1mi breast cancer treated with HDR brachytherapy to 30.3 Gy or 36.4 Gy delivered over 4 days. The 12-year rate of local recurrence was 9.3%. Good or excellent cosmesis was achieved in nearly 80% of patients.[29]

A larger multi-institutional phase III noninferiority trial randomly assigned 1184 patients with stage 0, I, and IIA breast cancer who underwent BCS to either SF-WBI or APBI. Patients randomly assigned to the APBI arm received HDR multicatheter brachytherapy to a dose of 32 Gy in 8 twice-daily fractions or 30.3 Gy in 7 twice daily fractions. The 5-year local recurrence rates were 0.92% in the SF-WBI arm and 1.44% in the APBI arm (P value, not significant), which was below the relevance margin of 3%. There was no significant difference in 5-year DFS or OS. Skin and subcutaneous tissue toxicity rates remained low in both arms. Long-term follow-up is needed to establish durable tumor control with APBI.[30]

Balloon catheter brachytherapy

The use of the MammoSite (Hologic, Bedford, MA) balloon applicator was approved by the US Food and Drug Administration in 2002. Compared with interstitial brachytherapy, balloon catheter brachytherapy allows for simplified catheter insertion. The American Society of Breast Surgeons MammoSite Registry Trial included 1449 patients treated at 97 participating institutions. Study inclusion criteria were age 45 years or older, tumor size 2 cm or less, invasive ductal carcinoma or ductal carcinoma in situ histology, and negative surgical margins. Technical guidelines, such as balloon-to-skin distance of 7 mm or more and cavity size, were also provided. After lumpectomy, patients were treated to a dose of 34 Gy in 10 fractions delivered twice daily. The 7-year actuarial rate of IBR was 5.8%. For patients with long-term data on cosmesis, good or excellent cosmetic outcome was achieved in more than 90%.[31]

Three-dimensional conformal radiation therapy

The major advantage of 3D-CRT APBI is its accessibility at a wider range of centers, as treatment is not limited to facilities with brachytherapy capabilities. Several randomized studies compared WBI with 3D-CRT APBI. The Christie Hospital Breast Conservation Trial randomly assigned 708 patients to WBI (40 Gy in 15 fractions) or tumor bed–only irradiation using electrons (40–42.5 Gy in 8 fractions). At a median follow-up of 5.4 years, patients with infiltrating ductal carcinoma had an IBR rate of 15% with APBI compared with 11% with WBI. For patients with infiltrating lobular carcinoma, the increase in IBR with APBI was significantly larger (34% APBI vs 8% WBI).[32] A similar study randomly assigned patients to WBI (40 Gy in 15 fractions) or partial-breast irradiation (55 Gy in 20 fractions with electrons). Although statistical analysis was limited because of poor accrual, the rate of IBR was higher with partial-breast irradiation (12% vs 4%; P value, not significant).[33]

The Canadian Randomized Trial of Accelerated Partial Breast Irradiation (RAPID) enrolled 2135 women age older than 40 years with node-negative invasive ductal carcinoma or DCIS measuring ≤3 cm. Patients were randomly assigned after BCS to WBI (either 42.5 Gy in 16 fractions or 50 Gy in 25 fractions with or without a boost) versus 3D-CRT APBI (38.5 Gy in 10 fractions delivered twice daily without a boost). The trial was closed to accrual in 2011, and final results are not yet available. However, an interim analysis found significantly inferior cosmetic outcomes in the APBI arm based on patient, nurse, and physician assessment. The rate of grade 3 toxicity was very low in both arms, but grade 1 and 2 toxicities were more common in the APBI arm.[34] In contrast, a long-term update of the RTOG 0319 trial, a smaller phase 1 and 2 trial evaluating 3D-CRT APBI, showed a 7-year IBR rate of 5.9% and a grade 3 adverse event rate of 7.7%. However, this study only evaluated 52 patients.[35]

Intraoperative radiation therapy

Intraoperative APBI (IO-APBI) is a newer technique that uses applicators to deliver low-energy photons immediately after lumpectomy. Although this treatment can be very convenient for patients and shows promising early results, long-term efficacy data are not yet available. An additional limitation to IO-APBI is the incomplete knowledge of tumor pathology at the time of surgery and treatment.

The TARGIT-A trial was a randomized, phase 3 noninferiority trial that included 3451 patients. Women were randomly assigned to conventional WBI (per each center's protocols) versus a single fraction of 20 Gy immediately after lumpectomy prescribed to the surface of the applicator. Postoperative WBI was permitted for predefined pathologic features at the discretion of the treating institution. The primary endpoint was local recurrence, and noninferiority of IO-APBI was defined as a less than 2.5% absolute difference. The 5-year local recurrence rate was 3.3% in the IO-APBI arm compared with 1.3% in the WBI arm, which met the noninferiority criteria. Toxicity was also similar between the 2 treatment arms.[36]

The ELIOT trial was an equivalence trial that randomly assigned 1305 patients to WBI (50 Gy in 25 fractions with a 10-Gy boost) versus IORT (21 Gy in 1 fraction). The 5-year IBR rate was 4.4% in the IORT group compared with 0.4% in the WBI group. Although this finding met the equivalence criteria, the rate of IBR after IORT was significantly higher than that after WBI.[37]

Consensus statements on accelerated partial breast irradiation

ASTRO released a consensus statement regarding the use of APBI after lumpectomy in 2009. Patients classified as suitable for APBI included those who were older than 60 years, had T1, N0 tumors, had positive estrogen receptor (ER) status, had no lymphovascular space invasion (LVSI), had widely (>2 mm) negative margins, and had no multicentric disease. The cautionary group included any patients with one of the following criteria: age less than 60, T2 tumor, pure DCIS less than 3 cm, close margins (<2 mm), focal LVSI, multifocal or multicentric disease, invasive lobular carcinoma, or ER negativity. Unsuitable patients included those with tumors greater than 3 cm, positive margins, positive lymph nodes, no axillary surgery, extensive LVSI, multicentricity, DCIS greater than 3 cm, and those with a BRCA 1 or 2 mutation. The Task Force did not specify a preferred APBI technique.[38]

After additional data on the efficacy of APBI became available, ASTRO released a revised consensus statement in 2016, which is summarized in **Table 3**. The suitable group was modified to include patients age 50 years or older and patients with

Table 3
Summary of American Society for Radiation Oncology consensus statement

Variable	Suitable	Cautionary	Unsuitable
Age, y	≥50	40–49 if otherwise suitable	<40
		≥50 if at least one cautionary feature is present	40–49 if cautionary criteria not met
Tumor size	≤2 cm	2.1–3.0 cm	>3 cm
N stage	pN0		pN1-3
Margins	≥2 mm	<2 mm	Positive
LVSI	None	Focal	Extensive
ER status	Positive	Negative	
Multicentricity	Clinically unifocal, microscopic multifocality allowed if total lesion size is ≤2 cm	Clinically unifocal, microscopic multifocality allowed if total lesion size is 2.1–3.0 cm	Clinically multifocal or microscopic multifocality with total lesion size >3.0 cm
Histology	Invasive ductal	Invasive lobular	
Pure DCIS	Allowed if screen-detected, low-intermediate grade, size ≤2.5 cm, negative margins ≥3 mm	≤3 cm and does not meet suitable criteria	
Nodal surgery	SLNB or ALND		None
Neoadjuvant therapy	No		Yes
BRCA1/2 mutation	No		Yes

Abbreviations: ALND, axillary lymph node dissection; SLNB, sentinel lymph node biopsy.

low-risk DCIS (low-intermediate grade, size ≤2.5 cm, ≥3 mm margins, as per RTOG 9804). The cautionary group was modified to include patients age 40 to 49 years if all other criteria in the suitable category were met.

Future Directions

Both HF-WBI and APBI represent more convenient and potentially cost-effective treatment modalities compared with SF-WBI. Although long-term efficacy data for HF-WBI are available, there are some remaining questions regarding the optimal candidates for HF-WBI, as previously discussed. Additionally, there is interest in further shortening the treatment regimen to provide greater convenience and cost savings.

The UK FAST trial randomly assigned 915 women age 50 years or older with node-negative early breast cancer to SF-WBI with 50 Gy in 25 daily fractions versus HF-WBI with 28.5 Gy or 30 Gy in 5 once-weekly fractions. Preliminary results showed similar rates of adverse effects in the breast between the 28.5-Gy and 50-Gy regimens. Tumor control rates have not yet been evaluated.[39] The FAST-Forward trial is a phase III randomized trial comparing 40 Gy in 15 daily fractions to 26 Gy or 27 Gy in 5 daily fractions. The trial enrolled 4100 patients with a primary endpoint of ipsilateral breast tumor control. Results are pending.[40]

The fractionation schemes of 42.5 Gy in 16 daily fractions from the Canadian trial and 40 Gy in 15 daily fractions from the START B trial are the most appropriate HF-WBI schemes outside of a clinical trial and are the most commonly used regimens in current day practice. Other smaller prospective phase II trials have evaluated alternate schemes that deliver equivalent radiobiologic doses with promising results. One series evaluating a 3-week regimen consisting of 36.63 Gy in 11 fractions to the whole breast followed by a lumpectomy bed boost in 4 fractions of 3.33 Gy showed high local control rates, low toxicity, and favorable cosmetic outcomes on short-term follow-up.[41] Another series showed the feasibility of using accelerated whole-breast intensity modulated RT in the prone position to reduce normal tissue exposure and spare the heart and lung. A dose of 40.5 Gy in 15 daily fractions was delivered to the whole breast with a concomitant boost of 0.5 Gy to the lumpectomy cavity, for a total dose of 48 Gy to the tumor bed.[42]

Data on the use of HF-WBI for postmastectomy irradiation and regional nodal irradiation remains limited. A recent phase II study evaluating a 3-week regimen for treatment of the chest wall and regional lymphatics showed favorable results.[11] The safety and efficacy of hypofractionation to the regional nodes is also being studied in a recently launched phase III randomized trial.[12] Until these data mature, SF-WBI will likely remain the most commonly used regimen for patients requiring regional nodal irradiation. An ongoing Trans-Tasman Radiation Oncology Group trial is investigating the role of HF-WBI for DCIS.[43]

Although the available efficacy data on APBI is encouraging, it is largely limited by inadequate follow-up. Two large randomized trials were recently closed to accrual, and, once mature, their results should help to establish the long-term efficacy and toxicity of APBI. The RAPID trial, as previously discussed, enrolled 2135 women with node-negative invasive ductal carcinoma or DCIS to WBI versus 3D-CRT APBI. The National Surgical Adjuvant Breast and Bowel B-39/RTOG 0413 trial is a randomized phase III study comparing SF-WBI with APBI using multicatheter interstitial brachytherapy, balloon catheter brachytherapy, or 3D-CRT APBI. This trial completed enrollment in 2013 and includes 4311 patients with stage 0, I, or II breast cancer with primary tumor size ≤3 cm and no more than 3 positive lymph nodes. Patients age 18 and older with unifocal invasive adenocarcinoma or DCIS were eligible. Negative lumpectomy margins and axillary evaluation were required. Once available, results from this trial and those from the recently closed RAPID trial may help address several questions regarding APBI, such as the appropriate patient age criteria, suitability for DCIS, and which technique provides the greatest long-term tumor control.[34,44]

SUMMARY

Adjuvant whole-breast irradiation after BCS has been an established standard of care to optimize local tumor control for decades. Although SF-WBI can achieve excellent durable tumor control with low toxicity and favorable cosmesis, a 5- to 7-week treatment regimen can be inconvenient for patients and may be an ineffective use of available resources.

HF-WBI presents an appealing alternate treatment regimen and may be considered the preferred standard of care in appropriately selected patients. The long-term data on APBI are more limited, but the available results suggest it is an effective alternative to WBI in certain subsets of patients.

REFERENCES

1. Fisher B, Anderson S, Bryant J, et al. Twenty-year follow-up of a randomized trial comparing total mastectomy, lumpectomy, and lumpectomy plus irradiation for the treatment of invasive breast cancer. N Engl J Med 2002;347(16):1233–41.
2. Veronesi U, Cascinelli N, Mariani L, et al. Twenty-year follow-up of a randomized study comparing breast-conserving surgery with radical mastectomy for early breast cancer. N Engl J Med 2002;347(16):1227–32.
3. Clarke M, Collins R, Darby S, et al. Effects of radiotherapy and of differences in the extent of surgery for early breast cancer on local recurrence and 15-year survival: an overview of the randomised trials. Lancet 2005;366(9503):2087–106.
4. Owen JR, Ashton A, Bliss JM, et al. Effect of radiotherapy fraction size on tumour control in patients with early-stage breast cancer after local tumour excision: long-term results of a randomised trial. Lancet Oncol 2006;7(6):467–71.
5. START Trialists' Group, Bentzen SM, Agrawal RK, Aird EG, et al. The UK Standardisation of Breast Radiotherapy (START) Trial A of radiotherapy hypofractionation for treatment of early breast cancer: a randomised trial. Lancet Oncol 2008; 9(4):331–41.
6. Haviland JS, Owen JR, Dewar JA, et al. The UK Standardisation of Breast Radiotherapy (START) trials of radiotherapy hypofractionation for treatment of early breast cancer: 10-year follow-up results of two randomised controlled trials. Lancet Oncol 2013;14(11):1086–94.
7. START Trialists' Group, Bentzen SM, Agrawal RK, Aird EG, et al. The UK Standardisation of Breast Radiotherapy (START) Trial B of radiotherapy hypofractionation for treatment of early breast cancer: a randomised trial. Lancet 2008; 371(9618):1098–107.
8. Whelan TJ, Pignol JP, Levine MN, et al. Long-term results of hypofractionated radiation therapy for breast cancer. N Engl J Med 2010;362(6):513–20.
9. Yarnold J, Ashton A, Bliss J, et al. Fractionation sensitivity and dose response of late adverse effects in the breast after radiotherapy for early breast cancer: long-term results of a randomised trial. Radiother Oncol 2005;75(1):9–17.
10. Smith BD, Bentzen SM, Correa CR, et al. Fractionation for whole breast irradiation: an American Society for Radiation Oncology (ASTRO) evidence-based guideline. Int J Radiat Oncol Biol Phys 2011;81(1):59–68.

11. Khan AJ, Poppe MM, Goyal S, et al. Hypofractionated postmastectomy radiation therapy is safe and effective: first results from a prospective Phase II trial. J Clin Oncol 2017;35(18):2037–43.

12. Conventional versus hypofractionated radiotherapy in node positive breast cancer. 2017. Available at: https://clinicaltrials.gov/ct2/show/NCT02690636. Accessed March 23, 2017.

13. Wapnir IL, Dignam JJ, Fisher B, et al. Long-term outcomes of invasive ipsilateral breast tumor recurrences after lumpectomy in NSABP B-17 and B-24 randomized clinical trials for DCIS. J Natl Cancer Inst 2011;103(6):478–88.

14. Holmberg L, Garmo H, Granstrand B, et al. Absolute risk reductions for local recurrence after postoperative radiotherapy after sector resection for ductal carcinoma in situ of the breast. J Clin Oncol 2008;26(8):1247–52.

15. EORTC Breast Cancer Cooperative Group, EORTC Radiotherapy Group, Bijker N, Meijnen P, Peterse JL, et al. Breast-conserving treatment with or without radiotherapy in ductal carcinoma-in-situ: ten-year results of European Organisation for Research and Treatment of Cancer randomized phase III trial 10853–a study by the EORTC Breast Cancer Cooperative Group and EORTC Radiotherapy Group. J Clin Oncol 2006;24(21):3381–7.

16. Cuzick J, Sestak I, Pinder SE, et al. Effect of tamoxifen and radiotherapy in women with locally excised ductal carcinoma in situ: long-term results from the UK/ANZ DCIS trial. Lancet Oncol 2011;12(1):21–9.

17. Williamson D, Dinniwell R, Fung S, et al. Local control with conventional and hypofractionated adjuvant radiotherapy after breast-conserving surgery for ductal carcinoma in-situ. Radiother Oncol 2010;95(3):317–20.

18. Hathout L, Hijal T, Théberge V, et al. Hypofractionated radiation therapy for breast ductal carcinoma in situ. Int J Radiat Oncol Biol Phys 2013;87(5):1058–63.

19. Wai ES, Lesperance ML, Alexander CS, et al. Effect of radiotherapy boost and hypofractionation on outcomes in ductal carcinoma in situ. Cancer 2011; 117(1):54–62.

20. Oar AJ, Boxer MM, Papadatos G, et al. Hypofractionated versus conventionally fractionated radiotherapy for ductal carcinoma in situ (DCIS) of the breast. J Med Imaging Radiat Oncol 2016;60(3):407–13.

21. Nilsson C, Valachis A. The role of boost and hypofractionation as adjuvant radiotherapy in patients with DCIS: a meta-analysis of observational studies. Radiother Oncol 2015;114(1):50–5.

22. ASTRO releases list of five radiation oncology treatments to question as part of national Choosing Wisely campaign. 2017. Available at: http://www.choosingwisely. org/astro-releases-list-of-five-radiation-oncology-treatments-to-question-as-part-of-national-choosing-wisely-campaign. Accessed March 23, 2017.

23. Volpp KG, Loewenstein G, Asch DA. Choosing wisely: low-value services, utilization, and patient cost sharing. JAMA 2012;308(16):1635–6.

24. Wang EH, Mougalian SS, Soulos PR, et al. Adoption of hypofractionated whole-breast irradiation for early-stage breast cancer: a National Cancer Data Base analysis. Int J Radiat Oncol Biol Phys 2014;90(5):993–1000.

25. Jagsi R, Falchook AD, Hendrix LH, et al. Adoption of hypofractionated radiation therapy for breast cancer after publication of randomized trials. Int J Radiat Oncol Biol Phys 2014;90(5):1001–9.

26. Bekelman JE, Sylwestrzak G, Barron J, et al. Uptake and costs of hypofractionated vs conventional whole breast irradiation after breast conserving surgery in the United States, 2008-2013. JAMA 2014;312(23):2542–50.

27. White J, Winter K, Kuske RR, et al. Long-term cancer outcomes from Study NRG Oncology/RTOG 9517: a phase 2 study of accelerated partial breast irradiation with multicatheter brachytherapy after lumpectomy for early-stage breast cancer. Int J Radiat Oncol Biol Phys 2016;95(5):1460–5.

28. Hattangadi JA, Powell SN, MacDonald SM, et al. Accelerated partial breast irradiation with low-dose-rate interstitial implant brachytherapy after wide local excision: 12-year outcomes from a prospective trial. Int J Radiat Oncol Biol Phys 2012;83(3):791–800.

29. Polgar C, Major T, Fodor J, et al. Accelerated partial-breast irradiation using high-dose-rate interstitial brachytherapy: 12-year update of a prospective clinical study. Radiother Oncol 2010;94(3):274–9.

30. Strnad V, Ott OJ, Hildebrandt G, et al. 5-year results of accelerated partial breast irradiation using sole interstitial multicatheter brachytherapy versus whole-breast irradiation with boost after breast-conserving surgery for low-risk invasive and in-situ carcinoma of the female breast: a randomised, phase 3, non-inferiority trial. Lancet 2016;387(10015):229–38.

31. Shah C, Badiyan S, Ben Wilkinson J, et al. Treatment efficacy with accelerated partial breast irradiation (APBI): final analysis of the American Society of Breast Surgeons MammoSite((R)) breast brachytherapy registry trial. Ann Surg Oncol 2013;20(10):3279–85.

32. Ribeiro GG, Magee B, Swindell R, et al. The Christie Hospital breast conservation trial: an update at 8 years from inception. Clin Oncol (R Coll Radiol) 1993;5(5):278–83.

33. Dodwell DJ, Dyker K, Brown J, et al. A randomised study of whole-breast vs tumour-bed irradiation after local excision and axillary dissection for early breast cancer. Clin Oncol (R Coll Radiol) 2005;17(8):618–22.

34. Olivotto IA, Whelan TJ, Parpia S, et al. Interim cosmetic and toxicity results from RAPID: a randomized trial of accelerated partial breast irradiation using three-dimensional conformal external beam radiation therapy. J Clin Oncol 2013; 31(32):4038–45.

35. Rabinovitch R, Moughan J, Vicini F, et al. Long-term update of NRG oncology RTOG 0319: a phase 1 and 2 trial to evaluate 3-dimensional conformal radiation therapy confined to the region of the lumpectomy cavity for stage I and II breast carcinoma. Int J Radiat Oncol Biol Phys 2016;96(5):1054–9.

36. Vaidya JS, Wenz F, Bulsara M, et al. Risk-adapted targeted intraoperative radiotherapy versus whole-breast radiotherapy for breast cancer: 5-year results for local control and overall survival from the TARGIT-A randomised trial. Lancet 2014;383(9917):603–13.

37. Veronesi U, Orecchia R, Maisonneuve P, et al. Intraoperative radiotherapy versus external radiotherapy for early breast cancer (ELIOT): a randomised controlled equivalence trial. Lancet Oncol 2013;14(13):1269–77.

38. Prosnitz LR, Horton J, Wallner PE. Accelerated partial breast irradiation: caution and concern from an ASTRO task force. Int J Radiat Oncol Biol Phys 2009;74(4):981–4.

39. FAST Trialists group, Agrawal RK, Alhasso A, Barrett-Lee PJ, et al. First results of the randomised UK FAST Trial of radiotherapy hypofractionation for treatment of early breast cancer (CRUKE/04/015). Radiother Oncol 2011;100(1):93–100.

40. UK Clinical Research Network Study Portfolio. FAST-Forward Study. 2017. Available at: https://www.ncbi.nlm.nih.gov/pmc/articles/PMC4152718/#B51. Accessed March 23, 2017.

41. Ahlawat S, Haffty BG, Goyal S, et al. Short-course hypofractionated radiation therapy with boost in women with stages 0 to IIIa breast cancer: a phase 2 trial. Int J Radiat Oncol Biol Phys 2016;94(1):118–25.

42. Formenti SC, Gidea-Addeo D, Goldberg JD, et al. Phase I-II trial of prone accelerated intensity modulated radiation therapy to the breast to optimally spare normal tissue. J Clin Oncol 2007;25(16):2236–42.

43. Radiation doses and fractionation schedules in non-low risk ductal carcinoma in situ (DCIS) of the breast (DCIS). 2017. Available at: https://clinicaltrials.gov/ct2/show/NCT00470236. Accessed March 23, 2017.

44. A Randomized Phase III Study of Conventional Whole Breast Irradiation (WBI) Versus Partial Breast Irradiation (PBI) for Women with Stage 0, I, or II Breast Cancer. 2017. Available at: http://rpc.mdanderson.org/rpc/credentialing/files/B39_Protocol1.pdf. Accessed March 23, 2017.

Surgical Intervention for Lymphedema

Kristalyn Gallagher, DO*, Kathleen Marulanda, MD, MS, Stephanie Gray, MD

KEYWORDS

- Lymphedema • Surgery • Lymph node transfer • Axillary reverse mapping
- LYMPHA • Lymphovenous anastomosis • Vascularized lymph node transfer
- Liposuction

KEY POINTS

- Lymphedema is a chronic, progressive disease with no curative treatment.
- Surgical treatment options are effective at managing early and late stage lymphedema.
- Standardized methods for quantifying lymphedema, universal reporting standards, and an increased amount of high-quality evidence are necessary to advance understanding and management of lymphedema.

INTRODUCTION

Lymphedema is a chronic, progressive disease that affects approximately 140 to 200 million people worldwide.[1,2] There is no curative treatment and palliation is challenging. The incidence is difficult to quantify as early stage lymphedema is often underreported until it necessitates intervention. The etiology includes congenital malformations (primary) and direct injury to the lymphatic channels (secondary). Oncologic treatment for solid tumors is the leading cause of secondary lymphedema in the developed world. In the upper extremity, it is most often associated with breast cancer treatment. Patients with breast cancer who have undergone axillary lymph node dissection and/or radiotherapy are a particularly susceptible group, with reported lymphedema rates as high as 65% to 70%.[3,4] Other causes of secondary lymphedema include trauma, neoplastic obstruction, or inflammatory destruction of the lymphatics. Obesity-induced lymphedema occurs in super obese patients with body mass indexes of greater than 50 to 60 kg/m^2 stemming from overwhelmed or damaged lymphatics secondary to increased adipose tissue and fibrosis.[5,6]

Lymphedema can manifest as mild to severe arm swelling, pain, dysfunction, disfigurement, lipodermatosclerosis, skin ulceration, cellulitis, and rarely lymphangiosarcoma. Treatment of lymphedema includes both nonsurgical and surgical strategies.

Disclosure Statement: The authors have nothing to disclose.
Department of Surgery, The University of North Carolina at Chapel Hill, Campus Box 7213, 1150 POB, 170 Manning Drive, Chapel Hill, NC 27599-7123, USA
* Corresponding author.
E-mail address: Kristalyn_gallagher@med.unc.edu

Surg Oncol Clin N Am 27 (2018) 195–215
http://dx.doi.org/10.1016/j.soc.2017.08.001
1055-3207/18/© 2017 Elsevier Inc. All rights reserved.

Nonsurgical management involves meticulous skin care, limb elevation, lifelong external compression therapy (both static and pneumatic), and physical therapy with manual lymph drainage and massage to minimize symptoms. Surgical options have been reserved for failure of conservative management historically, but recent data suggest early intervention with surgical techniques may reduce incidence of symptom progression.[7–9] Preventative surgical techniques have been described to reduce the initial disruption of the lymphatics and maintain function. Microsurgical techniques, including lymphaticovenous anastomosis (LVA), vascularized lymph node transfer (VLNT), and lymphaticolymphatic bypass aim to restore the underlying physiologic impairment. Additional surgical interventions such as liposuction and surgical excision remove affected tissues to effectively decrease the drainage load. The successful selection of surgical therapy depends on the stage of lymphedema with LVA and VLNT more suitable for fluid-predominant disease and suction-assisted protein lipectomy (SAPL) for solid disease. Open debulking and reductive procedures are used for management of late-stage solid lymphedematous disease.

ANATOMY AND PATHOPHYSIOLOGY

Lymphedema is an abnormal accumulation of protein-rich interstitial fluid within the interstitial space. It can occur anywhere in the body, most commonly in the lower extremity, followed by the upper extremity and genitalia. Disruptions in the interstitial pressures lead to an imbalance between the arterial capillary inflow, an increased demand for lymphatic outflow, and the decreased capacity of the lymphatic circulation.[10–12]

Secondary lymphedema occurs because of surgical, inflammatory, neoplastic, or traumatic destruction of the dermal lymphatics and their outflow tracts. During early stage lymphedema, compensatory mechanisms including lymphatic regeneration make up for the initial insult. At later stages, the lymphatic capillaries become overwhelmed and damaged leading to fibrosis, thickened basement membranes, and loss of permeability of the lymphatic capillaries.[11] This breakdown allows protein to leak into the interstitial tissues, which increases the tissue colloid osmotic pressure. Water then accumulates in the interstitial space. The edematous tissues signal increased numbers of fibroblasts, adipocytes, keratinocytes, and inflammatory cells. These cell types cause increased collagen deposition, adipose accumulation, chronic inflammation, and fibrosis of the skin and subcutaneous tissues.[11,13] Clinical manifestations include nonpitting edema with overlying skin changes. Stasis of the protein-rich fluid makes the subcutaneous tissues prone to recurrent bacterial and fungal infections, which ultimately leads to progressive damage of the lymphatics.[14]

The enlarged and edematous limb can subsequently cause debilitating and chronic pain, decreased quality of life (QoL), psychosocial issues, increased infection risk, higher medical costs, and loss in productive days for those afflicted with the disease.[15,16] Although the incidence, onset, and progression of lymphedema differ greatly among patients, there are several associated risk factors that have been identified. These risk factors include obesity (body mass index $\geq$30 kg/m^2), number of nodes resected during oncologic surgery, radiation therapy, high rates of paclitaxel use, infection, and underlying genetic makeup.[16,17]

CLINICAL PRESENTATION

Patients who have undergone breast cancer treatment with surgery, radiation, and/or chemotherapy have a lifetime risk of lymphedema occurrence[17,18] and should be monitored with a low threshold of suspicion. Most patients become symptomatic within 8 months of surgery and 75% will present in the first 3 years.[17]

The two most commonly used staging systems for lymphedema are the International Society of Lymphology and Campisi systems (**Table 1**). Both systems agree that lymphedema can be classified as subclinical, mild (early), moderate (intermediate), or severe (advanced). The symptoms of lymphedema by stage are listed in **Table 2**. Early lymphedema typically presents with subjective symptoms, most commonly heaviness in the affected limb without any appreciable swelling or edema.[10,19–21] These symptoms may be present for months or years before any detectable physical change occurs. As interstitial fluid accumulates, patients experience increased extremity circumference followed by pitting edema that usually worsens at the end of the day (**Fig. 1**). A 2 cm or greater difference in arm circumference or a 200 mL limb volume difference between affected and nonaffected arms is considered to meet diagnostic criteria for lymphedema, although no universal criteria exist.[22] Early symptoms are initially alleviated with compressive garments, limb elevation, and physical therapy with manual lymph drainage and massage to minimize symptoms. As the disease progresses, irreversible, nonpitting edema develops. Patients report increased firmness, decreased functionality, and disfigurement.[20,23] Significant swelling and increased limb volume severely impair limb mobility and cause chronic debilitating pain that impedes activities of daily living. This disease

Table 1
ISL and Campisi staging systems for comparison with proposed treatment

		ISL Staging and Description		Campisi Staging and Description	Proposed Surgical Treatment
Subclinical	0	No swelling, changes found only on imaging.			None CDT
Mild	I	Accumulation of fluid with high protein content, which subsides with limb elevation. Usually lasts ≤24 h.	Ia	No overt swelling despite impaired lymph drainage	CDT LVA or VLNT
			Ib	Reversible swelling with limb elevation	
Moderate	IIa	Rarely resolves with limb elevation alone.	II	Mild persistence of swelling with elevation	LVA or VLNT SAPL
	IIb	Loss of pitting owing to progression of dermal fibrosis. Sometimes called spontaneously irreversible lymphedema.	III	Persistent swelling with recurrent lymphangitis	
Severe	III	Lymphostatic elephantiasis. No pitting; develop trophic skin changes (fat deposits, acanthosis, and warty overgrowths).	IV	Fibrotic changes with columnlike limb	SAPL Surgical excision
			V	Elephantiasis with limb deformation including widespread lymphostatic warts	

Abbreviations: CDT, complex decongestive therapy; ISL, International Society of Lymphology; LVA, lymphaticovenous anastomosis; SAPL, suction-assisted protein lipectomy; VLNT, vascularized lymph node transfer.
Data from Refs.[19,24,27]

Table 2
Symptoms of lymphedema by stage

Stage		Symptoms
Subclinical	0	• Heaviness • Tightness • Firmness • Pain • Aching • Soreness • Numbness • Limb fatigue • Limb weakness • Impaired limb mobility • Absence of swelling
Early (mild)	I	• Above symptoms • Presence of swelling that decreases with compression or elevation
Moderate (Intermediate)	II	• Above symptoms • Disfigurement • Early skin changes • With or without cellulitis or infections • Presence of swelling that does not decrease with compression or elevation
Severe (Advanced)	III	• Above symptoms • Disability • Recurrent cellulitis or infections • Late skin changes (hyperkeratosis, hyperpigmentation, papillomas, induration)

Data from Refs.[10,19–21,23–26]

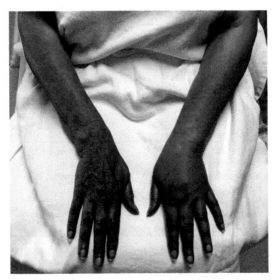

Fig. 1. Clinical presentation of lymphedema.

progression results in an undeniable decline in QoL. Disfiguring skin changes including hyperpigmentation and skin infections also arise secondary to chronic venostasis in the affected limb.[10,19,20,24–26] Very rarely, this results in Stewart-Treves syndrome or angiosarcoma. Conservative palliation for advanced disease is exceedingly difficult.

The severity of disease is closely mirrored to a multifactorial decline in both objective and subjective symptoms, thereby making it difficult to accurately stage or define lymphedema. As such, no standardized staging system exists; the two predominantly used systems, the International Society of Lymphology and the Campisi (see **Table 1**), are limited owing to their heavy reliance on physical examination findings. Supplemental imaging studies and QoL evaluations are necessary to provide a more comprehensive assessment.[19,24,27] This step is crucial, because the outcome, effectiveness of treatment, and risk of recurrence greatly depend on the stage of lymphedema at presentation.[28]

CLINICAL MONITORING

Early detection and intervention lead to increased effectiveness of management therapies, fewer invasive procedures, and a decreased financial burden.[7,29,30] Prospective surveillance is recommended for at least 1 year postoperatively. For improved diagnostic accuracy, preoperative baseline assessments are established and monitored serially to determine disease progression and therapeutic response. Early detection and treatment can lead to reversal and prevention of progression.[7–9]

Limb size and volume measurements are typically used to quantitatively characterize the disease. The most commonly used criteria define lymphedema as a 10% change in limb volume measured by perometry or a 2-cm change in arm circumference.[31]

The ideal measuring tool should be simple and easily reproducible for serial measurements. Water displacement is considered the gold standard owing to its high sensitivity and specificity for quantifying overall limb volume, but owing to its burdensome technique it is rarely performed.[31] Tape measurements of arm circumference at 10 cm intervals along the limb are most frequently used owing to low cost and simplicity. Preferably, serial measurements are performed by the same operator to minimize variability. An increase in size between measurements (>10 cm or >10%) is found to correlate with subclinical lymphedema. Additional techniques available include perometry, a noninvasive optoelectronic device that uses infrared light to quantify limb volume, and bioelectrical impedance, which measures the flow of electrical currents to indirectly determine the limb volume. Notably, a recent study by Deltombe and colleagues[32] found that perometry is superior to both water displacement and arm circumference tests, but applicability remains limited owing to its high cost.[33]

Symptoms are frequently reported before any measurable physical changes, and continue to worsen in parallel with increasing volume.[34] The Functional Assessment of Cancer Therapy questionnaire including breast cancer and arm function subscales (FACT B+4), the Lymphedema and Breast Cancer Questionnaire, and the Morbidity Screening Tool[35] are used to assess QoL. These questionnaires evaluate symptoms including swelling and heaviness within the past year, which are the 2 most predictive factors associated with objective measurements.[31] High-quality evidence regarding lymphedema-specific symptoms remains scarce and most questionnaires are not specific to breast cancer–related lymphedema.

DIAGNOSTIC IMAGING

Lymphography was historically used, but is seldom used currently owing to technical difficulties with cannulization of the lymphatic vessels and morbidity associated with administration of oil-based contrast agents.[36] Current guidelines recommend lympho-scintigraphy as the gold standard to assess the caliber and anatomic location of lymphatic vessels, functional status, and disease severity. Radionuclide dye is injected intradermally via the interdigital space and taken up by the lymphatic system to visualize dynamic flow, areas of blockage, and dermal backflow. Disadvantages of this technique include prolonged radionuclide uptake, poor image quality, and limited visibility of small vessels owing to relatively poor spatial resolution.[35,36] Additional adjunct imaging modalities have been described including duplex ultrasound, which identifies tissue spaces and fluid accumulation, and computed tomography scan/MRI, which can delineate lymphatic abnormalities at multiple tissue levels.[37,38]

In recent years, the development of near-infrared fluorescence (NIRF) imaging has significantly enhanced noninvasive in vivo imaging capabilities.[35] NIRF imaging is a highly sensitive, quick and reproducible technique, which typically uses indocyanine green (ICG) as an optical contrast agent. In contrast with lymphoscintigraphy, NIRF imaging provides immediate, high-resolution images that assess contractile lymphatic flow volume and velocity, as well as finely detailed images of the lymphatic anatomy, including lymph nodes and surrounding collateral lymphatic network. Mihara and col-leagues[39] found that, unlike lymphoscintigraphy, NIRF imaging can definitively diag-nose early stage lymphedema. NIRF imaging is equally beneficial intraoperatively when performing microsurgical procedures, and postoperatively to evaluate postther-apeutic response. Further research may support the potential use of NIRF imaging as a screening diagnostic tool.[40]

NONSURGICAL MANAGEMENT OF LYMPHEDEMA

Lymphedema has traditionally been managed with nonoperative methods, primarily complex decongestive therapy, which consists of manual lymph drainage with mas-sage, compression garments, meticulous hygiene, and physical therapy to decrease swelling and improve mobility. Patients are required to be active lifelong participants in their care and, therefore, the success of complex decongestive therapy is highly dependent on patient compliance and engagement.

Surgical options have emerged to avoid a lifetime commitment to compressive ther-apy and the potential to achieve a definitive cure. Currently, there is no widely accepted consensus for the role for surgical management, optimal timing of surgery, which surgical procedure to perform, or which surgical technique is preferred. Never-theless, it is generally recognized that earlier initiation of treatment is preferred, given the progressive nature of the disease, which will only continue to deteriorate the lym-phovascular system over time.[41–43]

PREVENTATIVE SURGICAL TECHNIQUES

Surgical techniques such as sentinel lymph node biopsy (SLNB), axillary reverse mapping (ARM), and Lymphovascular anastamosis ("LYMPHA") have been developed to prevent or minimize the disruption of lymphatic flow from the upper extremity during breast cancer surgery.[44–46]

Sentinel Lymph Node Biopsy

SLNB is a technique by which the tumor's most proximal draining lymph node(s) are identified with radioactive dye and/or isosulfan blue and excised. Reported rates of lymphedema range from 1% to 7% after SLNB.[45] Recent data from ACOSOG (Amer-ican College of Surgeons Oncology Group) Z0011, ACOSOG Z1071, SENTINA (Sentinel-Lymph-Node Biopsy in Patients With Breast Cancer Before and After

Neoadjuvant Chemotherapy), AMAROS (Comparison of Complete Axillary Lymph Node Dissection With Axillary Radiation Therapy in Treating Women With Invasive Breast Cancer), and OTOSAR (Optimal Treatment of the Axilla - Surgery or Radiotherapy) clinical trials show the usefulness of minimizing axillary surgery even in the setting of selective patients with node-positive disease in the axilla.[46–52]

Axillary Reverse Mapping

ARM is a procedure where isosulfan blue is injected into the proximal arm, identifying and sparing the lymphatic drainage of the arm in patients with breast cancer who undergo axillary lymph node dissection or SLNB.[23,44,53,54] If ARM is used during SLNB, the radioisotope (Tc-99m) is injected into the breast and the blue dye is injected into the arm.

The ARM technique was initially described by Klimberg and colleagues[53,54,55] in 2007 as a way to directly visualize arm lymphatics and preserve them to minimize injury. A volume of 2 to 5 mL of isosulfan blue is injected subcutaneously into the volar aspect of the upper arm in the medial bicipital sulcus (**Fig. 2**) before incision. The blue dye travels through the arm lymphatics highlighting them for visualization during axillary surgery (**Fig. 3**). Multiple studies have demonstrated statistically significant improvement in lymphedema rates when the ARM technique is used (33% vs a range of 4%–9% in ARM groups).[55–59] Tausch and colleagues[60] reported identification of arm nodes, but did not show a statistically significant difference in prevention of lymphedema at 19 months of follow-up. In 2015, Yue and colleagues[61] performed a prospective feasibility study on 265 patients and showed reduction in lymphedema (33.7% in the control group and 5.93% in the ARM group; $P<.001$). They used both blue dye and radioisotope (Tc-99m-Nano-coll). Most studies have reported the feasibility of the procedure without long-term outcomes. Currently there is no large, multicenter trial assessing the effectiveness of this technique.

The ARM technique was developed with the hypothesis that the arm and breast lymphatic drainage systems are separate. Metastatic disease has been reported in 8.7% to 25% of ARM nodes. The involvement of the ARM node increases with the increased axillary burden of disease (more common in N2 and N3 disease). The possibility of crossover nodes should be discussed with patients preoperatively. If a lymph node is dyed blue and there is strong clinical suspicion for involvement, the node

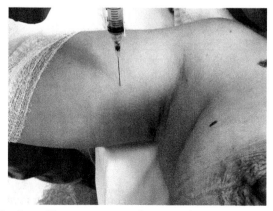

Fig. 2. Injection site for axillary reverse mapping procedure: 3 to 5 mL of isosulfan blue is injected subcutaneously in the volar surface of the upper extremity.

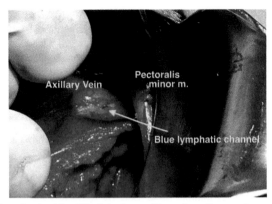

Fig. 3. Blue arm lymphatics identified during axillary dissection and preserved.

should be removed along with the remaining axillary nodes. The oncologic resection should not be compromised to minimize the risk of lymphedema (**Fig. 4**).

Lymphovascular Anastomosis Technique

The lymphovascular anastomosis ("LYMPHA") technique performed at the time of initial axillary dissection has shown a statistically significant reduction in the development of lymphedema at 18 months (30% vs 4.05%; $P<.01$).[45] This technique was originally described by Boccardo in 2009. Isosulfan blue is injected into the volar aspect of the ipsilateral upper arm before incision (see **Fig. 2**). During axillary dissection, the blue lymphatics are identified and the afferent lymphatics are clipped near insertion into the node. After dissection, the afferent lymphatics are directly anastomosed into a collateral branch of the axillary vein with microsurgical technique.[45]

SURGICAL TECHNIQUES

Surgical treatment options are divided into two general categories, reductive versus physiologic procedures. In this section, we focus on the physiologic procedures, which aim to assuage the physiologic disturbances that result from increased adipose volume and fibrosis in the affected limb. Microsurgical procedures, including LVA and VLNT, target the fluid component that predominates at earlier stages of the disease (**Fig. 4**).

Lymphaticovenous Anastomosis

LVA, first described in 1969, is a microsurgical procedure that effectively bypasses diseased lymphatics and restores adequate lymphatic drainage via direct drainage into the venous system.[19,62] Serial anastomoses are typically created between small lymphatics and subdermal venules, preferably less than 1 cm in diameter, along the entirety of the upper extremity. The minimally invasive approach allows multiple anastomoses to be created via a single 1- to 2-cm incision. The procedure is typically performed under locoregional anesthetic, which may be better suited for candidates with extensive comorbidities.

Indications
LVA is indicated after failed management of conservative therapy, and early International Society of Lymphology stage II disease with evidence of partial lymphatic obstruction.[27] Functional lymphatic vessels, albeit partially functional, are required

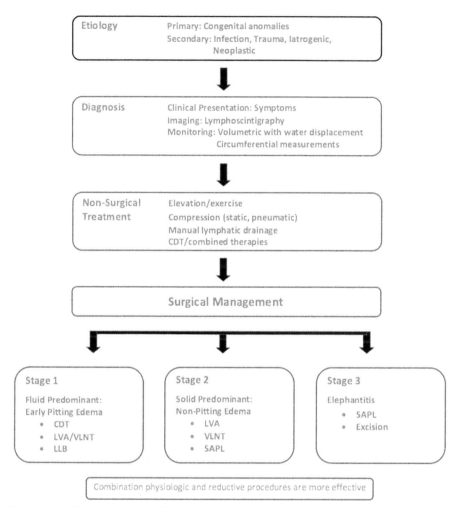

Fig. 4. Algorithm for managing lymphedema. CDT, complex decongestive therapy; LVA, lymphaticovenous anastomosis; LLB, lymphaticolymphatic bypass; SAPL, suction-assisted protein lipectomy; VLNT, vascularized lymph node transfer.

to create an effective anastomosis with durable patency; complete occlusion of the lymphatics is an absolute contraindication to LVA. Studies have shown that the earlier LVA is introduced, the greater the success of the procedure,[63] likely owing to the decreased presence of irreversibly damaged vessels. Guided by a similar premise, it was previously absolutely contraindicated to perform LVA on patients with primary lymphedema given the concern for hypoplastic vessels. However, studies have shown that certain types of primary lymphedema are adequately treated with LVA.[64]

Lymphoscintigraphy
Superior results have been reported when perioperative lymphatic mapping is used[65] to identify lymphatic vessels and determine functionality. ICG lymphoscintigraphy is a simple tool, frequently used to locate functional lymphatics, determine severity of disease, and identify optimal placement for surgical incisions.[41,66–69] Intraoperatively, the

dye illuminates functional lymphatics as it travels through the surgical field, which has been shown to increase the number of anastomoses created[70] despite an overall shorter length of operation.

Postoperative anastomotic patency is subsequently monitored with lymphoscintigraphy; the rate of radiotracer clearance provides an indirect measure of lymphatic flow.

Technique

There is no consensus in the literature regarding timing, location, number, or configuration of anastomoses when performing a LVA; these decisions are primarily dictated by surgeon preference. However, the likelihood of successful outcomes is determined primarily on the surgeon's ability to identify suitable venules and lymphatic vessels within the affected limb. Ideally, both vessels should be of similar diameter, preferably less than 0.8 mm, in close proximity to one another, and with minimal to no venous backflow after division.[24,71] Smaller veins are preferred because of the greater risk of increased intraluminal pressure, and subsequent risk of venous reflux associated with larger veins.

The number and location of anastomoses varies and is highly dependent on the presence of functional and accessible vessels; both proximal and distal placements have been widely reported. Stepped anastomosis creates multiple bypasses at various levels of the affected extremity (ie, wrist, forearm, and arm in the upper extremity),[72] which aims to improve success rates by providing additional routes for lymphatic drainage. Previously, Huang and colleagues[73] demonstrated that increased number of anastomoses provided better results. However, that has been refuted in a large study by O'Brien and colleagues, as well as a large prospective trial[63] which showed no difference in results based on number of anastomoses.[64,70] A variety of configurations may similarly be used including end-to-end, end-to-side, or side-to-end anastomoses without significant difference in outcomes. If anatomy permits, it is always preferred to create multiple lymphaticovenous anastomoses via a single incision.

Results

LVA has been proven to be an efficacious treatment option for patients that have failed nonoperative management. It is associated with a decrease in the overall incidence of severe cellulitis, compression garment discontinuation, and a subjective improvement in symptoms and QoL, compared with women who received conservative management alone.[19,74,75] In a systematic review of high-quality studies, 5 studies reported QoL outcomes, and found 91.7% symptom improvement, 94.5% average satisfaction rate, 90% improved QoL, and 50% subjective improvement in patients who underwent LVA.[42,63,76–78]

However, studies have shown that the success of LVA is primarily restricted to early stage disease; this is presumably owing to the ongoing presence of functional lymphatics that are subsequently irreversibly damaged in advanced disease. Chang and colleagues[63] found that, after LVA, stage I and II patients experienced a 61% volumetric reduction compared with 17% volumetric reduction in stage III patients after 1 year of follow-up. In another study, no limb volume reduction was seen in stage III patients.[72] Rates of recurrence are also closely associated with clinical staging. Poumellec and colleagues[72] reported 19.3% recurrence rates; however, all recurrences were isolated to patients with stages III and IV lymphedema. This finding further supports the notion that LVA is better suited for patients with early stage lymphedema.

Complications

Complications are uncommon after lymphaticovenous bypass, with rates reported at 5.9%.[27] Although the incidence is rare, known complications are infection, lymphatic fistula, partial skin ulceration, and wound dehiscence.[24,43,77] Given the low incidence of complications, LVA seems to be a safe and feasible procedure.

Vascularized Lymph Node Transfer

VLNT is a microsurgical procedure, in which a soft tissue flap containing lymphatic tissue and its associated arteriovenous supply is relocated from a donor site to the affected axilla. The reintroduction of healthy lymphatic tissue aims to restore function in the impaired limb, but the exact mechanism remains unclear. One theory hypothesizes that the transferred lymph nodes serve as a "sponge" that absorbs lymphatic fluid that is, then redistributed back into the lymphovenous circulatory system. A second theory suggests that lymphangiogenesis, primarily driven by vascular endothelial growth factor, leads to increased lymphatic vessel formation.[63,79]

Indications

Indications for VLNT include stages II to V lymphedema (Capisi staging system), absolute occlusion of lymphatic pathways verified on imaging (MRI or lymphoscintigraphy), fibrosis preventing lymphaticovenous bypass, brachial plexus neuropathy, chronic infections in the affected limb (ie, repeated episodes of cellulitis), and failed conservative management.[80–82] Conversely, some studies support the use of VLNT in early-stage lymphedema owing to the progressive course of the disease. Although lymph node transfer is not curative, early intervention may reduce the accumulation of excess lymphatic fluid and thereby, inhibit the positive feedback cycle that drives the progression of lymphedema.[71,79,83]

Technique

The recipient site may be selected as the axilla, elbow, or wrist of the affected limb. Axillary dissection may prove to be more challenging in patients who have undergone prior radiation therapy owing to significant scar tissue formation. However, wrist placement is less cosmetically pleasing owing to protrusion of the tissue and the possible need for skin grafting. Cheng and colleagues[82] suggests that wrist placement is more suitable for functionality, but the elbow provides improved aesthetic results. Ultimately, selection depends on surgeon preference, because recipient site selection has not been shown to impact outcomes. The most crucial part of axillary dissection is to ensure wide removal of all scar tissue; it is necessary to remove the obstruction to allow for good flow through the underlying lymphatics and to have sufficient space for placement of harvested lymph nodes.[84,85] An external neurolysis should also be performed if a neuroma is identified during dissection to avoid development of postoperative pain.[80,83] After careful identification of the thoracodorsal vessels, attention can be turned to the lymph node flap.

Lymphodynamic evaluation is conducted preoperatively with the aid of multiple imaging modalities. ICG assesses the severity of dermal backflow, and locates any viable and functional lymphatic vessels in the region. If an adequate amount of adequately functioning vessels is identified preoperatively, then a lymphovenous shunt may be considered, and the more invasive VLNT procedure can be avoided. Additionally, the presence of lymphatic drainage obstruction can be confirmed on Tc99 lymphoscintigraphy. Lymphoscintigraphy does not provide good information about the spatial and temporal resolution of the lymphatic system and involves exposure to radiation. If available, MRI and dynamic magnetic lymphangiography are preferred owing to the increased sensitivity and specificity to identify anatomic and functional variations.

The optimal donor site remains unclear, but the most common location is the inguinal region; it is based off the branches of the superficial circumflex iliac or superficial inferior epigastric vessels. Groin flaps are chosen owing to their abundance of lymph nodes in a well-understood anatomic region, an easily hidden scar, and a dual role in total breast reconstruction.[24] Dissection is delineated by 3 borders: the inguinal ligament (caudal), the muscular aponeurosis (deep), and the cribriform fascia (superficial). It is recommended that the surgeon not dissect lymph nodes beyond the caudal and deep borders to avoid inadvertent removal of deeper lymph nodes to minimize the risk of donor site lymphedema.[86] Less commonly, the submental, supraclavicular, thoracic, and omental tissues are used as donor sites. The submental and supraclavicular nodes require tedious dissection owing to nearby lymphatic ducts and branches of the marginal mandibular nerve. Although the omental nodes are the least likely to develop donor site iatrogenic lymphedema, the need for abdominal surgery poses additional risks.

Anastomosis selection varies depending on the flap of choice; the superficial circumflex iliac vessels are typically used in isolated VLNT, versus combined VLNT with microvascular breast reconstruction, in which the deep inferior epigastric vessels are preferred. Currently, no strict guidelines exist to determine which vessels should be used for optimal results. A recent study by Nguyen and colleagues[87] created an algorithm for transferring vascularized inguinal lymph nodes during autologous abdominal free flaps (AFP), specifically deep inferior epigastric perforator or transverse rectus abdominis myocutaneous flaps; the goal was to provide an alternative vasculature selection to the commonly used thoracodorsal vessels, which may be crucial later if the initial flap fails. Nguyen and colleagues address 3 different scenarios: (1) hemiabdominal flap for bilateral mastectomy or prior midline incision—ipsilateral VLNT, ipsilateral AFP, thoracodorsal pedicle; (2) unilateral reconstruction without prior violation of the midline—contralateral VLNT, ipsilateral AFP, internal mammary artery pedicle; and (3) a history of prior surgery with subsequent division of superficial vessels—VLNT ipsilateral, AFP contralateral, and internal mammary artery pedicle. Their study demonstrated promising results with 79% of patients reporting improved symptoms, and reduction of excess limb volume from 21% preoperatively down to 10% at 1 year of follow-up.

Results

VLNT has been shown to have successful outcomes with decreases in limb circumference and limb volume, as well as improvement in patient function and QoL. A large systematic review by Carl and colleagues[27] found a 33% excess volume reduction and 16.1% absolute circumference reduction after lymph node transfer. Notably, patients report a substantial improvement in limb functionality before any self-perceived changes in limb appearance, suggesting that even a slight decrease in size may prove beneficial with regard to limb mobility, and inevitably, better QoL. These functional improvements were reported as early as 1 month postoperatively, and continued throughout the first year of follow-up. Similarly, psychosocial issues including appearance, symptoms and mood also improved.[88–91] Studies have shown that patients who undergo lymph node transfer report 91.7% symptom improvement, 94.5% average satisfaction rate, 90% improved QoL, and 50% subjective improvement.[42,63,76–78] Despite the promising results, particularly in late-stage disease, VLNT is not a curative therapy. Patients are recommended to continue conservative therapies, including compressive bandages, elastic garments, and manual lymph drainage postoperatively.

Complications

The success rates for volume reduction, compression therapy discontinuation, and improved QoL are similar to those reported for LVA; however, the complication rates of donor site seroma, lymphocele, infection, delayed wound closure, and donor site lymphedema make VNLT a higher risk surgery.[62] VLNT is also associated with longer durations of hospital stay, longer duration of operation, and greater anesthetic requirements (general vs local) when compared with LVA.[92] A large, retrospective review of all high-quality studies demonstrated a 30.1% complication rate after lymph node transfer.[27] This finding is further supported by Vignes and colleagues,[90] who found an equally high complication rate at 38%. Similar findings are reported after combined VLNT and microvascular breast reconstruction with 25% recipient site complications (delayed wound healing, partial mastectomy flap necrosis, and abdominal flap venous thrombosis) and 20% donor site complications (abdominal wound healing or dehiscence, abdominal hernia, and groin seroma).[87] The most dreaded complication after lymph node transfer is iatrogenic lymphedema at the donor site. Despite low rates reported in the literature, it remains a significant concern among clinicians.[85,90,93–95] Studies have shown that, even with modified conservative surgical techniques, lymphoscintigraphy findings demonstrate subclinical disruptions in lymphatic flow postoperatively.[96] Given these findings, studies recommend supportive modalities including reverse mapping, ICG, and lymphoscintigraphy to maximally mitigate the risk of iatrogenic lymphedema. It should be noted, however, that complications are reported inconsistently across the literature, even among high-quality studies.

COMBINATION PROCEDURES

The combination of physiologic procedures with reductive surgery, which allows for removal of the chronic adipose and fibrotic tissue disrupting the lymphatic system, is the most effective treatment for severe lymphedema. Multiple combinations of excisional and physiologic procedures have been used, including VLNT with suction-assisted lipectomy, VLNT with microvascular breast reconstruction, and some surgeons have also attempted LVA with VLNT.[87,92,94,97–100] Limb volume reduction was reported to be as high as 91% after liposuction with VLNT.[97] Owing to its low risk profile, liposuction is an appealing adjunct treatment option, particularly in patients with nonpitting edema. Studies have shown that, after LVA, 16.0% of patients benefit from additional liposuction postoperatively. Likewise, when VLNT is used as the primary approach, additional reductive procedures are needed in 31.6% of patients.[27] The promising outcomes after combination therapy may represent an opportunity to minimize the need for serial invasive surgical interventions and simultaneously yield better outcomes. Nevertheless, similar to lymph node transfer, high rates of complications are associated with excisional procedures, as high as 39.3%,[27] and therefore, careful patient selection is required with the procedure reserved for those with severe disease.

LIPECTOMY

SAPL involves the removal of fat and fibrosis with suction technique.[23–26,62,101] Lipectomy addresses the solid component (fibrosis and hypertrophied subcutaneous adipose tissue) that typically presents later as chronic, nonpitting lymphedema of an extremity after the fluid component has been conservatively drained.[19,75] Patients often complain of discomfort and dysfunction in the affected arm despite conservative management.[102] Indications for lipectomy include stage II and III disease that has failed conservative management. Contraindications include active cancer, infection, wounds, or insufficient conservative management.[103] If there is more than 4 to 5 mm of pitting edema in the affected extremity, the patient should attempt conservative measures rather than undergo liposuction, because liposuction is a method to remove fibrotic adipose tissue, not fluid.[102]

During suction-assisted protein lipectomy, a tourniquet is first applied to the affected extremity to minimize the amount of fluid present in the operative field.[103] Liposuction is performed with suction cannulas through multiple incisions that are 3 mm long. Starting distal to the tourniquet, liposuction is performed circumferentially and in a longitudinal direction to the extremity to minimize damage to the remaining lymphatics.[104] This process is continued until liposuction is performed past the point of the tourniquet and the maximal amount of adipose tissue is removed. The incisions are left open to drain externally. A sterilized compression sleeve and glove are applied for hemostasis and minimization of edema. Perioperative antibiotics are generally given for 5 to 10 days. The patient is instructed to wear their compression sleeve and glove at all times.[102]

Studies have found that, in patients with lymphedema from breast cancer therapy, a statistically significant volume reduction of almost 1 L on average was achieved and maintained at 12 months.[19] Additionally, there is a significant improvement in QoL and decrease in infection rates.[62,65,101] However, lipectomy does not treat the underlying cause of lymphedema, namely lymphatic stasis and obstruction. Lifelong compression therapy, lymphedema therapist treatment, and/or lymphovascular anastomosis or VLNT must be used as adjuncts to prevent the reaccumulation of lymphedema. Lifelong compression therapy involves continuous use of a sleeve and glove on the affected arm, which requires strict patient compliance. Lymphedema therapy generally involves a combination of manual reduction, physical therapy, and yoga, which is also heavily reliant on patient compliance and motivation.[105] LVA and VLNT are microsurgical procedures that may be performed after the volume reductions from SAPL have stabilized and the patient has sufficiently healed from the first surgery. LVA and VLNT help to prevent fluid reaccumulation and reduce compression garment use after SAPL has removed the solid component of the lymphedema.[106]

SURGICAL EXCISION

Surgical excision or radical debulking for severe lymphedema was first described in 1912 as the Charles procedure. Several modifications of the Charles procedure have also been reported. Indications for this procedure include advanced (end-stage) fibrosclerotic lymphedema not amenable to other procedures, recurrent episodes of cellulitis, and severe disfigurement or dysfunction, and an inability to exclude sarcoma on the affected extremity.[23–26,62,106–109] The major disadvantage is that superficial skin lymphatic collaterals are removed or further obliterated.[20,24,25] Additionally, there is significant morbidity, scarring, and risk of skin graft failure with these operations. When lymphedema recurs at the hand or foot, regrafting and finger or toe amputations may prove necessary.

During the Charles procedure, longitudinal skin incisions are made along the length of lymphedema. The excess skin and subcutaneous tissue of the lymphedematous limb are excised circumferentially down to the level of the deep fascia.[20,25,62] Care is taken not to injure the deep fascia. Split thickness skin grafts are then harvested from the excised skin and are implanted onto the deep fascial layer. Sterile dressings are applied and the skin flaps are monitored postoperatively for adequate blood supply and infection.

Given the risks and morbidities listed, several versions of the modified Charles procedure were developed for severe lymphedema treatment. In the first modified Charles procedure, the initial debulking procedure is performed. A portion of the split thickness skin graft is deepithelialized and is buried into the deep subcutaneous tissues. The goal of this modification is to connect the deep subfascial lymphatics with the superficial dermal lymphatics, thereby facilitating lymph drainage.[110] Other modifications include use of negative pressure dressings, perpendicular cross-incisions, and combination procedures with liposuction and VLNT to decrease the amount of skin removed and allow primary closure.[100,107–109,111]

SUMMARY

Breast cancer–related lymphedema is a lifelong disease that is difficult to treat and requires multimodal therapy. A systematic review by Carl and colleagues[27] using MINORS criteria to distinguish high-quality studies attempted to create an algorithm for management of lymphedema. The microsurgical technique LVA at the time of axillary lymph node dissection has been proposed as a primary preventative treatment for arm lymphedema. The after treatments are suggested according to the International Society of Lymphedema Staging System. Conservative measures such as physiotherapy and compression garments are appropriate for stage 0 (subclinical) lymphedema. LVA or VLNT procedures are best suited for early stage I lymphedema (soft, pitting edema with little to no fibrosis). Suction-assisted protein liposuction should be considered for moderate stage II (nonpitting edema with fibrosis) and severe stage III lymphedema (nonpitting edema with severe fibrosis and hypertrophic skin changes). Surgical excision (the Charles procedure and its modifications) should be reserved for severe stage III lymphedema with severe disfigurement or disuse.[23,24] Most patients do report decreased edema and improved QoL after surgical intervention; however, compression garments or physiotherapy are still recommended postoperatively to maintain or further reduce limb volume.

Further research must be conducted in establishing best practices in lymphedema prevention and treatment. A standardized staging system for lymphedema would allow for accurate comparison of outcomes based on intervention type. There are also inconsistent methods of recording surgical outcomes and reporting outcomes and QoL indicators. At this time, there are limited large, randomized, controlled trials in the lymphedema literature that focus specifically on breast cancer related lymphedema. Much of the data come from observational studies that combine data from both upper extremity and lower extremity lymphedema. Lack of consistent quantitative reporting prevents comprehensive conclusions regarding which surgical approaches are associated with the greatest subjective improvements. Even the studies that did include QoL outcomes and reported overall improvement in function, symptom severity, and aesthetics after surgery, these data cannot be reliably used because they are inconsistently documented among the studies.

REFERENCES

1. Földi M, Földi E, editors. Földi's textbook of lymphology: for physicians and lymphedema therapists. 2nd edition. Mosby Elsevier; 2006.
2. Greene AK, Slavin SA, Brorson H, editors. Lymphedema. Cham (Switzerland): Springer International Publishing; 2015.
3. McLaughlin SA. Lymphedema: separating fact from fiction. Oncology (Williston Park) 2012;26(3):242–9. Available at: http://www.ncbi.nlm.nih.gov/pubmed/22545305.
4. Shah C, Vicini FA. Breast cancer-related arm lymphedema: incidence rates, diagnostic techniques, optimal management and risk reduction strategies. Int J Radiat Oncol Biol Phys 2011;81(4):907–14.
5. Greene AK, Grant FD, Slavin SA. Lower-extremity lymphedema and elevated body-mass index. N Engl J Med 2012;366(22):2136–7.

6. Greene AK. Diagnosis and management of obesity-induced lymphedema. Plast Reconstr Surg 2016;138(1):111e–8e.
7. Stout Gergich NL, Pfalzer LA, McGarvey C, et al. Preoperative assessment enables the early diagnosis and successful treatment of lymphedema. Cancer 2008;112(12):2809–19.
8. Boccardo FM, Ansaldi F, Bellini C, et al. Prospective evaluation of a prevention protocol for lymphedema following surgery for breast cancer. Lymphology 2009; 42(1):1–9. Available at: http://www.ncbi.nlm.nih.gov/pubmed/19499762.
9. Box RC, Reul-Hirche HM, Bullock-Saxton JE, et al. Physiotherapy after breast cancer surgery: results of a randomised controlled study to minimise lymphoedema. Breast Cancer Res Treat 2002;75(1):51–64. Available at: http://www.ncbi.nlm.nih.gov/pubmed/12500934.
10. Fu MR. Breast cancer-related lymphedema: symptoms, diagnosis, risk reduction, and management. World J Clin Oncol 2014;5(3):241.
11. Rockson SG. Lymphedema. Am J Med 2001;110(4):288–95. Available at: http://www.ncbi.nlm.nih.gov/pubmed/11239847.
12. Ridner SH. Breast cancer lymphedema: pathophysiology and risk reduction guidelines. Oncol Nurs Forum 2002;29(9):1285–93.
13. Hespe GE, Nitti MD, Mehrara BJ. Pathophysiology of lymphedema. In: Greene AK, Slavin SA, Brorson H, editors. Lymphedema. Cham (Switzerland): Springer International Publishing; 2015. p. 9–18.
14. Ryan TJ. Lymphatics and adipose tissue. Clin Dermatol 1995;13(5):493–8. Available at: http://www.ncbi.nlm.nih.gov/pubmed/8665460.
15. Paskett ED, Naughton MJ, McCoy TP, et al. The epidemiology of arm and hand swelling in premenopausal breast cancer survivors. Cancer Epidemiol Biomarkers Prev 2007;16(4):775–82.
16. Shih Y-CT, Xu Y, Cormier JN, et al. Incidence, treatment costs, and complications of lymphedema after breast cancer among women of working age: a 2-year follow-up study. J Clin Oncol 2009;27(12):2007–14.
17. Petrek JA, Senie RT, Peters M, et al. Lymphedema in a cohort of breast carcinoma survivors 20 years after diagnosis. Cancer 2001;92(6):1368–77. Available at: http://www.ncbi.nlm.nih.gov/pubmed/11745212.
18. DiSipio T, Rye S, Newman B, et al. Incidence of unilateral arm lymphoedema after breast cancer: a systematic review and meta-analysis. Lancet Oncol 2013; 14(6):500–15.
19. Granzow JW, Soderberg JM, Kaji AH, et al. An effective system of surgical treatment of lymphedema. Ann Surg Oncol 2014;21(4):1189–94.
20. International Society of Lymphology. The diagnosis and treatment of peripheral lymphedema. 2009 Consensus Document of the International Society of Lymphology. Lymphology 2009;42(2):51–60. Available at: http://www.ncbi.nlm.nih.gov/pubmed/19725269.
21. Armer JM, Radina ME, Porock D, et al. Predicting breast cancer-related lymphedema using self-reported symptoms. Nurs Res 2003;52(6):370–9. Available at: http://www.ncbi.nlm.nih.gov/pubmed/14639083.
22. Armer JM, Stewart BR. Post-breast cancer lymphedema: incidence increases from 12 to 30 to 60 months. Lymphology 2010;43(3):118–27. Available at: http://www.ncbi.nlm.nih.gov/pubmed/21226414.
23. Merchant SJ, Chen SL. Prevention and management of lymphedema after breast cancer treatment. Breast J 2015;21(3):276–84.
24. Allen RJ, Cheng M-H. Lymphedema surgery: patient selection and an overview of surgical techniques. J Surg Oncol 2016;113(8):923–31.

25. Granzow JW, Soderberg JM, Kaji AH, et al. Review of current surgical treatments for lymphedema. Ann Surg Oncol 2014;21(4):1195–201.
26. Cormier JN, Rourke L, Crosby M, et al. The surgical treatment of lymphedema: a systematic review of the contemporary literature (2004-2010). Ann Surg Oncol 2012;19(2):642–51.
27. Carl H, Walia G, Bello R, et al. Systematic review of the surgical treatment of extremity lymphedema. J Reconstr Microsurg 2017;33:212.
28. Szuba A, Cooke JP, Yousuf S, et al. Decongestive lymphatic therapy for patients with cancer-related or primary lymphedema. Am J Med 2000;109(4):296–300. Available at: http://www.ncbi.nlm.nih.gov/pubmed/10996580.
29. Loudon Petrek JL. Lymphedema in women treated for breast cancer. Cancer Pract 2000;8(2):65–71. Available at: http://www.ncbi.nlm.nih.gov/entrez/query.fcgi?cmd=Retrieve&db=PubMed&dopt=Citation&list_uids=11898179.
30. Cinar N, Seckin U, Keskin D, et al. The effectiveness of early rehabilitation in patients with modified radical mastectomy. Cancer Nurs 2008;31(2):160–5.
31. Armer JM, Stewart BR. A comparison of four diagnostic criteria for lymphedema in a post-breast cancer population. Lymphat Res Biol 2005;3(4):208–17.
32. Deltombe T, Jamart J, Recloux S, et al. Reliability and limits of agreement of circumferential, water displacement, and optoelectronic volumetry in the measurement of upper limb lymphedema. Lymphology 2007;40(1):26–34. Available at: http://www.ncbi.nlm.nih.gov/pubmed/17539462.
33. Ridner SH, Dietrich MS. Development and validation of the lymphedema symptom and intensity survey-arm. Support Care Cancer 2015. http://dx.doi.org/10.1007/s00520-015-2684-y.
34. Cormier JN, Xing Y, Zaniletti I, et al. Minimal limb volume change has a significant impact on breast cancer survivors. Lymphology 2009;42(4):161–75. Available at: http://www.ncbi.nlm.nih.gov/pubmed/20218084.
35. Shaitelman SF, Cromwell KD, Rasmussen JC, et al. Recent progress in the treatment and prevention of cancer-related lymphedema. CA Cancer J Clin 2015; 65(1):55–81.
36. O'Donnell TF, Rasmussen JC, Sevick-Muraca EM. New diagnostic modalities in the evaluation of lymphedema. J Vasc Surgery Venous Lymphat Disord 2017; 5(2):261–73.
37. Bernas MJ, Askew RL, Armer JM, et al. Lymphedema: how do we diagnose and reduce the risk of this dreaded complication of breast cancer treatment? Curr Breast Cancer Rep 2010;2(1):53–8.
38. Liu NF, Wang CG. The role of magnetic resonance imaging in diagnosis of peripheral lymphatic disorders. Lymphology 1998;31(3):119–27. Available at: http://www.ncbi.nlm.nih.gov/pubmed/9793922.
39. Mihara M, Hara H, Araki J, et al. Indocyanine green (ICG) lymphography is superior to lymphoscintigraphy for diagnostic imaging of early lymphedema of the upper limbs. PLoS One 2012;7(6):e38182.
40. Rasmussen JC, Tan I-C, Marshall MV, et al. Human lymphatic architecture and dynamic transport imaged using near-infrared fluorescence. Transl Oncol 2010; 3(6):362–72. Available at: http://www.ncbi.nlm.nih.gov/pubmed/21151475.
41. Kitai T, Inomoto T, Miwa M, et al. Fluorescence navigation with indocyanine green for detecting sentinel lymph nodes in breast cancer. Breast Cancer 2005;12(3): 211–5. Available at: http://www.ncbi.nlm.nih.gov/pubmed/16110291.
42. Demirtas Y, Ozturk N, Yapici O, et al. Supermicrosurgical lymphaticovenular anastomosis and lymphaticovenous implantation for treatment of unilateral lower extremity lymphedema. Microsurgery 2009;29(8):609–18.

43. Narushima M, Mihara M, Yamamoto Y, et al. The intravascular stenting method for treatment of extremity lymphedema with multiconfiguration lymphaticovenous anastomoses. Plast Reconstr Surg 2010;125(3):935–43.

44. Ochoa D, Klimberg VS. Surgical strategies for prevention and treatment of lymphedema in breast cancer patients. Curr Breast Cancer Rep 2015;7(1):1–7.

45. Feldman S, Bansil H, Ascherman J, et al. Single institution experience with lymphatic microsurgical preventive healing approach (LYMPHA) for the primary prevention of lymphedema 2015;22(10):3296–301.

46. Giuliano AE, Hunt KK, Ballman KV, et al. Axillary dissection vs no axillary dissection in women with invasive breast cancer and sentinel node metastasis: a randomized clinical trial. JAMA 2011;305(6):569–75.

47. Boughey JC. Sentinel lymph node surgery after neoadjuvant chemotherapy in patients with node-positive breast cancer. JAMA 2013;310(14):1455.

48. Boughey JC, Suman VJ, Mittendorf EA, et al. Factors affecting sentinel lymph node identification rate after neoadjuvant chemotherapy for breast cancer patients enrolled in ACOSOG Z1071 (Alliance). Ann Surg 2015;261(3):547–52.

49. Kuehn T, Bauerfeind I, Fehm T, et al. Sentinel-lymph-node biopsy in patients with breast cancer before and after neoadjuvant chemotherapy (SENTINA): a prospective, multicentre cohort study. Lancet Oncol 2013;14(7):609–18.

50. Donker M, van Tienhoven G, Straver ME, et al. Radiotherapy or surgery of the axilla after a positive sentinel node in breast cancer (EORTC 10981-22023 AMAROS): a randomised, multicentre, open-label, phase 3 non-inferiority trial. Lancet Oncol 2014;15(12):1303–10.

51. Sávolt Á, Péley G, Polgár C, et al. Eight-year follow up result of the OTOASOR trial: The Optimal Treatment Of the Axilla – Surgery Or Radiotherapy after positive sentinel lymph node biopsy in early-stage breast cancer. Eur J Surg Oncol 2017;43(4):672–9.

52. Sávolt Á, Musonda P, Mátrai Z, et al. Optimal treatment of the axilla after positive sentinel lymph node biopsy in early invasive breast cancer. Early results of the OTOASOR trial. Orv Hetil 2013;154(49):1934–42.

53. Tummel E, Ochoa D, Korourian S, et al. Does axillary reverse mapping prevent lymphedema after lymphadenectomy? Ann Surg 2016;265(5):987–92.

54. Ochoa D, Korourian S, Boneti C, et al. Axillary reverse mapping: five-year experience. Surgery 2014;156(5):1261–8.

55. Thompson M, Korourian S, Henry-Tillman R, et al. Axillary Reverse Mapping (ARM): a new concept to identify and enhance lymphatic preservation. Ann Surg Oncol 2007;14(6):1890–5.

56. Nos C, Kaufmann G, Clough KB, et al. Combined axillary reverse mapping (ARM) technique for breast cancer patients requiring axillary dissection. Ann Surg Oncol 2008;15(9):2550–5.

57. Gennaro M, Maccauro M, Sigari C, et al. Selective axillary dissection after axillary reverse mapping to prevent breast-cancer-related lymphoedema. Eur J Surg Oncol 2013;39(12):1341–5.

58. Han JW, Seo YJ, Choi JE, et al. The efficacy of arm node preserving surgery using axillary reverse mapping for preventing lymphedema in patients with breast cancer. J Breast Cancer 2012;15(1):91–7.

59. Boneti C, Korourian S, Bland K, et al. Axillary reverse mapping: mapping and preserving arm lymphatics may be important in preventing lymphedema during sentinel lymph node biopsy. J Am Coll Surg 2008;206(5):1038–42.

60. Tausch C, Baege A, Dietrich D, et al. Can axillary reverse mapping avoid lymphedema in node positive breast cancer patients? Eur J Surg Oncol 2013; 39(8):880–6.

61. Yue T, Zhuang D, Zhou P, et al. A prospective study to assess the feasibility of axillary reverse mapping and evaluate its effect on preventing lymphedema in breast cancer patients. Clin Breast Cancer 2015;15(4):301–6.

62. Lee GK, Perrault DP, Bouz A, et al. Surgical treatment modalities for lymphedema. J Aesthet Reconstr Surg 2016;2(2).

63. Chang DW, Suami H, Skoracki R. A prospective analysis of 100 consecutive lymphovenous bypass cases for treatment of extremity lymphedema. Plast Reconstr Surg 2013;132(5):1305–14.

64. O'Brien BM, Mellow CG, Khazanchi RK, et al. Long-term results after microlymphaticovenous anastomoses for the treatment of obstructive lymphedema. Plast Reconstr Surg 1990;85(4):562–72. Available at: http://www.ncbi.nlm.nih.gov/pubmed/2315396.

65. Leung N, Furniss D, Giele H. Modern surgical management of breast cancer therapy related upper limb and breast lymphoedema. Maturitas 2015;80(4): 384–90.

66. Suami H, Chang DW, Yamada K, et al. Use of indocyanine green fluorescent lymphography for evaluating dynamic lymphatic status. Plast Reconstr Surg 2011;127(3):74e–6e.

67. Unno N, Inuzuka K, Suzuki M, et al. Preliminary experience with a novel fluorescence lymphography using indocyanine green in patients with secondary lymphedema. J Vasc Surg 2007;45(5):1016–21.

68. Ogata F, Narushima M, Mihara M, et al. Intraoperative lymphography using indocyanine green dye for near-infrared fluorescence labeling in lymphedema. Ann Plast Surg 2007;59(2):180–4.

69. Yamamoto T, Matsuda N, Doi K, et al. The earliest finding of indocyanine green lymphography in asymptomatic limbs of lower extremity lymphedema patients secondary to cancer treatment: the modified dermal backflow stage and concept of subclinical lymphedema. Plast Reconstr Surg 2011;128(4): 314e–21e.

70. Chang DW. Lymphaticovenular bypass for lymphedema management in breast cancer patients: a prospective study. Plast Reconstr Surg 2010;126(3):752–8.

71. Koshima I, Narushima M, Yamamoto Y, et al. Recent advancement on surgical treatments for lymphedema. Ann Vasc Dis 2012;5(4):409–15.

72. Poumellec M-A, Foissac R, Cegarra-Escolano M, et al. Surgical treatment of secondary lymphedema of the upper limb by stepped microsurgical lymphaticovenous anastomoses. Breast Cancer Res Treat 2017;162(2):219–24.

73. Li X, Huang H, Lin Q, et al. Validation of a breast cancer nomogram to predict lymphedema in a Chinese population. J Surg Res 2017;210:132–8.

74. Cornelissen AJM, Kool M, Lopez Penha TR, et al. Lymphatico-venous anastomosis as treatment for breast cancer-related lymphedema: a prospective study on quality of life. Breast Cancer Res Treat 2017. http://dx.doi.org/10.1007/s10549-017-4180-1.

75. Basta MN, Gao LL, Wu LC. Operative treatment of peripheral lymphedema. Plast Reconstr Surg 2014;133(4):905–13.

76. Auba C, Marre D, Rodríguez-Losada G, et al. Lymphaticovenular anastomoses for lymphedema treatment: 18 months postoperative outcomes. Microsurgery 2012;32(4):261–8.

77. Ayestaray B, Bekara F, Andreoletti J-B. Patent blue-enhanced lymphaticovenular anastomosis. J Plast Reconstr Aesthet Surg 2013;66(3):382–9.

78. Damstra RJ, Voesten HGJ, van Schelven WD, et al. Lymphatic venous anastomosis (LVA) for treatment of secondary arm lymphedema. A prospective study of 11 LVA procedures in 10 patients with breast cancer related lymphedema and a critical review of the literature. Breast Cancer Res Treat 2009;113(2):199–206.

79. Suami H, Chang DW. Overview of surgical treatments for breast cancer-related lymphedema. Plast Reconstr Surg 2010;126(6):1853–63.

80. Becker C, Assouad J, Riquet M, et al. Postmastectomy lymphedema: long-term results following microsurgical lymph node transplantation. Ann Surg 2006; 243(3):313–5.

81. Dayan JH, Dayan E, Kagen A, et al. The use of magnetic resonance angiography in vascularized groin lymph node transfer: an anatomic study. J Reconstr Microsurg 2014;30(1):41–5.

82. Cheng M-H, Chen S-C, Henry SL, et al. Vascularized groin lymph node flap transfer for postmastectomy upper limb lymphedema: flap anatomy, recipient sites, and outcomes. Plast Reconstr Surg 2013;131(6):1286–98.

83. Becker C, Vasile JV, Levine JL, et al. Microlymphatic surgery for the treatment of iatrogenic lymphedema. Clin Plast Surg 2012;39(4):385–98.

84. Blum KS, Hadamitzky C, Gratz KF, et al. Effects of autotransplanted lymph node fragments on the lymphatic system in the pig model. Breast Cancer Res Treat 2010;120(1):59–66.

85. Viitanen TP, Mäki MT, Seppänen MP, et al. Donor-site lymphatic function after microvascular lymph node transfer. Plast Reconstr Surg 2012;130(6):1246–53.

86. Silva AK, Chang DW. Vascularized lymph node transfer and lymphovenous bypass: novel treatment strategies for symptomatic lymphedema. J Surg Oncol 2016;113(8):932–9.

87. Nguyen AT, Chang EI, Suami H, et al. An algorithmic approach to simultaneous vascularized lymph node transfer with microvascular breast reconstruction. Ann Surg Oncol 2015;22(9):2919–24.

88. Travis EC, Shugg S, McEwan WM. Lymph node grafting in the treatment of upper limb lymphoedema: a clinical trial. ANZ J Surg 2015;85(9):631–5.

89. Dionyssiou D, Demiri E, Tsimponis A, et al. A randomized control study of treating secondary stage II breast cancer-related lymphoedema with free lymph node transfer. Breast Cancer Res Treat 2016;156(1):73–9.

90. Vignes S, Blanchard M, Yannoutsos A, et al. Complications of autologous lymph-node transplantation for limb lymphoedema. Eur J Vasc Endovasc Surg 2013; 45(5):516–20.

91. Belcaro G, Errichi BM, Cesarone MR, et al. Lymphatic tissue transplant in lymphedema–a minimally invasive, outpatient, surgical method: a 10-year follow-up pilot study. Angiology 2008;59(1):77–83.

92. Akita S, Mitsukawa N, Kuriyama M, et al. Comparison of vascularized supraclavicular lymph node transfer and lymphaticovenular anastomosis for advanced stage lower extremity lymphedema. Ann Plast Surg 2015;74(5):573–9.

93. Lin C-H, Ali R, Chen S-C, et al. Vascularized groin lymph node transfer using the wrist as a recipient site for management of postmastectomy upper extremity lymphedema. Plast Reconstr Surg 2009;123(4):1265–75.

94. Saaristo AM, Niemi TS, Viitanen TP, et al. Microvascular breast reconstruction and lymph node transfer for postmastectomy lymphedema patients. Ann Surg 2012;255(3):468–73.

95. Pons G, Masia J, Loschi P, et al. A case of donor-site lymphoedema after lymph node-superficial circumflex iliac artery perforator flap transfer. J Plast Reconstr Aesthet Surg 2014;67(1):119–23.

96. Sulo E, Hartiala P, Viitanen T, et al. Risk of donor-site lymphatic vessel dysfunction after microvascular lymph node transfer. J Plast Reconstr Aesthet Surg 2015;68(4):551–8.

97. Nicoli F, Constantinides J, Ciudad P, et al. Free lymph node flap transfer and laser-assisted liposuction: a combined technique for the treatment of moderate upper limb lymphedema. Lasers Med Sci 2015;30(4):1377–85.

98. Qi F, Gu J, Shi Y, et al. Treatment of upper limb lymphedema with combination of liposuction, myocutaneous flap transfer, and lymph-fascia grafting: a preliminary study. Microsurgery 2009;29(1):29–34.

99. Koshima I, Narushima M, Mihara M, et al. Lymphadiposal flaps and lymphaticovenular anastomoses for severe leg edema: functional reconstruction for lymph drainage system. J Reconstr Microsurg 2016;32(1):50–5.

100. Sapountzis S, Ciudad P, Lim SY, et al. Modified Charles procedure and lymph node flap transfer for advanced lower extremity lymphedema. Microsurgery 2014;34(6):439–47.

101. Greene AK, Maclellan R. Management of lymphedema with suction-assisted lipectomy. Plast Reconstr Surg 2014;134:36.

102. Brorson H, Svensson B, Ohlin K. Suction-assisted lipectomy. In: Greene AK, Slavin SA, Brorson H, editors. Lymphedema. Cham (Switzerland): Springer International Publishing; 2015. p. 313–24.

103. Schaverien M, Munnoch D. Chapter-02 Liposuction for chronic lymphedema of the upper limb. In: Giuseppe AD, Shiffman MA, editors. New frontiers in plastic and cosmetic surgery. New Delhi, India: Jaypee Brothers Medical Publishers (P) Ltd; 2015. p. 13–22.

104. Frick A, Baumeister RGH, Hoffmann JN. Liposuction technique and lymphatics in liposuction. In: Shiffman MA, Giuseppe AD, editors. Liposuction. Berlin: Springer Berlin Heidelberg; 2016. p. 179–83.

105. Hsiao P-C, Hong R, Chou W, et al. Role of physiotherapy and patient education in lymphedema control following breast cancer surgery. Ther Clin Risk Manag 2015;11:319.

106. Granzow JW, Soderberg JM, Dauphine C. A novel two-stage surgical approach to treat chronic lymphedema. Breast J 2014;20(4):420–2.

107. Jabbar F, Hammoudeh ZS, Bachusz R, et al. The diagnostic and surgical challenges of massive localized lymphedema. Am J Surg 2015;209(3):584–7.

108. van der Walt JC, Perks TJ, Zeeman BJ, et al. Modified Charles procedure using negative pressure dressings for primary lymphedema. Ann Plast Surg 2009; 62(6):669–75.

109. Maruccia M, Chen H-C, Chen S-H. Modified Charles' procedure and its combination with lymph node flap transfer for advanced lymphedema. In: Greene AK, Slavin SA, Brorson H, editors. Lymphedema. Cham (Switzerland): Springer International Publishing; 2015. p. 289–99.

110. Mavili ME, Naldoken S, Safak T. Modified Charles operation for primary fibrosclerotic lymphedema. Lymphology 1994;27(1):14–20. Available at: http://www.ncbi.nlm.nih.gov/pubmed/8207967.

111. Louton RB, Terranova WA. The use of suction curettage as adjunct to the management of lymphedema. Ann Plast Surg 1989;22(4):354–7.

Breast Cancer Disparities

How Can We Leverage Genomics to Improve Outcomes?

Melissa B. Davis, PhD[a], Lisa A. Newman, MD, MPH[b],*

KEYWORDS

- Disparities • Genetics • Genomics • African ancestry

KEY POINTS

- Advances in breast cancer genomics will provide important insights regarding explanations for variations in incidence, as well as disparate outcomes, between African American and white American breast cancer patients.
- Germline genomics are essential in genetic counseling and risk assessment programs; somatic or tumor-based genomics will be critical in defining prognostic and therapeutic algorithms.
- It is imperative that the oncology community be prepared to apply these technologies equitably to diverse patient populations.

BACKGROUND

Disparities in breast cancer risk and outcome related to racial-ethnic identity in the United States have been documented by population-based statistics from the Surveillance, Epidemiology, and End Results (SEER) Program over the past several decades. These patterns are further supported by data from a variety of health care systems and oncology programs. Variations in the breast cancer burden of African Americans (AA) women compared with white American (WA) women have been the subject of rigorous study[1] because of the magnitude of the observed differences and are the focus of this article. **Table 1** summarizes these divergent patterns.

Breast cancer mortality rates are higher for AA compared with WA women, and this is at least partly explained by a more advanced stage distribution, with AA women being diagnosed more frequently with larger, node-positive disease. Breast cancer incidence

Disclosure: This work was partially supported by Susan G. Komen for the Cure through Komen Scholars Leadership Grant HFHS F11047 (LAN).
a Henry Ford Cancer Institute, 2799 West Grand Boulevard, Detroit, MI 48202, USA; b Breast Oncology Program, Department of Surgery, Henry Ford Health System, Henry Ford Cancer Institute, International Center for the Study of Breast Cancer Subtypes, 2799 West Grand Boulevard, Detroit, MI 48202, USA
* Corresponding author.
E-mail address: lnewman1@hfhs.org

Table 1
Breast cancer in African Americans and European or White Americans

		African American	White American
Population-based incidence rates (per 100,000), female breast cancer	Overall, age-standardized	122.9	124.4
	Age-stratified		
	35–39 y	70.6	59.9
	40–44 y	118.2	122.2
	45–49 y	180.4	188.1
	50–54 y	231.6	220.3
	55–59 y	270.7	260.4
	60–64 y	332.0	332.4
	65–69 y	399.5	428.7
Population-based mortality rates (per 100,000), female breast cancer	Overall, age-standardized	28.2	20.3
	Age-stratified		
	35–39 y	10.2	5.8
	40–44 y	22.1	11.5
	45–49 y	30.7	18.3
	50–54 y	47.3	27.3
	55–59 y	57.4	36.6
	60–64 y	71.3	49.2
	65–69 y	80.4	62.2
Stage distribution at diagnosis, female breast cancer	Localized	53%	64%
	Regional	35%	28%
	Distant	8%	5%
	Unknown	4%	3%
5-y cause-specific survival, female breast cancer	All stages	80%	89%
	Localized	93%	96%
	Regional	78%	87%
	Distant	24%	34%
TNBC population-based incidence rates, female breast cancer		27.2	14.4
Population-based incidence rates, male breast cancer		2.04	1.25

Abbreviation: TNBC, triple-negative breast cancer.
Data from Refs.[4,5,72]

rates historically have been lower for AA compared with WA women, and variations in incidence (eg, increasing and declining rates before vs after the 2003 Women's Health Initiative,[2] with findings linking postmenopausal hormone replacement therapy with elevated breast cancer risk) typically occurred in parallel. Most recently, however, breast cancer incidence rates have risen disproportionately among AA women and have now converged with those of WA women.[3] This escalation in the breast cancer burden of the AA community has resulted in a widening of the mortality gap between AA and WA women, which is now a 42% difference.[3] Socioeconomic disadvantages (eg, living below the poverty level, and being underinsured or not insured) that are more prevalent in the AA community undoubtedly contribute to outcome disparities by creating health care access barriers associated with delays in diagnosis and comprehensive treatment. Several lines of evidence, however, indicate that other factors related to tumor biology, the environment, and/or ancestral genetics are likely also contributing to the cause of breast cancer's disparate impact on the AA population. These various characteristics, which cannot be ascribed to socioeconomic resources, include

1. Younger age distribution of breast cancer in AA women. Population-based incidence rates of breast cancer are higher for AA compared with WA women younger than age 40 years.[4]
2. Distribution of breast cancer phenotypes in AA women. Frequency and population-based incidence rates of tumors that are negative for the estrogen receptor (ER), the progesterone receptor (PR), and HER2/neu (HER2), commonly called triple-negative breast cancer (TNBC), are approximately 2-fold higher for AA compared with WA women.[5]
   a. Studies from Great Britain[6,7] and Switzerland[8] reveal that prevalence of TNBC is higher among women with African ancestry compared with those with British, European, or Asian heritage.
   b. The association between African ancestry and TNBC appears to be specific for western sub-Saharan African heritage because the highest frequencies of this phenotype have been reported among Ghanaians,[9–11] Nigerians,[12,13] and Malians,[14] with relatively lower frequencies in East African countries, such as Ethiopia,[11] and northern African countries, such as Egypt,[15,16] Morocco,[17,18] and Algeria.[19] These geographically defined correlations are relevant because the forced population migration of the colonial-era trans-Atlantic slave trade brought millions of Africans from western sub-Sharan Africa to North America and, therefore, contemporary AA communities have less shared ancestry with eastern and northern Africans.[1] Furthermore, a SEER-based study looked at breast cancer patients from Africa but residing in the United States and found higher frequencies of ER-negative tumors among the West Africans (most from Nigeria) but lower frequencies of ER-negative tumors among eastern Africans (most from Ethiopia).[20]
3. Meta-analysis of studies reporting breast cancer outcomes in AA compared with WA women after controlling for socioeconomic status reveals a nearly 30% higher mortality rate among AA patients (mortality hazard 1.27; 95% confidence interval, 1.18–1.38).[21]
4. Multiple phase III clinical trials (including the Southwest Oncology Group, the Eastern Cooperative Oncology Group, and the Women's Health Initiative), which would be expected to disentangle socioeconomic status from racial-ethnic identity because of the tightly regulated randomization and management structure, reveal that AA identity remains a statistically significant risk factor for increased mortality.[22–25]
5. Higher population-based incidence rates of male breast cancer in the AA community.

Geographic ancestry is strongly correlated with shared genetic inheritance; therefore, the clear associations of West African geographic ancestry with tumor phenotype and clinical outcomes are a strong indication that genetics plays a major role in these trends.

Advances in genomic technologies that now allow full characterization of germline and somatic DNA sequence, patterns of DNA modifications, and gene expression signatures hold great promise in defining the complex and multifactorial cause of breast cancer disparities, thereby launching opportunities to improve outcomes for all.

GERMLINE GENOMICS

Most of what we know about breast cancer genetics has been defined in the context of European ancestry. Once genomic technologies are applied to West African populations and we are able to establish the breast cancer risk alleles in this ancestral background, our ability to investigate the genetic components of risk in African and AA women will be greatly enhanced. The study of an individual's inherited genome can inform the discussion of breast cancer disparities related to African ancestry in several ways: (1) genetic testing of African ancestry families to evaluate the frequency of mutations in genes known to associated with breast cancer risk, (2) quantification of African ancestry through genotyping to evaluate Ancestry Informative Markers (AIMs), (3) application of genome-wide association studies (GWASs) in African ancestry populations to identify novel loci associated with breast cancer susceptibility, and (4) the study of epigenetics with race-specific or ethnicity-specific modification of the inherited genome.

Hereditary Susceptibility Syndromes in African Ancestry Families

Technology allowing for the sequencing of germline, inherited DNA sequences within genes has revolutionized breast cancer genetics and genetic counseling. These advances have resulted in the identification of a spectrum of genes associated with familial breast cancer. A comprehensive review of breast cancer hereditary susceptibility syndromes is beyond the scope of this article, which summarizes the data available thus far regarding BRCA1 and BRCA2 mutations identified in African ancestry families.

Interesting parallels are observed in the breast cancer burden of AA patients and BRCA1 mutation–associated breast cancer, prompting questions regarding the existence of BRCA founder mutations related to African ancestry. Interpretation of older studies was limited by the relatively sparse genetic testing information available in African ancestry families, resulting in high rates of identification of variants of unknown significance. More recent studies, however, have been successful in reporting prevalence of BRCA disease–associated mutations in families with African ancestry. These reports include the identification of novel founder mutations associated with Bahamian heritage, present in nearly one-quarter of Bahamian breast cancer patients,[26,27] and another founder mutation detected in one-quarter of black South African breast cancer patients.[28] Other founder mutations have also been identified related to West African ancestry.[29,30] The spectrum of BRCA mutations identified in international African ancestry populations is reviewed by Oluwagbemiga and colleagues,[31] as well as by Karami and Mehdipour.[32] Selected results from these studies and reports of BRCA testing in African Americans are summarized in **Table 2**, revealing BRCA mutations in 7% to 56% of high-risk breast cancer patients.

Zhang and colleagues[33] further demonstrated the importance of complete gene sequencing for BRCA1 and BRCA2 among high-risk African ancestry individuals because recurrent mutations identified in an African ancestry population will not

Table 2
Frequency of BRCA mutations in African ancestry populations

Study, y	Study Site	Main Findings (Sample Size, Study Population)
Trottier et al,[27] 2016	Nassau, Bahamas	Bahamian BRCA founder mutations identified in 2.8% high-risk Bahamian women and 0.09% general population of Bahamian women (20/705 unaffected Bahamians with family history of breast or ovarian cancer; 1/1089 unaffected Bahamians unselected for age, family history)
Churpek et al,[98] 2015	Chicago, Illinois	BRCA deleterious mutations identified in 18% (52/289 AA high-risk subjects: personal or family history of breast cancer; TNBC)
Francies et al,[73] 2015	Johannesburg, South Africa	BRCA deleterious mutations identified in 7% (6/85 black South African breast cancer subjects diagnosed younger than 50 y old and/or with TNBC)
Pal et al,[74] 2015	Florida Cancer Registry	BRCA deleterious mutations identified in 12.4% (49/396 AA breast cancer subjects from Florida younger than 50 y old)
Akbari et al, 2014[26]	Bahamas (multiple islands)	BRCA mutations identified in 27% (58/214 Bahamian breast cancer subjects unselected for age or family history; 53/58 were Bahamian BRCA founder mutations)
Sharma et al,[75] 2014	Kansas City, Kansas	BRCA1 large genomic rearrangement mutations identified in 7% (2/30 AA TNBC subjects)
Biunno et al,[76] 2014	Central Sudan	BRCA1 mutations in 56% (33/59 premenopausal Sudanese breast cancer subjects with point mutations, including 1/33 deleterious and 8/33 unknown significance)
Greenup et al,[77] 2013	Duke University, North Carolina, and University of California San Francisco	BRCA deleterious mutations identified in 20% (17/83 AA TNBC subjects including 9/17 BRCA1 and 8/17 BRCA2 mutations)
Pal et al,[78] 2013	Florida Cancer Registry	BRCA mutations identified in 41% as pathogenic; 35% as VUS (3/46 pathogenic variants; 16/46 VUS; all AA breast cancer subjects diagnosed younger than 50 y old)
Judkins et al,[79] 2012	Myriad Genetic Laboratories, Inc (predominantly cases from USA)	BRCA deleterious mutations in 29.4% African ancestry (519/1767 African ancestry women with suspected hereditary susceptibility found to have BRCA1/2 mutations, including 476/519 sequence mutations and 43/519 large genomic rearrangements)
Zhang et al,[33] 2012	University of Ibadan, Nigeria University of Chicago Cancer Risk Clinic, Illinois Barbados National Cancer Study	BRCA1 recurrent mutations in 3.1% Nigerians (11/356 Nigerian breast cancer subjects) BRCA1 mutations in 0.8% AA (2/260 AA breast cancer subjects found to harbor the BRCA1 recurrent mutations identified in the Nigerian cohort) BRCA1 mutations in 0% Barbadians (0/118 Barbadian breast cancer subjects found to harbor the BRCA1 recurrent mutations identified in the Nigerian cohort)

(continued on next page)

Table 2 *(continued)*		
Study, y	Study Site	Main Findings (Sample Size, Study Population)
Van der Merwe et al,[28] 2012	Western Cape, South Africa	BRCA2 founder mutation identified in 25% (4/16 black western South Africa breast cancer subjects)
Fackenthal et al,[80] 2012	Ibadan, Nigeria	BRCA deleterious mutations identified in 11.1% (48/434 unselected Nigerian breast cancer subjects, including 31/48 BRCA1 and 17/48 BRCA2 mutations)
Donenberg et al, 2011[81]	Bahamas (multiple islands)	BRCA mutations identified in 23% (49/214 Bahamian subjects unselected for age or family history)
Zhang et al,[82] 2010	Ibadan, Nigeria	BRCA1 large genomic rearrangement in 0.3% (1/352 Nigerian breast cancer subjects unselected by age or family history)
Zhang et al,[29] 2009	Ibadan, Nigerian	BRCA1 founder mutation in 1.1% (4/365 unrelated Yoruban Nigerian breast cancer subjects)
John et al,[83] 2007	Northern California Breast Cancer Family Registry	BRCA1 deleterious mutations in 1.3% (8/178 AA breast cancer subjects with high-risk for hereditary susceptibility; 0/163 AA breast cancer subjects with suspected sporadic disease; all diagnosed younger than 65 y old)
Awadelkarim et al,[84] 2007	Wad Medani, Sudan	BRCA deleterious mutations in 14% (5/35 Sudanese breast cancer subjects diagnosed younger than 40 y old, including 2/5 BRCA1 mutations and 3/5 BRCA2 mutations [including 1/3 male])
Malone et al,[85] 2006	Women's CARE Study	BRCA deleterious mutations in 4% cases and 0.9% controls[a] (26/483 cases with BRCA mutation including 10/26 BRCA1 and 16/26 BRCA2; all AA breast cancer subjects diagnosed 35–64 y old) (3/213 AA controls with BRCA2 mutation)
Fackenthal et al,[86] 2005	Ibadan, Nigeria	BRCA deleterious mutations in 3%; VUS in 72% (29/39 BRCA mutations in Nigerian breast cancer subjects diagnosed younger than 40 y old, including 1 BRCA2 deleterious truncating mutation)
Nanda et al,[87] 2005	University of Chicago, Mayo Clinic, and University of California San Francisco	BRCA deleterious mutations identified in 28%; VUS in 44% (7/43 pathogenic BRCA1 and 5/43 BRCA2 mutations; 19/43 VUS; all AA families with high-risk for hereditary susceptibility)
Gao et al,[88] 2000	Ibadan, Nigeria	BRCA deleterious mutations in 4%; VUS in 23% (3/70 pathogenic mutations and 18/70 VUS; all Nigerian premenopausal breast cancer subjects)
Yawitch et al,[89] 2000	South Africa	BRCA1 commonly recurring mutations in 0% (0/206 black South African breast cancer subjects)
Gao et al,[90] 2000	University of Chicago and University of Texas Southwestern (Dallas)	BRCA deleterious mutations identified in 18% (5/28 AA breast cancer subjects with family history of breast and/or ovarian cancer, including 1/5 BRCA1 and 4/5 BRCA2 mutations)

(continued on next page)

Table 2 (continued)		
Study, y	Study Site	Main Findings (Sample Size, Study Population)
Panguluri et al,[91] 1999	Howard University Cancer Center, Washington DC	BRCA1 deleterious mutations in 4%; VUS in 11% (2/45 AA deleterious BRCA1 mutations and 5/45 VUS; all AA breast cancer subjects from families with high-risk for hereditary susceptibility)
Newman et al,[99] 1998	Carolina Breast Cancer Study, North Carolina	BRCA1 deleterious mutations in 0% (0/88 AA breast cancer subjects and 0/79 AA controls)
Gao et al,[92] 1997	University of Chicago Cancer Risk Clinic, Illinois	BRCA1 mutations identified in 56% (5/9 AA breast cancer subjects with suspected hereditary susceptibility)

Abbreviation: VUS, variant of unknown significance.
[a] Reported proportions weighted to account for sample tested as representing entire study cohort.

necessarily be found in other African ancestry populations. These investigators identified recurrent BRCA1 mutations in Nigerian breast cancer patients, but these particular mutations were uncommon among AA and Barbadian breast cancer patients. Genetic counseling and testing is clearly warranted in African ancestry families and expanded results will likely characterize a broader spectrum of deleterious mutations in the BRCA genes.

Ancestry Informative Markers

The AA population represents a heavily admixed community in terms of geographically defined ancestry. Various individuals may self-identify as being AA based on community ties, physical appearance or pigmentation, and familial or personal preferences, but the extent of African versus European or Native American contributions to ancestry can differ substantially between these individuals. Ancestral background can be inferred and quantified by genotyping to evaluate genetic markers associated with substantial differences in allele frequency between geographically defined populations. These genetic patterns, AIMs, can be assessed through the study of uniparental heritage via maternally linked mitochondrial DNA (mtDNA) or Y-linked chromosomal markers. Alternatively, they can be analyzed via autosomal short tandem repeats or single nucleotide polymorphisms (SNPs), with the latter being the most commonly used. Africa is a large, diverse continent and African ancestry can be further stratified by region. The potential value of AIMs to better characterize the genetics of disease associated with racial-ethnic identity has been reviewed extensively.[34–38]

Recent reports have yielded provocative findings with regard to potential novel applications for AIMs in evaluating breast cancer risk. Rao and colleagues[39] studied mtDNA in 92 subjects with TNBC (31 of whom self-identified as AA), and found discordance between self-reported race or ethnicity and genetic ancestry in 13% of cases. Davis and colleagues[40] have reported on African ancestry-specific isoform expression of the atypical chemokine receptor 1 (ACKR1)/Duffy antigen receptor for chemokines (DARC) as being associated with ancestry-specific inflammatory response, with potential implications for several disease processes, including breast cancer.

Genome-Wide Association Studies

GWASs have been used extensively to characterize breast cancer risk associated with various patient populations. In the study of breast cancer burden associated with race or ethnicity, GWASs have been applied with self-reported identity, as well as in conjunction with AIMs and genetic admixture mapping. In an effort to strengthen sample sizes and power calculations, several large AA cohorts have been assembled for these analyses, such as those of the Black Women's Health Study, the Women's Circle of Health Study, the Carolina Breast Cancer Study (CBCS), the Multiethnic Cohort; and various collaborations of these, as well as additional cohorts (eg, African American Breast Cancer Epidemiology and Risk [AMBER] Consortium; the African Diaspora Study [known as the ROOT Study]; and the African American Breast Cancer Consortium [AABC]). Some of these analyses have identified genetic susceptibility loci for specific breast cancer subtypes in AA women, such as SNP rs8170 associated with TNBC in AA patients,[41] 3 novel regions associated with ER-positive disease in AA patients,[42] a novel gene (FBXL22) associated with ER-negative disease in AA patients,[43] and 3q26.21 as a novel susceptibility locus associated with African ancestry ER-negative breast cancer.[44]

Epigenetics

Epigenetics refers to modification of the primary or inherited genome without alteration of the actual DNA sequence. Most commonly, these epigenetic events occur as DNA methylation or histone modification. Epigenetic changes can influence gene expression and they can be stable, heritable, or reversible. Epigenetics have been implicated in the initiation, promotion, and metastasis of breast cancer, as reviewed by Wu and colleagues.[45] Several investigators have demonstrated that epigenetics may also contribute to breast cancer disparities. Genome-wide methylation patterns have been associated with ER-negative breast cancer in AA patients,[46] have been found to differ in benign breast tissue from WA and AA women,[47] and global DNA methylation has been associated with ancestral admixture variation in breast cancer risk.[48]

Epigenetics may also play a unique role in breast cancer disparities by acting as an intermediary between the genetics of racial-ethnic identity and racial-ethnic identity as a sociopolitical construct.[49] Cumulative stressors over a lifetime, such as poverty and psychosocial adversity, have been theorized to cause biological dysregulation (called allostatic load) that may influence a variety of medical hazards.[49–51] Measures of allostatic load have been found to be elevated among AA individuals,[52] and disparities in allostatic load have been implicated in health disparities between the AA and WA communities.[53] An analysis of the National Health and Nutrition Examination Survey found that allostatic load among AA women was disproportionately associated with breast cancer risk.[54] Epigenetics have been proposed as a method for quantifying stress response and possible allostatic load,[49,55,56] thereby serving as a potential surrogate measure for the effect of socioeconomic disadvantages on breast cancer disparities associated with race or ethnicity.

SOMATIC GENOMICS

In contemporary breast cancer clinical care, immunohistochemistry is routinely used to define breast cancer phenotype based on expression of the protein biomarkers ER, PR, and HER2. Combinations of these results are have prognostic value and predict for response to targeted therapies. The diversity of breast cancer biology is further underscored by gene expression studies that identify an even more complex spectrum of tumor mutations and subtypes, also associated with a range of prognostic risks. Differences in the somatic mutational landscape and tumor subtype represent additional genomic factors that might contribute to breast cancer disparities between AA and WA patients.

Table 3 summarizes data from various studies that have reported on the somatic genomic landscape of tumors from AA and WA breast cancer patients, demonstrating unique and diverse gene signatures in the tumors of AA patients. The Cancer Genome

Table 3
Studies reporting on the landscape of somatic mutations and tumor subtypes in breast cancers of African American and white American subjects

Study	Cases Studied	Selected Findings
Martin et al,[93] 2009	Baltimore, MD 18 AA (72% ER-negative) 17 WA (29% ER-negative)	• Prominent interferon signal in tumors of African American subjects • Phosphoserine phosphatase-like expressed more highly in tumor epithelium and stroma of AA subjects • Thymopoietin expressed more highly in stroma of AA subjects • Chemokine ligands 10 and 11 expressed more strongly in tumor stroma of AA subjects
Field et al,[94] 2012	Clinical Breast Care Project 26 AA (38% TNBC) 26 WA (35% TNBC)	• Crystallin beta B2, lactotransferrin, and L-3-phosphoserine-phosphatase homologue expressed more strongly in AA subjects
Grunda et al,[95] 2012	Birmingham, AL 11 AA (45% ER-negative) 11 WA (9% ER-negative)	• AA subjects more likely to have aberrant G1/S cell-cycle regulatory genes • AA subjects more likely to have decreased expression of cell adhesion genes • AA subjects more likely to have low or no expression of ESR1, PGR, ERBB2 and estrogen pathway genes
Stewart et al,[57] 2013	The Cancer Genome Atlas 53 AA (19% TNBC) 574 WA (12% TNBC)	• Increase in number of differentially expressed genes between AA and WA subjects with each stage of tumor progression • Resistin (a gene that is linked to obesity, insulin resistance, and breast cancer) was expressed more than 4 times higher in AA cases, but was lowest in AA TNBC tumors. • Increased expression of p53 and BRCA1 subnetwork components in AA tumors
Lindner et al,[67] 2013	Yale TNBC Cohort 50 AA 69 WA	• Major transcriptional signature of proliferation found to be upregulated in AA cases • Differential activation of insulin-like growth factor 1 and a signature of BRCA1 deficiency in AA cases • TNBC subtyping revealed AA cases more likely to have basal subtype compared with WA cases

(continued on next page)

Table 3
(continued)

Study	Cases Studied	Selected Findings
Kroenke et al,[60] 2014	Pathways and Life after Cancer Epidemiology Cohorts 128 AA (30% TNBC) 1176 WA (11% TNBC)	• PAM50 subtyping revealed increased frequency of basal subtype among AA compared with WA cases (41% vs 17%)
Sweeney et al,[61] 2014	Pathways and Life after Cancer Epidemiology Cohorts 115 AA[a] 913 WA[a] 12% of entire cohort with TNBC; frequencies not reported by race or ethnicity	• PAM50 subtyping revealed increased frequency of basal subtype among AA cases; odds ratio for having basal vs Luminal A subtype (with WA as referent group) 4.38 (95% confidence interval 2.29–8.39)
Keenan et al,[58] 2015	The Cancer Genome Atlas 159 AA (17% TNBC) 711 WA (8% TNBC)	• PAM50 subtyping revealed increased frequency of basal subtype in AA cases (39% vs 19%) and fewer luminal A tumors (17% vs 35%) • TNBC subtyping revealed increased frequency of basal-like 1 and mesenchymal stem-like tumors in AA vs WA cases; no LAR tumors in the AA cases • Greater intratumoral heterogeneity among AA vs WA cases
Ademuyiwa et al,[59] 2017	The Cancer Genome Atlas 183 AA (33% TNBC) 764 WA (15% TNBC)	• PAM50 subtyping revealed increased frequency of basal subtype in AA cases (35% vs 16%) • Median counts of somatic tumor mutations higher in AA vs WA cases overall • No significant differences in median mutation counts for AA TNBC compared with WA TNBC cases
Huo et al,[100] 2017	The Cancer Genome Atlas 154 AA 776 WA	• PAM50 subtyping: increased frequency of basal subtype in AA cases (36% versus 15%; p<0.0001) • AA cases with more TP53 and fewer PIK3CA mutations compared to WA (52% versus 31%; $p = 2.5 \times 10^{-5}$ and 24% versus 36%; $p = 0.012$, respectively)

[a] Estimated from percentage distributions provided.

Atlas has been interrogated by several investigators[57–59] and PAM50 has been used extensively for tumor subtyping.[58–61] As noted previously, TNBC is twice as common among AA compared with WA patients; the adverse prognosis of TNBC is related to approximately 80% belonging to the inherently aggressive basal breast cancer subtype defined by gene expression profiling.[62] Not surprisingly, therefore, PAM50 subtyping studies have also confirmed higher rates of basal subtype tumors among AA breast cancer patients. Most recently, Huo et al have utilized Ancestry Informative Markers to distinguish African ancestry from European ancestry breast cancer

Table 4
Findings from selected studies reporting on outcomes in African American compared with White American breast cancer subjects, after accounting for gene expression subtype

Study	Source	Subject Sample (n)		Follow-up	Results	AA Outcome Worse?
		AA	WA			
Kroenke et al,[60] 2014	Kaiser Permanente Northern California and Utah Cancer Registry	128 (38 TNBC, 53 basal-like, 32 luminal A)	1176 (129 TNBC, 205 basal-like, 268 luminal A)	NR	• Hazard ratio recurrence (adjusted for age and stage): *Basal:* 0.81 (0.10–6.49) *Luminal A:* 1.45 (0.59–3.55)	Basal: no Luminal A: yes
Keenan et al,[58] 2015	The Cancer Genome Atlas	159 (27 TNBC, 62 basal-like, 27 luminal A)	711 (58 TNBC, 132 basal-like, 247 luminal A)	AA: 29.9 mo WA: 24.4 mo	• Hazard ratio tumor recurrence (adjusted for age, stage, and *TNBC:* 1.47 (0.68–3.14) *Basal:* 1.48 (0.67–3.27) *All PAM50 Subtypes:* 1.35 (0.62–2.95)	TNBC: no Basal: no
Tao et al,[96] 2015	California Cancer Registry	9738 (1896 TNBC, 4813 HR-positive, HER2-not overexpressed)	93,760 (8589 TNBC, 59,341 HR-positive, HER2-not overexpressed)	3.5 y	• Mortality hazard ratio (adjusted for age, tumor size, nodal status, SES): TNBC: 1.21 (1.06–1.37) *HR-positive, HER2-not overexpressed:* 1.27 (1.12–1.43) *ER/PR-negative, HER2-positive:* 1.09 (0.85–1.39)	TNBC: yes ER-positive: yes HER2-positive: no
Ademuyiwa et al,[59] 2017	The Cancer Genome Atlas	61 (all TNBC)	114 (all TNBC)	6 y	• Disease-free survival worse for AA compared with WA subjects with basal-like tumors (*P*<.0001) but no significant differences for AA compared with WA subjects with TNBC	Basal-like: yes TNBC: no
D'Arcy et al,[97] 2015	Publically available datasets	57 (all luminal A)	108 (all luminal A)	NR	• No survival analyses but AA luminal A cases with higher expression of poor prognosis genes and lower expression of good prognosis genes	NA

(samples sizes estimated based upon reported frequencies if values not provided).
Abbreviations: SES, socioeconomic status; HR, hormone receptor (ER and/or PR); NA, not applicable; NR, not reported.

patients whose tumors have been analyzed through The Cancer Genome Atlas, also demonstrating an association between African ancestry and basal breast tumors. Gene expression studies have not yet completely clarified explanations for breast cancer disparities. As shown in **Table 4**, inconsistent results have been demonstrated in various studies reporting on outcome disparities between AA and WA patients, even after accounting for tumor subtype.

TNBCs themselves have diverse genetic pathways. Lehman and colleagues[63] first characterized these triple-negative subtypes by analyses of gene expression profiles from 21 publically available datasets that included 587 TNBC cases. They identified 6 different subtypes: 2 basal-like, 1 immunomodulatory, 1 mesenchymal, 1 mesenchymal stem-like, and 1 luminal androgen receptor subtype. Similarly, Burstein and colleagues[64] identified 4 TNBC subtypes based on gene expression profiles from 198 cases from Baylor College of Medicine: luminal androgen receptor, mesenchymal, basal-like immune suppressed, and basal-like immune-activated subtype. These different patterns have been shown to be associated with prognostic, as well as predictive, therapeutic value. The luminal androgen receptor subtype tends to respond poorly to neoadjuvant chemotherapy[65,66] and may be amenable to endocrine manipulation through anti-androgen therapy. Unfortunately, neither the Lehmann and colleagues[63] nor the Burstein and colleagues[64] studies included meaningful samples of triple-negative tumors from women with African ancestry. Lindner and colleagues[67] evaluated 136 tumors from the Yale TNBC cohort (including 50 AA patients) and found basal-like subtypes to be more common among the AA cases. Using the Cancer Genome Atlas, Keenan and colleagues[58] also found that TNBC tumors from AA were more likely to have the basal-like and mesenchymal triple-negative subtypes. The luminal androgen receptor TNBC subtype appears to be less common in AA patients.

The American Joint Committee's 8th edition of their cancer staging system, will be implemented by tumor registries in 2018 and a major shift is that the new breast cancer staging system will account for results from commercially available gene expression profiles,[68] such as the 21-gene recurrence score, also known as Oncotype DX (Genomic Health, Redwood City, CA, USA). This change represents an opportunity to evaluate disparities related to race or ethnicity in the use of Oncotype testing as a quality of care metric. Thus far, inconsistent results have been reported. The CBCS revealed no disparities in guideline-concordant use of the Oncotype test between AA and WA patients.[69] Two other studies (from the California Cancer Registry[70] and the Virginia Tumor Registry[71]) both found disproportionately lower use of Oncotype testing in AA patients.

SUMMARY

Advances in breast cancer genomics will definitely provide important insights regarding explanations for variations in incidence, as well as disparate outcomes between AA and WA breast cancer patients. Germline genomics are essential in genetic counseling and risk-assessment programs; somatic or tumor-based genomics will be critical in defining prognostic and therapeutic algorithms. It is, therefore, imperative that the oncology community be prepared to apply these technologies equitably to diverse patient populations.

REFERENCES

1. Newman LA, Kaljee LM. Health disparities and triple-negative breast cancer in African American women: a review. JAMA Surg 2017;152(5):485–93.

2. Chlebowski RT, Hendrix SL, Langer RD, et al. Influence of estrogen plus progestin on breast cancer and mammography in healthy postmenopausal women: the Women's Health Initiative Randomized Trial. JAMA 2003;289(24):3243–53.

3. DeSantis CE, Fedewa SA, Goding Sauer A, et al. Breast cancer statistics, 2015: Convergence of incidence rates between black and white women. CA Cancer J Clin 2016;66(1):31–42.

4. U.S. Cancer Statistics Working Group. United States cancer statistics: 1999–2013 incidence and mortality web-based report. Atlanta (GA): U.S. Department of Health and Human Services, Centers for Disease Control and Prevention and National Cancer Institute; 2016. Available at: www.cdc.gov/uscs. Accessed September 6, 2016.

5. Kohler BA, Sherman RL, Howlader N, et al. Annual report to the nation on the status of cancer, 1975-2011, featuring incidence of breast cancer subtypes by race/ethnicity, poverty, and state. J Natl Cancer Inst 2015;107(6):djv048.

6. Bowen RL, Duffy SW, Ryan DA, et al. Early onset of breast cancer in a group of British black women. Br J Cancer 2008;98(2):277–81.

7. Copson E, Maishman T, Gerty S, et al. Ethnicity and outcome of young breast cancer patients in the United Kingdom: the POSH study. Br J Cancer 2014; 110(1):230–41.

8. Rapiti E, Pinaud K, Chappuis PO, et al. Opportunities for improving triple-negative breast cancer outcomes: results of a population-based study. Cancer Med 2017;6(3):526–36.

9. Der EM, Gyasi RK, Tettey Y, et al. Triple-negative breast cancer in Ghanaian women: the Korle Bu Teaching Hospital experience. Breast J 2015;21(6):627–33.

10. Ohene-Yeboah M, Adjei E. Breast cancer in Kumasi, Ghana. Ghana Med J 2012;46(1):8–13.

11. Jiagge E, Jibril AS, Chitale D, et al. Comparative analysis of breast cancer phenotypes in African American, White American, and West Versus East African patients: correlation between African ancestry and triple-negative breast cancer. Ann Surg Oncol 2016;23(12):3843–9.

12. Agboola AJ, Musa AA, Wanangwa N, et al. Molecular characteristics and prognostic features of breast cancer in Nigerian compared with UK women. Breast Cancer Res Treat 2012;135(2):555–69.

13. Nwafor CC, Keshinro SO. Pattern of hormone receptors and human epidermal growth factor receptor 2 status in sub-Saharan breast cancer cases: Private practice experience. Niger J Clin Pract 2015;18(4):553–8.

14. Ly M, Antoine M, Dembele AK, et al. High incidence of triple-negative tumors in sub-Saharan Africa: a prospective study of breast cancer characteristics and risk factors in Malian women seen in a Bamako university hospital. Oncology 2012;83(5):257–63.

15. Aiad HA, Wahed MM, Asaad NY, et al. Immunohistochemical expression of GPR30 in breast carcinoma of Egyptian patients: an association with immunohistochemical subtypes. APMIS 2014;122(10):976–84.

16. Salhia B, Tapia C, Ishak EA, et al. Molecular subtype analysis determines the association of advanced breast cancer in Egypt with favorable biology. BMC Womens Health 2011;11:44.

17. Rais G, Raissouni S, Aitelhaj M, et al. Triple negative breast cancer in Moroccan women: clinicopathological and therapeutic study at the National Institute of Oncology. BMC Womens Health 2012;12:35.

18. Bennis S, Abbass F, Akasbi Y, et al. Prevalence of molecular subtypes and prognosis of invasive breast cancer in north-east of Morocco: retrospective study. BMC Res Notes 2012;5:436.

19. Cherbal F, Gaceb H, Mehemmai C, et al. Distribution of molecular breast cancer subtypes among Algerian women and correlation with clinical and tumor characteristics: a population-based study. Breast Dis 2015;35(2):95–102.

20. Jemal A, Fedewa SA. Is the prevalence of ER-negative breast cancer in the US higher among Africa-born than US-born black women? Breast Cancer Res Treat 2012;135(3):867–73.

21. Newman LA, Griffith KA, Jatoi I, et al. Meta-analysis of survival in African American and white American patients with breast cancer: ethnicity compared with socioeconomic status. J Clin Oncol 2006;24(9):1342–9.

22. Albain KS, Unger JM, Crowley JJ, et al. Racial disparities in cancer survival among randomized clinical trials patients of the Southwest Oncology Group. J Natl Cancer Inst 2009;101(14):984–92.

23. Hershman DL, Unger JM, Barlow WE, et al. Treatment quality and outcomes of African American versus white breast cancer patients: retrospective analysis of Southwest Oncology studies S8814/S8897. J Clin Oncol 2009;27(13):2157–62.

24. Sparano JA, Wang M, Zhao F, et al. Race and hormone receptor-positive breast cancer outcomes in a randomized chemotherapy trial. J Natl Cancer Inst 2012; 104(5):406–14.

25. Chlebowski RT, Chen Z, Anderson GL, et al. Ethnicity and breast cancer: factors influencing differences in incidence and outcome. J Natl Cancer Inst 2005; 97(6):439–48.

26. Akbari MR, Donenberg T, Lunn J, et al. The spectrum of BRCA1 and BRCA2 mutations in breast cancer patients in the Bahamas. Clin Genet 2014;85(1):64–7.

27. Trottier M, Lunn J, Butler R, et al. Prevalence of founder mutations in the BRCA1 and BRCA2 genes among unaffected women from the Bahamas. Clin Genet 2016;89(3):328–31.

28. van der Merwe NC, Hamel N, Schneider SR, et al. A founder BRCA2 mutation in non-Afrikaner breast cancer patients of the Western Cape of South Africa. Clin Genet 2012;81(2):179–84.

29. Zhang B, Fackenthal JD, Niu Q, et al. Evidence for an ancient BRCA1 mutation in breast cancer patients of Yoruban ancestry. Fam Cancer 2009;8(1):15–22.

30. Mefford HC, Baumbach L, Panguluri RC, et al. Evidence for a BRCA1 founder mutation in families of West African ancestry. Am J Hum Genet 1999;65(2): 575–8.

31. Oluwagbemiga LA, Oluwole A, Kayode AA. Seventeen years after BRCA1: what is the BRCA mutation status of the breast cancer patients in Africa? - a systematic review. Springerplus 2012;1(1):83.

32. Karami F, Mehdipour P. A comprehensive focus on global spectrum of BRCA1 and BRCA2 mutations in breast cancer. Biomed Res Int 2013;2013:928562.

33. Zhang J, Fackenthal JD, Zheng Y, et al. Recurrent BRCA1 and BRCA2 mutations in breast cancer patients of African ancestry. Breast Cancer Res Treat 2012; 134(2):889–94.

34. Mersha TB, Abebe T. Self-reported race/ethnicity in the age of genomic research: its potential impact on understanding health disparities. Hum Genom 2015;9:1.

35. Zeng X, Chakraborty R, King JL, et al. Selection of highly informative SNP markers for population affiliation of major US populations. Int J Legal Med 2016;130(2):341–52.

36. Shriver MD, Parra EJ, Dios S, et al. Skin pigmentation, biogeographical ancestry and admixture mapping. Hum Genet 2003;112(4):387–99.

37. Tian C, Hinds DA, Shigeta R, et al. A genomewide single-nucleotide-polymorphism panel with high ancestry information for African American admixture mapping. Am J Hum Genet 2006;79(4):640–9.

38. Stefflova K, Dulik MC, Barnholtz-Sloan JS, et al. Dissecting the within-Africa ancestry of populations of African descent in the Americas. PLoS One 2011; 6(1):e14495.

39. Rao R, Rivers A, Rahimi A, et al. Genetic Ancestry using Mitochondrial DNA in patients with Triple-negative breast cancer (GAMiT study). Cancer 2017;123(1): 107–13.

40. Davis MB, Walens A, Hire R, et al. Distinct Transcript Isoforms of the Atypical Chemokine Receptor 1 (ACKR1)/Duffy Antigen Receptor for Chemokines (DARC) Gene Are Expressed in Lymphoblasts and Altered Isoform Levels Are Associated with Genetic Ancestry and the Duffy-Null Allele. PLoS One 2015; 10:e0140098.

41. Palmer JR, Ruiz-Narvaez EA, Rotimi CN, et al. Genetic susceptibility loci for subtypes of breast cancer in an African American population. Cancer Epidemiol Biomarkers Prev 2013;22(1):127–34.

42. Ruiz-Narvaez EA, Sucheston-Campbell L, Bensen JT, et al. Admixture mapping of African-American Women in the AMBER consortium identifies new loci for breast cancer and estrogen-receptor subtypes. Front Genet 2016;7:170.

43. Haddad SA, Ruiz-Narvaez EA, Haiman CA, et al. An exome-wide analysis of low frequency and rare variants in relation to risk of breast cancer in African American Women: the AMBER Consortium. Carcinogenesis 2016;37(9):870–7.

44. Huo D, Feng Y, Haddad S, et al. Genome-wide association studies in women of African ancestry identified 3q26.21 as a novel susceptibility locus for oestrogen receptor negative breast cancer. Hum Mol Genet 2016;112(4):387–99.

45. Wu Y, Sarkissyan M, Vadgama JV. Epigenetics in breast and prostate cancer. Methods Mol Biol 2015;1238:425–66.

46. Ambrosone CB, Young AC, Sucheston LE, et al. Genome-wide methylation patterns provide insight into differences in breast tumor biology between American women of African and European ancestry. Oncotarget 2014;5(1):237–48.

47. Song MA, Brasky TM, Marian C, et al. Racial differences in genome-wide methylation profiling and gene expression in breast tissues from healthy women. Epigenetics 2015;10(12):1177–87.

48. Cappetta M, Berdasco M, Hochmann J, et al. Effect of genetic ancestry on leukocyte global DNA methylation in cancer patients. BMC Cancer 2015;15:434.

49. Williams DR, Mohammed SA, Shields AE. Understanding and effectively addressing breast cancer in African American women: unpacking the social context. Cancer 2016;122(14):2138–49.

50. Gruenewald TL, Seeman TE, Karlamangla AS, et al. Allostatic load and frailty in older adults. J Am Geriatr Soc 2009;57(9):1525–31.

51. Seeman T, Epel E, Gruenewald T, et al. Socio-economic differentials in peripheral biology: cumulative allostatic load. Ann N Y Acad Sci 2010;1186:223–39.

52. Geronimus AT, Hicken M, Keene D, et al. "Weathering" and age patterns of allostatic load scores among blacks and whites in the United States. Am J Public Health 2006;96(5):826–33.

53. Beckie TM. A systematic review of allostatic load, health, and health disparities. Biol Res Nurs 2012;14(4):311–46.

54. Parente V, Hale L, Palermo T. Association between breast cancer and allostatic load by race: National Health and Nutrition Examination Survey 1999-2008. Psychooncology 2013;22(3):621–8.

55. Romens SE, McDonald J, Svaren J, et al. Associations between early life stress and gene methylation in children. Child Dev 2015;86(1):303–9.

56. Juster RP, Russell JJ, Almeida D, et al. Allostatic load and comorbidities: A mitochondrial, epigenetic, and evolutionary perspective. Dev Psychopathol 2016; 28(4pt1):1117–46.

57. Stewart PA, Luks J, Roycik MD, et al. Differentially expressed transcripts and dysregulated signaling pathways and networks in African American breast cancer. PLoS One 2013;8(12):e82460.

58. Keenan T, Moy B, Mroz EA, et al. Comparison of the genomic landscape between primary breast cancer in African American versus white women and the association of racial differences with tumor recurrence. J Clin Oncol 2015; 33(31):3621–7.

59. Ademuyiwa FO, Tao Y, Luo J, et al. Differences in the mutational landscape of triple-negative breast cancer in African Americans and Caucasians. Breast Cancer Res Treat 2017;161(3):491–9.

60. Kroenke CH, Sweeney C, Kwan ML, et al. Race and breast cancer survival by intrinsic subtype based on PAM50 gene expression. Breast Cancer Res Treat 2014;144(3):689–99.

61. Sweeney C, Bernard PS, Factor RE, et al. Intrinsic subtypes from PAM50 gene expression assay in a population-based breast cancer cohort: differences by age, race, and tumor characteristics. Cancer Epidemiol Biomarkers Prev 2014;23(5):714–24.

62. Newman LA, Reis-Filho JS, Morrow M, et al. The 2014 Society of Surgical Oncology Susan G. Komen for the Cure Symposium: triple-negative breast cancer. Ann Surg Oncol 2015;22(3):874–82.

63. Lehmann BD, Bauer JA, Chen X, et al. Identification of human triple-negative breast cancer subtypes and preclinical models for selection of targeted therapies. J Clin Invest 2011;121(7):2750–67.

64. Burstein MD, Tsimelzon A, Poage GM, et al. Comprehensive genomic analysis identifies novel subtypes and targets of triple-negative breast cancer. Clin Cancer Res 2015;21(7):1688–98.

65. Masuda H, Baggerly KA, Wang Y, et al. Differential response to neoadjuvant chemotherapy among 7 triple-negative breast cancer molecular subtypes. Clin Cancer Res 2013;19(19):5533–40.

66. Lehmann BD, Jovanovic B, Chen X, et al. Refinement of triple-negative breast cancer molecular subtypes: implications for neoadjuvant chemotherapy selection. PLoS One 2016;11(6):e0157368.

67. Lindner R, Sullivan C, Offor O, et al. Molecular phenotypes in triple negative breast cancer from African American patients suggest targets for therapy. PLoS One 2013;8(11):e71915.

68. Giuliano AE, Connolly JL, Edge SB, et al. Breast Cancer-Major changes in the American Joint Committee on Cancer eighth edition cancer staging manual. CA Cancer J Clin 2017;67(4):290–303.

69. Roberts MC, Weinberger M, Dusetzina SB, et al. Racial variation in the uptake of oncotype DX testing for early-stage breast cancer. J Clin Oncol 2016;34(2): 130–8.

70. Cress RD, Chen YS, Morris CR, et al. Underutilization of gene expression profiling for early-stage breast cancer in California. Cancer Causes Control 2016;27(6):721–7.

71. Ricks-Santi LJ, McDonald JT. Low utility of Oncotype DX in the clinic. Cancer Med 2017;6(3):501–7.

72. Surveillance Research Program, Available at: https://seer.cancer.gov/faststats/selections. Accessed April 2, 2017.

73. Francies FZ, Wainstein T, De Leeneer K, et al. BRCA1, BRCA2 and PALB2 mutations and CHEK2 c.1100delC in different South African ethnic groups diagnosed with premenopausal and/or triple negative breast cancer. BMC Cancer 2015;15:912.

74. Pal T, Bonner D, Cragun D, et al. A high frequency of BRCA mutations in young black women with breast cancer residing in Florida. Cancer 2015;121(23): 4173–80.

75. Sharma P, Klemp JR, Kimler BF, et al. Germline BRCA mutation evaluation in a prospective triple-negative breast cancer registry: implications for hereditary breast and/or ovarian cancer syndrome testing. Breast Cancer Res Treat 2014;145(3):707–14.

76. Biunno I, Aceto G, Awadelkarim KD, et al. BRCA1 point mutations in premenopausal breast cancer patients from Central Sudan. Fam Cancer 2014;13(3): 437–44.

77. Greenup R, Buchanan A, Lorizio W, et al. Prevalence of BRCA mutations among women with triple-negative breast cancer (TNBC) in a genetic counseling cohort. Ann Surg Oncol 2013;20(10):3254–8.

78. Pal T, Bonner D, Kim J, et al. Early onset breast cancer in a registry-based sample of African-American women: BRCA mutation prevalence, and other personal and system-level clinical characteristics. Breast J 2013;19(2):189–92.

79. Judkins T, Rosenthal E, Arnell C, et al. Clinical significance of large rearrangements in BRCA1 and BRCA2. Cancer 2012;118(21):5210–6.

80. Fackenthal JD, Zhang J, Zhang B, et al. High prevalence of BRCA1 and BRCA2 mutations in unselected Nigerian breast cancer patients. Int J Cancer 2012; 131(5):1114–23.

81. Donenberg T, Lunn J, Curling D, et al. A high prevalence of BRCA1 mutations among breast cancer patients from the Bahamas. Breast Cancer Res Treat 2011;125(2):591–6.

82. Zhang J, Fackenthal JD, Huo D, et al. Searching for large genomic rearrangements of the BRCA1 gene in a Nigerian population. Breast Cancer Res Treat 2010;124(2):573–7.

83. John EM, Miron A, Gong G, et al. Prevalence of pathogenic BRCA1 mutation carriers in 5 US racial/ethnic groups. JAMA 2007;298(24):2869–76.

84. Awadelkarim KD, Aceto G, Veschi S, et al. BRCA1 and BRCA2 status in a Central Sudanese series of breast cancer patients: interactions with genetic, ethnic and reproductive factors. Breast Cancer Res Treat 2007;102(2):189–99.

85. Malone KE, Daling JR, Doody DR, et al. Prevalence and predictors of BRCA1 and BRCA2 mutations in a population-based study of breast cancer in white and black American women ages 35 to 64 years. Cancer Res 2006;66(16): 8297–308.

86. Fackenthal JD, Sveen L, Gao Q, et al. Complete allelic analysis of BRCA1 and BRCA2 variants in young Nigerian breast cancer patients. J Med Genet 2005; 42(3):276–81.

87. Nanda R, Schumm LP, Cummings S, et al. Genetic testing in an ethnically diverse cohort of high-risk women: a comparative analysis of BRCA1 and BRCA2 mutations in American families of European and African ancestry. JAMA 2005;294(15):1925–33.

88. Gao Q, Adebamowo CA, Fackenthal J, et al. Protein truncating BRCA1 and BRCA2 mutations in African women with pre-menopausal breast cancer. Hum Genet 2000;107(2):192–4.

89. Yawitch TM, van Rensburg EJ, Mertz M, et al. Absence of commonly recurring BRCA1 mutations in black South African women with breast cancer. S Afr Med J 2000;90(8):788.

90. Gao Q, Tomlinson G, Das S, et al. Prevalence of BRCA1 and BRCA2 mutations among clinic-based African American families with breast cancer. Hum Genet 2000;107(2):186–91.

91. Panguluri RC, Brody LC, Modali R, et al. BRCA1 mutations in African Americans. Hum Genet 1999;105(1–2):28–31.

92. Gao Q, Neuhausen S, Cummings S, et al. Recurrent germ-line BRCA1 mutations in extended African American families with early-onset breast cancer. Am J Hum Genet 1997;60(5):1233–6.

93. Martin DN, Boersma BJ, Yi M, et al. Differences in the tumor microenvironment between African-American and European-American breast cancer patients. PLoS One 2009;4(2):e4531.

94. Field LA, Love B, Deyarmin B, et al. Identification of differentially expressed genes in breast tumors from African American compared with Caucasian women. Cancer 2012;118(5):1334–44.

95. Grunda JM, Steg AD, He Q, et al. Differential expression of breast cancer-associated genes between stage- and age-matched tumor specimens from African- and Caucasian-American Women diagnosed with breast cancer. BMC Res Notes 2012;5:248.

96. Tao L, Gomez SL, Keegan TH, et al. Breast cancer mortality in African-American and non-Hispanic white women by molecular subtype and stage at diagnosis: a population-based study. Cancer Epidemiol Biomarkers Prev 2015;24(7):1039–45.

97. D'Arcy M, Fleming J, Robinson WR, et al. Race-associated biological differences among Luminal A breast tumors. Breast Cancer Res Treat 2015;152(2):437–48.

98. Churpek JE, Walsh T, Zheng Y, et al. Inherited predisposition to breast cancer among African American women. Breast Cancer Res Treat 2015;149:31–9.

99. Newman B, Mu H, Butler LM, et al. Frequency of breast cancer attributable to BRCA1 in a population-based series of American women. JAMA 1998;279:915–21.

100. Huo D, Hu H, Rhie SK, et al. Comparison of Breast Cancer Molecular Features and Survival by African and European Ancestry in The Cancer Genome Atlas. JAMA Oncology 2017.

Moving?

Make sure your subscription moves with you!

To notify us of your new address, find your **Clinics Account Number** (located on your mailing label above your name), and contact customer service at:

Email: journalscustomerservice-usa@elsevier.com

800-654-2452 (subscribers in the U.S. & Canada)
314-447-8871 (subscribers outside of the U.S. & Canada)

Fax number: 314-447-8029

Elsevier Health Sciences Division
Subscription Customer Service
3251 Riverport Lane
Maryland Heights, MO 63043

*To ensure uninterrupted delivery of your subscription, please notify us at least 4 weeks in advance of move.